BRADY

The Long-Term Care
Nursing Assistant

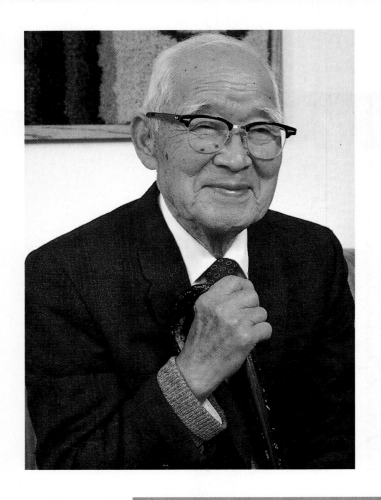

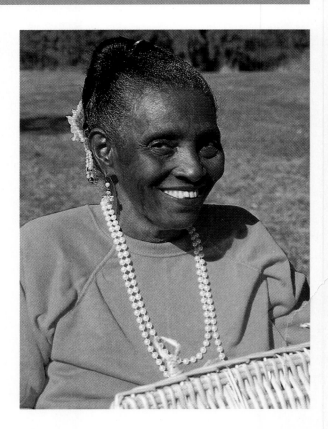

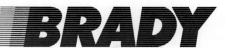

The Long-Term Care
Nursing Assistant

Peggy A. Grubbs
Barbara A. Blasband

BRADY
Prentice Hall
Englewood Cliffs, New Jersey 07632

Library of Congress Cataloging-in-Publication Data

Grubbs, Peggy A..
    The long-term care nursing assistant / Peggy A. Grubbs, Barbara A.
Blasband.
        p.   cm.
    Includes bibliographical references and index.
    ISBN 0-8359-4926-5
    1. Long-term care of the sick. 2. Nurses' aides. 3. Nursing home
care. I. Blasband, Barbara A. II. Title.
    [DNLM: 1. Long-Term Care--methods--nurses' instruction.
2. Nursing Care--methods. 3. Nurses' Aides. WY 152 G885L 1995]
RT120.L64G78 1995
610.73'61--dc20
DNLM/DLC
for Library of Congress   94-18668
                                                               CIP

Developmental Managing Editor: *Marilyn Meserve*
Production Editors: *Cathy O'Connell/Eileen O'Sullivan*
Formatter: *Kerry Reardon*
Brady Production Manager: *Patrick Walsh*
Director of Production/Manufacturing: *Bruce Johnson*
Photography Editor: *Michal Heron*
Interior Design: *Strategic Design Group*
Interior Art: *Network Graphics/North Market Street
                Graphics/Mark LaSalle*
Cover Design: *Mary Jo Defranco*
Cover Photo: *Richard Logan*
Prepress/Manufacturing Buyer: *Ilene Sanford*
Acquisitions Editor: *Mark Hartman/Barbara Krawiec*
Editorial Assistant: *Louise Fullam*
Color Separator: *TSI Graphics*
Printer/Binder: *Webcrafters*

Printed in the United States of America

10 9 8 7 6 5 4 3 2 1

ISBN 0-8359-4926-5

Prentice-Hall International (UK) Limited, *London*
Prentice-Hall of Australia Pty. Limited, *Sydney*
Prentice-Hall Canada Inc., *Toronto*
Prentice-Hall Hispanoamericana, S.A., *Mexico*
Prentice-Hall of India Private Limited, *New Delhi*
Prentice-Hall of Japan, Inc., *Tokyo*
Simon & Schuster Asia Pte. Ltd., *Singapore*
Editora Prentice-Hall do Brasil, Ltda., *Rio de Janeiro*

NOTICE

The procedures described in this textbook are based on consultation with nursing authorities. The author and publisher have taken care to make certain that these procedures reflect currently accepted clinical practice; however, they cannot be considered absolute recommendations.

The material in this textbook contains the most current information available at the time of publication. However, federal, state and local guidelines concerning clinical practices, including without limitation, those governing infection control and universal precautions, change rapidly. The reader should note, therefore, that new regulations may require changes in some procedures.

It is the responsibility of the reader to familiarize himself or herself with the policies and procedures set by federal, state and local agencies as well as the institution or agency where the reader is employed. The authors and the publishers of this textbook, and the supplements written to accompany it, disclaim any liability, loss or risk resulting directly or indirectly from the suggested procedures and theory, from any undetected errors, or from the reader's misunderstanding of the text. It is the reader's responsibility to stay informed of any new changes or recommendations made by any federal, state and local agency as well as by his or her employing health care institution or agency.

Dedication

*We dedicate this book to our nursing
assistant students, who by sharing
their joys and concerns,
motivated us to write this textbook.*

Thank you.

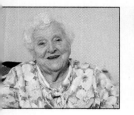

Brief
Contents

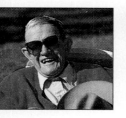

Contents

UNIT ONE: Introduction to Long-Term Care: The Facility
and the Nursing Assistant

UNIT TWO: Infection Control and Safety Considerations

UNIT SEVEN: Care of the Resident with Special Needs

List of Procedures

List of Guidelines

Foreword

In the early 1980s, there arose a national concern about the quality of care being provided for the elderly residents of the country's nursing homes. Florida shared that concern, and in an effort to improve the quality of care in our state, the legislature enacted a law that required certification of nursing assistants who were employed in long-term care facilities.

Prior to the enactment of this legislation, the objectives of formal educational programs developed for the preparation of nursing assistants were directed primarily toward training a practitioner for the acute care setting. Textbooks were written to meet these objectives.

The enactment of the nursing certification legislation was specific in its mandate for formal educational preparation. In Hillsborough County, Florida, the school district began offering nursing assistant programs in the nursing homes. As we developed the curriculum for the program, we began to search for a textbook. We wanted a book that was designed precisely for use by nursing assistant students in nursing homes, was thorough in procedural content, recognized the biopsychosocial aspect of the care provided for residents, emphasized the integral nature of restorative and rehabilitative procedures, and met the unique learning skills and abilities for the population for which it was written. Through the years, we have continued to look for such a textbook.

After reviewing *The Long-Term Care Nursing Assistant*, I believe our search has ended. The text meets all our criteria. In addition, the tone of the book is a constant reminder of the emphasis that must always be placed on the emotional aspect of care that is given to the elderly resident. Showing respect, building independence, and maintaining the resident's self-esteem, essential elements of quality care, are concepts that are explicit and implied in every chapter.

In 1985, at a seminar held by the National Citizens' Coalition for Nursing Home Reform, 450 residents from nursing homes in 15 cities stated that they wanted nursing aides who treated them with dignity, sympathy, and patience. In a 1975 book entitled *A Home Is Not a Home*, Janet Tullock, who had been a nursing home resident for 17 years, wrote, "Erosion of self-respect was never done intentionally, but neither was it intentionally prevented."

I envision a future where nursing assistants, who have been educated using *The Long-Term Care Nursing Assistant* as the textbook, will provide the kind of care that will instill a sense of well-being in the residents and cause them to say, "This home is my home."

L. June Saltzgaver R.N., Ph.D.
Supervisor, Health Occupations Education
Hillsborough District Schools
Florida

Preface

We, the authors of *The Long-Term Care Nursing Assistant,* are classroom teachers who interact with nursing assistants in long-term care on a daily basis. We have observed their problems and felt their frustration, as they searched for information that would enable them to deliver the highest quality of care. Many long-term care textbooks are adaptations of acute care texts, and only superficially address the circumstances and concerns of the nursing assistant in long-term care. This textbook is written for long-term care, and deals with the realities of that setting.

The unifying element of *The Long-Term Care Nursing Assistant* is restorative care, with emphasis on maintaining and regaining independence. Respect for the individuality of each resident and the well-being of the whole person are part of the continuing theme with the focus on the use of communication as a restorative measure. The restorative approach to meeting the resident's needs continues throughout the text.

The Long-Term Care Nursing Assistant emphasizes the integral role of the nursing assistant in providing resident care. It stresses a positive approach, as well as the challenges and rewards of caregiving. Guidelines are offered for taking care of oneself in this very demanding career. A writing style that speaks directly to the reader allows the student to identify with the material.

Special features for easier understanding include:

• Simple language, with clear, concise sentence structure accommodates students at various reading levels.

• Photographs are used generously to impact the reader on an emotional level, and allow identification with feelings and experiences.

• Numerous line drawings provide clear understanding of procedural steps.

• Thought-provoking discussion questions and innovative application exercises stimulate critical thinking, and involve the reader on a personal level. They help to verify understanding of the material.

• Easy to follow procedures are written in a simple style, beginning with a reminder to follow the steps that are basic to the provision of all care. This allows the student to focus on the actual procedural steps.

• Guidelines are offered in place of lengthy procedures when appropriate.

• Chapters and units address subject matter thoroughly, in context, rather than separating related topics.

• Specific, measurable objectives open each chapter and are easily referenced in headings and sub-headings.

• A vocabulary list contains key terms which are defined and highlighted in the text.

• The glossary contains all vocabulary words and important terms used in the text, and provides simple definitions.

• The index thoroughly references and cross-references subjects, allowing readers of various skill levels to readily access information.

The Long-Term Care Nursing Assistant is divided into 7 units, containing a total of 25 chapters. It is presented in a logical sequence, starting with an introduction to health care, and moving through an understanding of the resident's needs to procedures and techniques for meeting those needs. Each chapter is independent of the others, allowing the instructor to teach it in any order. The skills required by OBRA are presented early in the text. This provides a foundation for teaching either a short, concise nursing assistant program, or a longer, more detailed course.

Unit I: **Introduction to Long-Term Care: The Facility and the Nursing Assistant** explains the purpose and organization of the long-term care facility. It describes the health care team, the role of individual members of the team, and the function of the chain-of-command. A detailed explanation is given concerning the role of the nursing assistant. Employability skills are discussed, with emphasis on stress management and taking care of oneself. Legal responsibilities, ethical values and resident's rights are combined in one chapter. This unit introduces the unifying theme of the text—restorative care. Restorative measures and programs are defined, and the functions of the nursing assistant as a member of the restorative team are explained. Specific restorative measures and programs are described in more detail throughout the book.

Unit II: **Infection Control and Safety Considerations** addresses the protection, health, and safety of the residents. Infection control techniques, body mechanics and other safety measures are discussed. The psychosocial effects of isolation are explained, and a restorative approach is presented. Universal precautions as mandated by OSHA are emphasized. HIV and other bloodborne pathogens are discussed. Residents' rights and legal issues in regard to restraints are explained, and alternatives to restraints are emphasized. Fire prevention and emergency measures, such as CPR and the Heimlich Maneuver are discussed. Infection control and safety techniques introduced in this unit are included throughout the text, when appropriate.

Unit III: **Communication Skills Related to Long-Term Care** focuses on effective communication with residents, visitors and staff members. The dynamics of communication are described as a "bridge" that connects one human being with another. Resident care planning and the provision of quality care are shown to be dependent upon basic interpersonal communication skills, as well as thorough and timely observation, reporting and recording. Specific guidelines are provided for communicating with vision-, hearing- and speech-impaired residents. Basic medical terminology is presented in a simple, straight-forward manner. A list of commonly used abbreviations is included.

Unit IV: **The Resident in Long-Term Care** focuses on the geriatric resident and includes an explanation of the aging process. Basic body structure and function are presented in this unit. Uncomplicated line drawings of body systems enhance understanding. Changes of aging, and common problems of the elderly are grouped together for easier study and understanding. After differentiating between physical and psychosocial needs, the basic needs of human beings are presented in a manner that holds personal significance for most students. The importance of respect for individuality and concern for the whole person is approached through an explanation of the effects of life's experiences on aging individuals. This unit includes a discussion of the impact of psychosocial changes that occur in later life, and provides suggestions for restorative measures to be used in meeting psychosocial needs of the elderly resident. Sexuality, the need for love and affection, depression, aggressive behavior and confusion are addressed, with restorative care measures for each. A thorough presentation of care of the resident with Alzheimer's disease is included in this unit. Emphasis on the psychosocial aspect of care is incorporated throughout the text.

Unit V: **The Resident's Environment** addresses the resident's unit and bedmaking. It emphasizes the importance of a restorative environment. The care and use of equipment is discussed, as well as the responsibility of the nursing assistant in caring for the resident's unit. The emotional impact of admission is addressed, and the responsibilities of the nursing assistant in the admission, transfer and discharge of the resident are identified.

Unit VI: **Providing Basic Care** emphasizes a restorative approach for meeting the needs of the resident. It includes procedures for assisting the resident with mobility, personal care, hygiene, nutrition, fluids and elimination. It also includes restorative skin care and the measurement of vital signs.

Chapter 17, **Moving and Exercising Residents** is divided into three sections for easier study and understanding. Section I emphasizes the importance of exercise and activity. Section II includes procedures for moving, lifting and positioning the resident. Section III deals with ambulation, range of motion and other exercises.

This unit includes restorative dining, bowel and bladder retraining and range-of-motion exercises. Self-care and independence is stressed. Fluid balance and the role of the nursing assistant in preventing dehydration is discussed.

Unit VII: **Care of the Resident with Special Needs** includes special procedures such as care of the resident receiving oxygen, care of casts, weighing and measuring the resident, collecting specimens, hot and cold applications and the application of support stockings and bandages. Death and dying stresses the relationship between attitude toward death and the response to the dying resident. It addresses meeting the needs of the dying resident, the family and the other residents. Suggestions are offered to help staff members cope with their own stress.

While *The Long-Term Care Nursing Assistant* is specifically written for the nursing assistant in long-term care, it can be equally helpful to the nursing assistant in other settings. The thorough presentation of basic nursing skills will also be useful to L.P.N.'s as a remedial resource. The text meets OBRA guidelines and will accommodate state curriculums. It can be used in a regular school setting or in a nursing home training program. We, the authors, have written an instructor's manual and a student workbook to accompany the textbook. Lesson plans, chapter quizzes and a final exam are contained in the instructor's manual. The workbook includes worksheets, student activities and competency check-offs. Using both supplements will enhance and expedite the instructional process, while meeting the individual needs of the student.

To the student: Traditionally, textbooks are written for teachers. This book is written for you—it is centered around the nursing assistant student. Early on, we envisioned a textbook that would meet your specific needs. *The Long-Term Care Nursing Assistant* is that vision come true. Writing a textbook is hard work, it is often frustrating and stressful, but for us, it has been a labor of love.

Information is provided to assist both the student and the instructor. It is the instructor's responsibility to explain and enhance the material, but it is your responsibility to learn. It is with this thought in mind that we dedicate *The Long-Term Care Nursing Assistant* to you, the nursing assistant in long-term care.

Acknowledgments

We, the authors, would like to express our gratitude and appreciation to the people who provided support and assistance during this project. We would, first, like to thank the most important people in our lives—our families. Writing a textbook is a time-consuming process that often interferes with family dynamics. We appreciate your understanding.

For their love and encouragement, we wish to express our gratitude to our families:

My daughter, Cara, was mature enough to become a successful young adult while I devoted my time and energy to this project. My son, Jeff, listened, and encouraged me when I needed it most. My brother, Richard, and my Aunt Roberta, for helping me believe in myself when I had doubts. My parents, Frank and Jolene, for their pride in my success. Thanks to all of you.

Barbara A. Blasband

Special thanks to my children and their spouses: Lewis and Dolores, Wayne and Debbie, Sandy and Ray, Roger and Susan, Tom and Donna. You gave me support and understanding when I needed it most. Your belief in me, helped me believe in myself, and gave me strength when I thought the project would never end. And to my grandchildren for sharing me with the textbook: Michelle, David, Christopher, Nicholas, Melissa and Jessica.

Peggy A. Grubbs

Our colleagues and friends:

Dr. June Saltzgaver, our mentor and ardent supporter. Without her this book would have been an idea that never blossomed. Judy Thom and our co-workers at Learey Technical Center for their support and assistance. Linda McClamma for her support, advice and willingness to share her knowledge of the long-term care industry. Anne Rutherford who shared, not only her knowledge, but the hospitality of her house. Shirley Bracken, for her creative assistance in planning the art. Frank Hill for his advice and expertise in emergency care procedures.

Staff members, families, and residents of the following facilities:

Arbors at Brandon, Subacute and Rehabilitative Center of Brandon, Florida, an affiliate of Arbor Health Care Company

C.S.I. Inc., Lake Towers and Sun Terrace Health Care Convalescent Services Inc., of Sun City Center, Florida

Palm Gardens of Sun City, Florida, an affiliate of National Health Corp L.P.

Plant City Health Care Center, an affiliate of National Health Corp L.P.

The photography models:

Residents and their families; nurses, nursing assistants and other staff members; students; our families and friends. Thank you for your time and patience.

The Prentice Hall staff for all their expertise, assistance and patience:

Mark Hartman who believed in us, allowed us to be ourselves, and helped create a new and exciting concept.

Louise Fullam, who was always there with an answer.

Marilyn Meserve, who did her best to keep us organized.

Michal Heron, photographer, whose artistry and perfectionism helped us create images of the world of the long-term care resident.

Richard Logan, assistant photographer and peacemaker.

Reviewers

Barbara Acello, R.N.
Director of Education
H.E.A. Management Group
Denton, TX 76201

Sheila Chesanow, R.N., B.S.
Care Enterprises
Education Department
Chico, CA 95926

Margaret J. Denault, R.N.C., Med.
Staff Development
Heritage Hall Nursing and Rehabilitation Centers
Agawam, MA 01001

Clair Dickey
Staff Development Coordinator
Living Centers of America (Windsor Health Care Center)
Windsor, CO 80550

Cheryl L. Hoffman, B.S.N., R.N.C.
Education Department
St. Luke's Extended Care Center
Spokane, WA 99202

Ida A. Horvitz, Director
Continuing Education
University of Cincinnati
College of Nursing and Health
Cincinnati, OH 45221-0038

Beverly Long R.N.
Staff Development
Yuma Life Care Center
323 West Ninth Avenue
Yuma, CO 80759

Judith Pawloski
Child and Family Service of Washtenaw
Lifework Department
Ypsilanti, MI 48197

Dr. Rosanne Pruitt
College of Nursing
Clemson University
Clemson, SC 29634

Gail Shoulders Ph.D., R.N.
Gail Shoulders & Company
Toledo, OH 43609

Lana B. Simonds, R.N., M.S.N.
Nursing Quality Advisor
Living Centers of America
Greeley, CO 80634

Cynthia D. Voorhees
Medishare Health Education Learning Programs
Edison, NJ 08817

Julia Walters, R.N.
Staff Development
Annaburg Manor
Manassas, VA 22110

Introduction to the Long-Term Care Facility

OBJECTIVES

Upon completing this chapter, you will be able to do the following:

1. List two purposes of the long-term care facility.

2. Identify the purpose of federal and state regulations.

3. Describe the organization of the long-term care facility.

4. Explain the meaning and importance of the chain of command.

5. Identify four members of the health care team.

6. Identify the members of the nursing department and define their roles.

7. Explain the concept of the career ladder in health care.

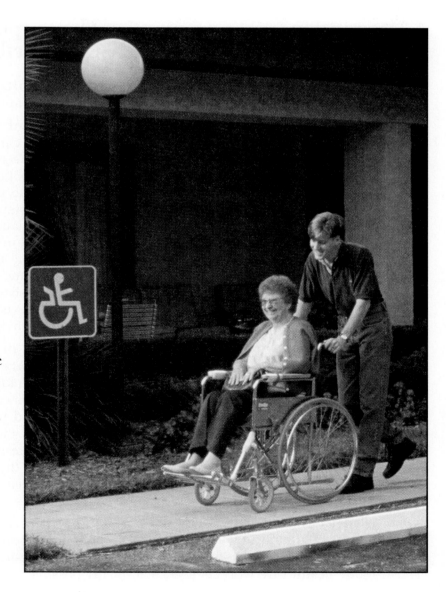

VOCABULARY

The following words or terms will help you to understand this chapter:

Long-term care facility (LTCF)
Resident
Geriatrics
Rehabilitation
Function
Restorative care

OBRA (Omnibus Budget Reconciliation Act)
Administrator
Chain of command
Health care team
Director of nurses (D.O.N.)

Assistant director of nurses (A.D.O.N.)
Registered nurse (R.N.)
Licensed practical nurse (L.P.N.)
Certified nursing assistant (C.N.A.)

A Description of Long-Term Care

A **long-term care facility (LTCF)** provides health care to people who are not able to care for themselves at home, but are not sick enough to be in a hospital. A long-term care facility may be called a skilled nursing facility, an intermediate care facility, an extended care facility, a convalescent center, or a nursing home. While the name of the facility may indicate the level of care that is given, many facilities provide several levels of care. Long-term care facilities share many of the same goals and serve similar groups of people.

A few of the people who are admitted to a long-term care facility stay only for a short time. However, many stay for years, and some remain for the rest of their lives. The facility becomes their home. A person who lives in a long-term care facility is called a **resident**. That person is a resident of the long-term care facility, just as you are a resident of your home.

Although long-term care facilities care for all age groups, many residents are elderly. The elderly who live in a long-term care facility are called geriatric residents. **Geriatrics** is the branch of medicine that is concerned with the problems and diseases of the elderly. Many health care workers specialize in geriatrics.

The Purpose of a Long-Term Care Facility

Three important purposes of a long-term care facility are as follows:

Provision of Care. The main purpose of any health care facility is to provide care based on the resident's needs. These needs may change. For example, a person who has had a stroke may be almost helpless and require assistance for most needs. Care would be planned to meet all those needs. As improvement occurs and strength is regained, the resident might be able to do more self-care, and would no longer require as much assistance. The plan of care would be changed as needed. Much of this care would be provided by nursing assistants.

Prevention of Injury or Disease. Prevention of injury or disease is an important purpose of a long-term care facility. The resident must be cared for in a safe manner. Safe practices and procedures prevent the spread of infection and disease. Protecting the resident is the responsibility of every employee. It is one of the major responsibilities of the nursing assistant. Practicing proper procedure protects the employee as well.

Rehabilitation and Restorative Care. **Rehabilitation** is a method that is used to bring the resident back to as nearly normal as possible. This includes physical, mental, emotional, and social functions. **Function**

means a purpose or action. **Restorative care** is the nursing care that is given to attain and maintain the highest level of function and independence. Although restorative care is discussed in detail in Chapter 4, throughout this textbook you will learn to use the restorative approach.

Federal and State Regulations: OBRA

The federal government sets certain regulations (standards or rules) that long-term care facilities must follow. Each state must enforce these regulations and may add others. Many of the tasks that nursing assistants do are required by regulations. For example, regulations determine the way that equipment must be used.

The purpose of these regulations is to protect the residents and ensure quality care. A state survey team inspects the facility and looks at the records. Members of the survey team talk to the staff and the residents. It is the responsibility of every employee to help meet the regulations. The nursing assistant plays a very important role in the delivery of quality care.

OBRA (Omnibus Budget Reconciliation Act) is a law that focuses on the care of the elderly in long-term care facilities. This federal law was enacted in 1987 and went into effect in 1990. OBRA provides for the safety, happiness, and well-being of the residents. Resident rights such as confidentiality and freedom of choice are specifically addressed. Quality of care is assured by requirements regarding nursing assistant training and the provision of licensed nursing personnel and social services. All departments are subject to OBRA. State laws and regulations may be even more strict than OBRA and must also be upheld.

Organization of the Long-Term Care Facility

Many long-term care facilities are owned by corporations. One corporation may own facilities that are located in different parts of the country. There are usually regional or district managers who are responsible for a certain number of facilities. Individuals may own one or two facilities and may manage one of them.

Each facility has an administrator. The **administrator** is responsible for the operation of the entire facility. All department heads report to the administrator, who is responsible to the owner, manager, or a board of trustees.

The person who is in charge of a department is called a department head. The facility is divided into several departments. These may include nursing, social services, activities, dietary, rehabilitation, medical records, business, housekeeping, and maintenance. A small facility might combine some of these departments, and a large facility may have additional departments. All departments are involved in the residents' care (see Fig. 1-1).

The Chain of Command

The **chain of command** is the order of authority and problem solving within a facility. Authority begins at the top and moves downward, as problems move upward. To follow the chain of command, employees should take problems, questions, and reports to the person directly above them on the chain. If the problem is not resolved, it continues to move upward, one level at a time. Each level is a link in the chain. Skipping links in the chain causes confusion and misunderstanding. Figure 1-3 gives an example of the chain of command in the nursing department. Each department follows a chain of command that keeps communication flowing smoothly in both directions.

The Health Care Team

The **health care team** includes all the people who provide care and services for the residents. The team works together to accom-

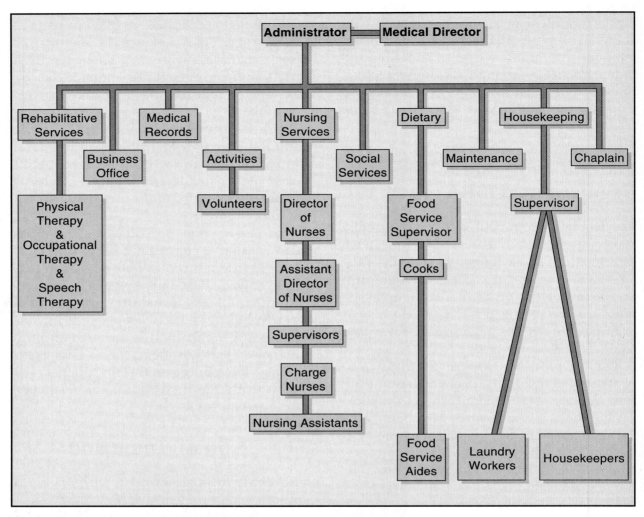

Fig. 1-1 An example of an organizational chart for a long-term care facility.

plish the job. Each team member is important in his or her own way. This team can be compared to a ball team in which each player has a position to play, and it takes all of them to win the game. Each person on the health care team has a job to do, and it takes all of them to deliver high-quality care. For example, the nursing assistant gives the resident a bath. Medicine that is ordered by the doctor is given by the nurse. The dietary department prepares meals, and the housekeeper cleans the rooms. All the team members work with the resident, and with each other, to deliver quality care (see Fig. 1-2). The nursing assistant is the member of the health care team who provides basic care for the residents on a daily basis.

The Nursing Department

Nursing is the largest department in any health care facility because it provides most of the direct patient care.

Responsibilities of Nurses. Nurses plan and provide the care of the residents. They must see that the plan of care is followed. Nurses teach, give medications, and provide treatments to the residents.

The **director of nurses (D.O.N.)** is responsible for the nursing department. Some facilities have an **assistant director of nurses (A.D.O.N.)** who helps the D.O.N. There also may be a staff development coordinator who is responsible for staff education. Some facilities have a nurse

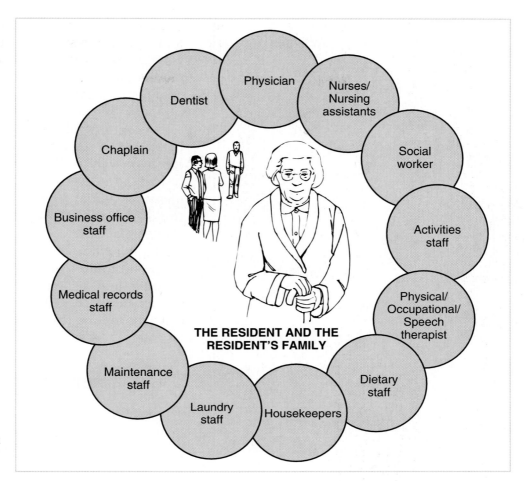

THE RESIDENT AND THE
RESIDENT'S FAMILY

Fig. 1-2
All members of the
health care team work
with the resident and
with each other.

practitioner who works with a physician and may write orders and do assessments. Most facilities have supervisors and charge nurses.

The nursing supervisor is usually responsible for one shift and reports to the D.O.N. or A.D.O.N. The charge nurse is responsible for one team or nursing station and may be called the team leader. The team leader reports to the nursing supervisor. The chain of command does not change, although the titles may vary from one facility to another.

Look at the nursing department chart (see Fig. 1-3). As you can see by the chart, the nursing assistant reports to the charge nurse, who determines your work assignment. If you have a question or a problem, you should take it to the charge nurse first. If the charge nurse can't help you, you should go to the supervisor or proceed up the chain as necessary.

Members of the Nursing Department.
The nursing department members include registered nurses (R.N.s), licensed practical nurses (L.P.N.s), and certified nursing assistants (C.N.A.s). In some states, the L.P.N. is called a licensed vocational nurse (L.V.N.). Individual responsibilities depend upon education and training.

Registered Nurse: The **registered nurse (R.N.)** is a person who is educated and licensed to plan, provide, and evaluate nursing care. Upon graduation from a two-, three-, or four-year program the student must take a state board examination to become an R.N.

Licensed Practical Nurse/Licensed Vocational Nurse: The **licensed practical nurse (L.P.N.)** is a person who is educated and licensed to assist the registered nurse in planning, providing, and evaluating nursing care. Upon completion of a 12 to 18 month

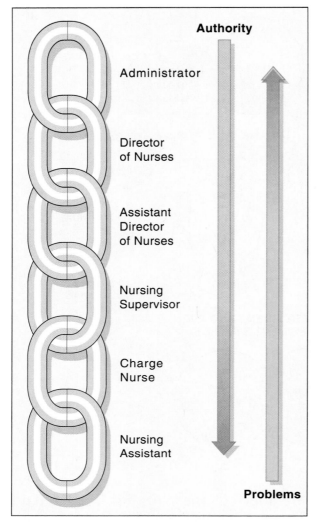

Authority

Administrator

Director of Nurses

Assistant Director of Nurses

Nursing Supervisor

Charge Nurse

Nursing Assistant

Problems

Fig. 1-3 An example of a nursing department chart. Always follow the chain of command.

training program, the student must pass a state board examination for licensure. The training is focused on technical nursing skills.

Certified Nursing Assistant: The **certified nursing assistant (C.N.A.)** assists the nurses in providing care for the residents. A nursing assistant may be called an aide, a nurses aide, or a patient care assistant. A male nursing assistant may use one of those titles, or he may be called an orderly.

In the past, nursing assistant education has varied from on-the-job training to state-approved certification classes. A federal law now requires that nursing assistants who work in long-term care facilities must complete a state-approved training program to demonstrate competency. A state examination may be required for certification.

The training of nursing assistants is very important because they provide most of the hands-on care to the residents. Helping the residents to eat, bathe, and dress are examples of activities in which a person's hands touch the resident's body. This is called "hands-on" care.

Many facilities have rehabilitation aides, hospitality aides, or area aides. The titles, training, and responsibilities vary from one facility to another. The role of the nursing assistant will be discussed in more detail in Chapter 2.

The Career Ladder

The C.N.A. position is the first rung of the health care career ladder. There are many job opportunities available in the health care field. With additional training and education, you can move into higher levels of employment. If you decide that you would like to enter some other branch of health care, your C.N.A. training will be a valuable asset.

Conclusion

Remember these important points:

1. Patients in long-term care facilities are called residents.

2. Geriatrics concerns the problems and diseases of the elderly.

3. Restorative care is the nursing care that encourages normal function and independence.

4. The purpose of federal and state regulations is to protect the residents and ensure quality care.

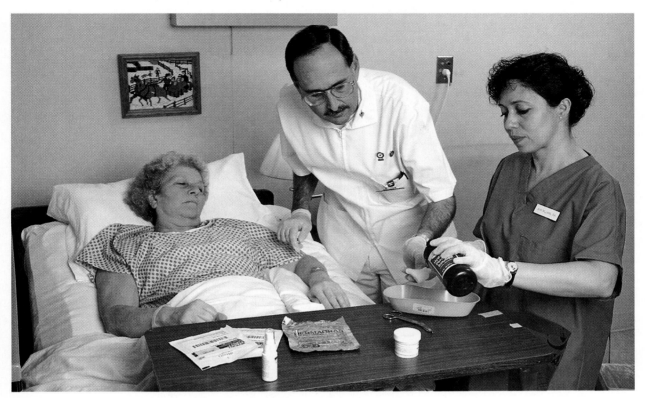

Fig. 1-4 The nursing assistant helps the nurse care for the resident.

5. Members of the health care team should always follow the chain of command.

6. The health care team includes all the people who provide care and services to the residents.

7. Members of the nursing department include R.N.s, L.P.N.s, and C.N.A.s

Discussion Questions

1. Why did you decide to work in a long-term care facility?

2. How do federal and state regulations protect the resident?

3. What problems might arise if you do not follow the chain of command?

Application Exercise

1. Each student should obtain a copy of the organizational chart of the facility in which he or she is working. If the student is not yet working or assigned to a facility, the instructor may collect some charts for this exercise.

As a group compare the differences in the charts.

 a. Discuss why some charts have more positions.

 b. List the different titles for the same job.

 c. Identify the chain of command in each chart.

 d. Discuss the responsibilities at each level of the chain.

The Nursing Assistant in the Long-Term Care Facility

OBJECTIVES

Upon completing this chapter, you will be able to do the following:

1. Describe the role and responsibilities of the nursing assistant in the long-term care facility.

2. Explain the nursing assistant's responsibilities in providing restorative care.

3. List six desirable qualities and characteristics of the nursing assistant.

4. List four areas of importance in caring for yourself.

5. Identify four measures to cope with stress.

6. Describe the procedure for conducting a job search, completing an application and participating in an interview.

7. Identify three skills that will improve job performance.

8. Identify the five basic steps that are used with all procedures.

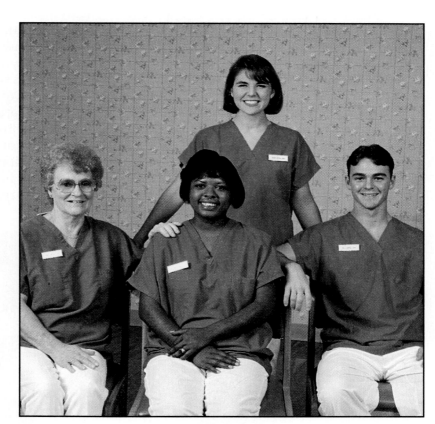

VOCABULARY

The following words or terms will help you to understand this chapter:

Responsibility
Activities of daily living
  (ADLs)
Job description

Empathy
Self-esteem
Stress
Personal hygiene

Employability skills
Procedure
Priority

The Role of the Nursing Assistant

It takes a very special kind of person to be a nursing assistant. Nursing assistants work very closely with residents and often develop special trusting relationships with them. Residents who have been separated from their families, and residents who have no families depend on those closest to them for emotional support. If you choose to be a nursing assistant, you may be the one person who makes a difference in their lives. The resident may actually think of you as a family member and look to you for love and affection. This can be the most rewarding job of your life.

Nursing assistants help nurses provide care for the residents of the long-term care facility. They work under the supervision of a nurse. They make beds, give baths, and provide care to promote physical comfort. Nursing assistants help to meet the residents' social, spiritual, and other emotional needs.

The role of the nursing assistant is changing. In the past, most nursing assistants were employed in hospitals. Today, there are many jobs available to nursing assistants in clinics, adult care centers, mental health centers, or assisted care facilities. However, the majority of nursing assistants work in home health or long-term care facilities.

The role of the nursing assistant in the long-term care facility is different from that of the nursing assistant in the hospital. There are more nurses to provide direct care in the hospital. The nursing assistant in the long-term care facility provides most of the hands-on care.

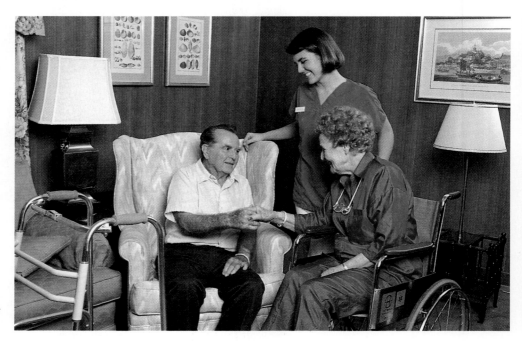

Fig. 2-1
The nursing assistant helps residents to meet their social needs.

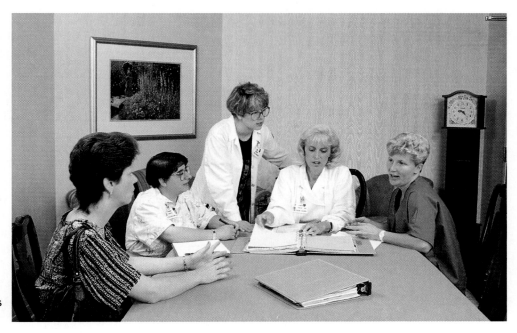

Fig. 2-2
The R.N.A. participates in care plan meetings.

The emphasis on restorative nursing has created another role for the nursing assistant. Although all nursing assistants are expected to provide restorative care, additional training may be obtained to specialize in rehabilitation. The nursing assistant who completes this training is called a restorative or rehabilitation nursing assistant (R.N.A.). The R.N.A. must be able to encourage and teach the residents. Restorative charting may require detailed notes. The R.N.A. participates in care plan meetings and provides progress reports. The presence of an R.N.A. in a facility does not take away the responsibility of the other nursing assistants. Restorative care must be provided by all staff members.

Other roles of the nursing assistant in long-term care, such as area aide or hospitality aide, are difficult to define. Their responsibilities and qualifications vary from one facility to another.

Responsibilities of the Nursing Assistant

A **responsibility** is a duty or obligation to do something. One of the most important responsibilities of a nursing assistant is to perform correctly certain tasks, skills, or procedures. Instructions for performing these tasks are included in this textbook. Many of them involve assisting the resident with activities of daily living.

Activities of daily living (ADLs) are activities that a person does every day in order to live. ADLs include personal care such as mouth care, bathing, hair care, skin care, foot and nail care, and shaving. Eating, drinking, getting dressed, and going to the bathroom are ADLs. Exercise, positioning, and moving are also ADLs that may require the nursing assistant's help.

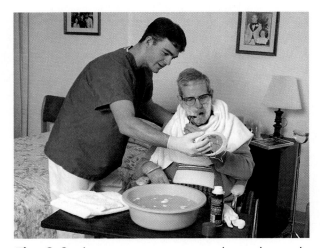

Fig. 2-3 The nursing assistant assists the residents with activities of daily living.

The nursing assistant is responsible for performing other tasks such as

- Making beds
- Straightening the resident's room or area
- Caring for equipment
- Measuring the resident's temperature, pulse, respiration, and blood pressure
- Measuring fluid intake and output
- Collecting specimens
- Performing urine tests
- Applying support hose
- Measuring height and weight
- Admitting, transferring, or discharging a resident
- Observing, reporting, and recording information

As a nursing assistant, you will be helping the nurse to perform these tasks, or you will do them alone. The nursing assistant always works under the supervision of a nurse.

Other responsibilities of the nursing assistant in the long-term care facility are the following:

- Assist the residents with restorative care.
- Treat the residents with respect.
- Respect the residents' privacy.
- Protect the residents from injury.
- Treat families and visitors with respect.
- Follow the policies of the facility.
- Attend educational programs for employees (inservices).
- Follow state and federal guidelines.
- Follow safety rules.
- Prevent the spread of infection.
- Maintain a professional appearance.
- Assist new employees.
- Be a loyal and dependable employee.
- Continue to learn.
- Develop reliable work habits.

A **job description** lists the tasks and responsibilities of a nursing assistant. The tasks may not be the same in every facility. There are some tasks that a nursing assistant is not allowed to do. Education, training, and governmental guidelines determine the appropriate responsibilities.

The nursing assistant may *not*

- Give medications
- Perform sterile procedures
- Suction a resident
- Start, adjust, or discontinue an IV
- Supervise the work of another nursing assistant

Providing Restorative Care

In the past, many long-term care facilities provided what was called "custodial care." Custodial care placed emphasis on meeting the needs of the body. Although the residents were kept clean, dry, and well fed, limited time was spent in attempts to restore normal function. Restorative care is not the same as custodial care. The objective of restorative care is to assist the resident toward independence and a return to as nearly normal function as possible. Restorative care is now the basis of all nursing care. Providing restorative care is one of the major responsibilities of the nursing assistant in long-term care. It is accomplished by encouraging the resident to function independently with as little assistance as possible. The resident will benefit more if allowed to help, although it may be quicker and easier to do the task yourself. Chapter 4 offers more detailed information about rehabilitation and restorative care. The restorative approach should be used in all the nursing tasks that you perform. That is the best way to assist the resident with rehabilitation.

Personal Qualities and Characteristics of the Nursing Assistant

Qualities and characteristics help form a person's attitude. While you are born with some qualities, others are learned. For example, can you usually be counted on to do what you are supposed to do? This is a quality called dependability. You can learn to be dependable, if that is not a quality that you already have. Dependability is one of the most important qualities of a nursing assistant. If you are dependable, your employer can count on your being at work when you are scheduled. You will carry out assignments in a timely manner. Your coworkers will also appreciate your dependability.

There are many qualities and characteristics in addition to dependability that are necessary to be a successful nursing assistant. It is important that you like caring for other people. You must have patience and self-control. Caring for sick people is not always easy. Some residents may be demanding, or they may be confused and have difficulty understanding. Slowness and uncertainty may cause frustration.

You will need to be sensitive and considerate. Think about how your words will sound before you speak. Be courteous and respectful and avoid hurting anyone's feelings. It is important to develop empathy. **Empathy** is the ability to realize how you would feel if you were in the other person's place. An example of empathy is saying to yourself, "If I couldn't be independent, I might be unhappy too."

The best nursing assistants are cooperative and willing to learn. You will be expected to develop many new skills, which must be performed correctly. You will have to be flexible to adjust to changes and new situations. It is important that you be honest and trustworthy. These qualities will help you to be the kind of person that can be respected by employers, coworkers, residents, and others. Their respect will also increase your self-esteem. **Self-esteem** is the opinion one has of oneself. If you feel good about yourself and think that you are a worthwhile person, then you have a high self-esteem.

A nursing assistant should have a cheerful, positive attitude. Your attitude will have a direct effect on your work. If you believe that what you are doing will succeed, it usually will. If you do not believe in success, failure is likely. Your attitude also affects the people with whom you work. When you think positively, you are more likely to have a positive influence on the residents and your coworkers. A happy person helps those around her to feel happy. Take pride in what you do, and you will be better satisfied with

your job. Remember that you are one of the most important members of the health care team.

Taking Care of Yourself

One of the most important people you will learn to care for is yourself. Taking care of yourself involves protecting your health, developing proper hygiene practices and presenting a good appearance.

Health. You have a responsibility to protect your own health. You cannot function safely as a nursing assistant unless you are physically and emotionally healthy. The following suggestions will help you to stay healthy.

Eat three well-balanced meals every day, beginning with a good breakfast, to prevent fatigue. It is better to eat a light lunch, so you don't get sleepy in the afternoon. Do not go on a diet without your doctor's approval. Many "crash" diets do not provide adequate nutrition. For a healthier form of energy, eat fresh fruit instead of "junk food" at break time.

A good night's sleep, for most adults, includes eight hours of rest. However, you should try to meet your own needs. If you have a lot of responsibilities away from work, you may not feel that you have time for rest. Sometimes, 30 minutes of relaxation is all you need to feel refreshed.

Regular exercise such as swimming, playing ball or walking, helps you feel and look better. Choose a form of exercise that you enjoy. After working all day you might think you are too tired, but exercise can help you relax and feel less tense.

Avoid using alcohol or drugs. These substances affect vision, balance, coordination, and judgment. A person on drugs or alcohol often makes mistakes. Never bring alcohol or drugs to the workplace. Do not come to work if you are under the influence of alcohol or drugs. You will endanger those you are caring for, as well as yourself.

See your doctor for a regular checkup. Follow the advice given, and start treatment promptly for colds or other health problems. This helps to prevent transmission of illness to the residents who are often frail and defenseless against disease. You are more likely to catch a disease if you are run down or over tired.

Stress. Learn to cope with stress. **Stress** is mental and physical tension or strain. Your job as a nursing assistant in a long-term care facility can be stressful. Your responsibilities include the health and well-being of the residents. You must perform with a high degree of accuracy at all times. Dealing with sickness and death is difficult. Your job is physically and emotionally demanding, and stress is unavoidable as you help others with their problems. You may have problems of your own. All these demands on your time can leave you feeling overwhelmed and out of control.

You cannot eliminate all the stress in your life, nor would you want to do so, because some stress is motivating. You can learn to manage stress by using the following tools:

STRESS-REDUCTION "TOOLS"

- Laughter: Take time for humor each day because laughter relieves tension.
- Talk: Talking to a friend relieves frustration and makes you feel less alone.
- Reason: Think the problem through before you start worrying.
- Assertiveness: Stand up for what you believe is right.
- Flexibility: Be willing to accept change.
- Relaxation: Do something you like. Have fun!
- Self-care: Be nice to yourself. Be aware of your own needs.
- Self-esteem: Give yourself credit for the good things you do.

Personal Hygiene. Personal hygiene is cleanliness and care of health. Cleanliness helps prevent disease. You look better and feel better when you are clean. Suggestions for personal hygiene include the following:

- Take a bath every day.
- Use deodorant to prevent underarm odor.
- Brush your teeth at least three times a day.
- Wash your hair at least once a week.
- Clean your fingernails daily, or as often as needed.

- Wash your hands frequently. Dirty hands carry germs.

Appearance. Appearance is the way you look. A nursing assistant should always have a neat, well-groomed appearance. Residents and visitors often judge the quality of care in a facility by the appearance of the employees. They may think that a nursing assistant who does not pay attention to personal appearance will not care how the residents look. Consider the following guidelines.

GUIDELINES FOR A NEAT APPEARANCE

- Practice correct posture. Stand straight with your head held high.
- Wear a clean uniform every day, following the dress code of your facility.
- Change your underclothes daily.
- Keep your shoes polished and your shoelaces clean. Wear shoes that fit well and are in good repair.
- Make sure that your stockings have no holes or runs in them.
- Wear your hair in a neat style, off your collar and out of your face. Pin up long hair.
- You may wear a watch and wedding band. Jewelry collects germs and can scratch the resident.
- Apply cosmetics and cologne lightly.
- Do not wear nail polish. Germs collect in chipped polish.
- Male nursing assistants should shave daily. Beards should be kept neatly trimmed.
- Avoid smoking while in uniform.

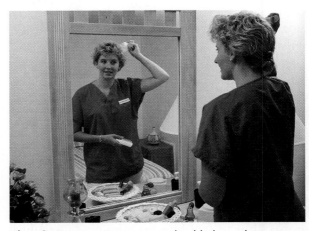

Fig. 2-4 A nursing assistant should always have a neat, well-groomed appearance.

Employability Skills

Employability skills are skills that are necessary to get a job and keep it. You may already have some of these skills, and you may have to learn others. The first important skill is how to find a job.

Job Search. The easiest way to find a job is by asking your friends and family, particularly those who are working in health care. You should check the "Help Wanted" advertisements in the classified section of the local newspaper. You can also get the names and addresses of facilities from the phone book.

Make a list of the places in which you are interested, including the address and telephone number of each facility. If you know the name of the person whom you should contact, add that to your list. Decide which facility you will apply to first. This decision will depend on several considerations such as working conditions, salary, and benefits. You may not learn this information until you are interviewed. The distance from your home to the facility and available transportation are major factors. It costs money and time to travel long distances. You might locate the facilities that are nearest to you and number them in order. Start with the facility that you have selected as number one and continue through the list as needed.

Job Application. It will save time and effort if you first make a call to the facility. You may be asked to come in to fill out an application, and you may be interviewed at that time. You should be neat and well groomed, even if you are only picking up an application form. Do not take anyone with you. Always be courteous and respectful, and answer the questions honestly. The impression you make upon application may determine whether you will be called for an interview. Figure 2-5 gives an example of an application.

You will need the following information to fill out the application:

- Educational background: When and where did you go to school? When did you gradu-

ate from high school or get a general education diploma (GED)? Be sure to include any additional education or training that you have had.

- Work experience: List your last three or four places of employment, including addresses and telephone numbers. List your duties and positions on these jobs.
- References: Include names, addresses, and telephone numbers of people who know you and will speak well of you. Ask your pastor or teacher, but do not list your relatives. You should not list a person as a reference unless you have permission from that person to do so.
- Documents: You will need your social security card, driver's license, and nursing assistant certificate. Carry copies of your certificate, as well as the original. After the interviewer sees the original, be sure to take it with you. Proof of continuing education will enhance your qualifications.

Job Interview. The meeting between an employer and an applicant to discuss a job is called an interview. The decision to hire a person is often made at this time.

GUIDELINES FOR A JOB INTERVIEW

- Be on time for the interview.
- Be prepared with the necessary information and documents.
- Present a neat, clean appearance.
- Communicate clearly.
- Show interest and enthusiasm.
- Be courteous and polite.
- Demonstrate self-confidence.
- Bring a pencil and note paper.

The interview is the time to ask questions about employee benefits. Benefits might include life insurance, medical and hospitalization insurance, and retirement or tuition reimbursement. Availability of a credit union is also very helpful. A credit union is a form of banking that offers many advantages to its members, including low-interest loans.

Job Performance. When you start a new job, you may be in orientation for a few

EMPLOYMENT APPLICATION
(Please print plainly)

Personal Information
Date:_____

1. Name_____
   (Last)   (First)   (Middle)

2. Soc. Sec. No.:_____

3. Present Address:_____
   (No.)   (Street)   (Apt. No.)

   _____
   (City)   (State)   (Zip)

4. Number of years at the above address:_____

5. Phone Number:_____
   (Area Code)   (Number)

Educational Background

Type of School	Name and Address	How Many Years Attended	Graduated	Course or Major
Grammar or Grade			__Yes __No	
High School			__Yes __No	
College			__Yes __No	

Work History (List in order, last or present employer first)

Dates From To	Name, Address and Telephone Number of Employer	Rate of Pay Start Finish	Supervisor's Name	Reason for Leaving
From To				

Describe in detail the
work you did:

Dates From To	Name, Address and Telephone Number of Employer	Rate of Pay Start Finish	Supervisor's Name	Reason for Leaving
From To				

Describe in detail the
work you did:

May we contact the employers listed above? _____ If not, indicate below which one(s) you do not wish
us to contact and why._____

Personal References
List three people who can give you personal references. (You may exclude former employees, relatives,
members of the clergy or persons whose title or business address might indicate your race, color, religion,
sex, age, national origin, ancestry or disability.)

Name and Occupation   Address   Telephone Number

1._____
   (Name)   (Occupation)

2._____
   (Name)   (Occupation)

3._____
   (Name)   (Occupation)

Fig. 2-5 A sample job application form.

days. During this time you will become familiar with the policies and procedures of the facility. Policies are guidelines for operating a facility. A **procedure** explains steps to be taken in performing a task. Procedures can be found in the procedure book located at each nurses' station. Don't be afraid to ask questions if you don't understand.

You will probably be on probation for a period of time. Probation provides the employer with an opportunity to evaluate your performance as a nursing assistant. Following probation the decision is made as to whether or not you will become a permanent employee. Evaluation is an ongoing process. Promotions and raises depend upon your evaluation. Developing the qualities and characteristics listed earlier in this chapter will help to make you a valued employee. Skills that improve job performance include

- Working with others
- Organizing your work
- Planning
- Prioritizing

Working with Others: One of the most important employability skills that you can develop is the ability to get along with others. As a member of the health care team, the nursing assistant works with many people to care for the residents. Care is delivered best when all work together as a team. Cooperation makes the job easier for everyone in the long-term care facility. Assist your coworkers whenever possible. Many procedures are more comfortable for the resident when employees work together. It is also safer, because there is less chance of accident or injury. However, do not expect others to do your work for you. You are responsible for completing your assignment.

Your assignment may not always be the same. The nurse makes the assignment at the beginning of the shift. The care of the residents is divided among the nursing assistants who are on duty each day. Some days your assignment may seem difficult, while at other times it may be easier. You must work where you are assigned. No matter where you are working in the facility,

never say, "That's not my resident." You must assist any resident whenever it is necessary.

A nursing assistant must learn to follow orders. Listen carefully, and question the nurse if you do not understand. Be sure the nurse knows if there is something that you cannot do. Always let the nurse know when you are leaving your work area for any reason.

Be polite and considerate. Do not argue, use abusive language, talk about other people, or criticize your employer. If you look at both sides of the situation, it will help you to control angry feelings. Personal problems should be left at home. Always follow the chain of command when you have problems or complaints.

Organizing Your Work: The job of the nursing assistant in a long-term care facility is not an easy one. There is a lot of work to be done, and organizing helps you get it done on time. Organization also reduces stress. It is frustrating to work hard all day and fail to finish, because you were not organized. Organization is a skill that can be learned and improved.

The key to organization is planning. Take time, before rounds, to plan your day. Spending a few minutes then will save time later. You should make rounds as soon as you get a report from the nurse. This means that you will briefly visit each of the residents that you have been assigned. Identify and take care of any immediate needs that they might have. Because this reassures the residents and makes them less anxious, they will be less likely to interrupt you while you do your planning.

Make a list of any procedures that must be done at scheduled times, such as "turn every two hours." Add planned events or visits to the list, and make a note of appointments the residents need to keep. Check the calendar for activities the residents might enjoy. Do not forget meetings or inservice classes that you are required to attend.

After you have completed your list, decide which items have priority. **Priority** means rating each task in its order of importance. Anything that must be done at a specific time must be high on your priority list. Procedures that have to be done by the end of your shift might be placed next on your list. Follow that order as closely as possible. Because priorities can change, you must be flexible. A new admission or sudden illness will change the order of priority. A priority list will help you complete the most important tasks on time.

Organizing your work involves managing your time. Estimate the time that each task will take. With experience you will have a general idea of the amount of time you will need. Be familiar with the roles of the other health care team members. Know the routine of your facility. For example, you will have to plan your schedule around mealtimes. Identify tasks that you can group together. While the resident is in the bathroom, you might be able to make the bed. Plan ahead for tasks that will require someone's help, or for which you will need special equipment.

Collecting supplies and equipment is an important part of being organized. Before you begin any procedure, determine what you will need to complete the task, and take the necessary supplies to the area in which you will be working. The job will be easier

and will be accomplished faster if you are prepared. For example, it is a waste of time to begin making a bed only to discover that you have forgotten the top sheet.

Planning and Prioritizing: Planning, prioritizing, time management, and collecting supplies lead to organization, a job performance skill well worth developing. There are five basic steps that you must take before you begin any procedure:

Five Basic Steps Before Beginning a Procedure

1. Wash your hands.
2. Collect the equipment.
3. Identify the resident.
4. Explain the procedure.
5. Provide privacy.

There will be times when you will need to change the steps slightly. For example, you would not "explain to the resident" if you were making a bed in an empty room. However, if you will learn these steps, and remember to follow them, you will be able to do your work in a safe, organized, and efficient manner. In this text, procedures will begin with a reminder to follow the basic steps.

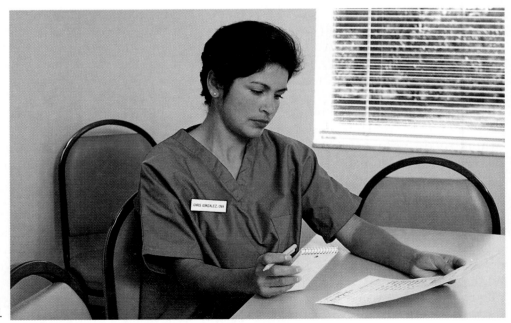

Fig. 2-6
A priority list will help you complete the most important tasks on time.

Conclusion

Remember these important points:

1. The nursing assistant always works under the supervision of a nurse.

2. Tasks and responsibilities are not the same at every facility. You will learn what is expected of you.

3. Dependability is an important quality for a nursing assistant.

4. Your attitude will have a direct effect on your work.

5. A nursing assistant must be physically and emotionally healthy.

6. Never come to work under the influence of drugs or alcohol.

7. Having high self-esteem helps you to cope with stress.

8. You look and feel better when you are clean and well groomed.

9. Residents and visitors often judge the care of the residents by the appearance of the employees.

10. Cooperation makes everybody's job easier.

11. Being organized helps you to avoid stress and get your work done on time.

12. Planning, prioritizing, managing time, and collecting supplies are important employability skills.

Discussion Questions

1. How do you feel about working as a nursing assistant?

2. Think about a restaurant that you have been in recently. Did the appearance of the employees affect your desire to eat there? How does that relate to this chapter?

3. List the qualities and characteristics that you now have that would make you a valued employee. Are there any others that you would like to develop?

4. How do you take care of yourself when you are feeling stressed?

Application Exercises

1. The instructor will invite a director of nurses from a long-term care facility to visit the class and discuss employability skills. Areas of discussion should include the following:

   a. What determines whom he or she hires?

   b. What does he or she consider to be important employability skills for a nursing assistant?

2. The class will participate in role playing a job interview. The instructor will role play the interviewer. The class will divide into three groups. Each group will select a student to be interviewed. The groups will meet for ten minutes to plan their strategies. The instructor will briefly interview each selected student. The student being interviewed may confer with other members of that group as needed. At the end of this exercise, the class will share comments and criticisms.

Ethical and Legal Concerns

OBJECTIVES

Upon completing this chapter, you will be able to do the following:

1. Identify four rules of ethics to be followed by the nursing assistant.

2. Describe four examples of legal problems that may affect nursing assistant responsibilities.

3. Identify six rights of the resident in a long-term care facility.

4. Describe three types of elderly abuse.

5. Explain how the nursing assistant can prevent elderly abuse.

6. Describe the function of the Ombudsmen Committee.

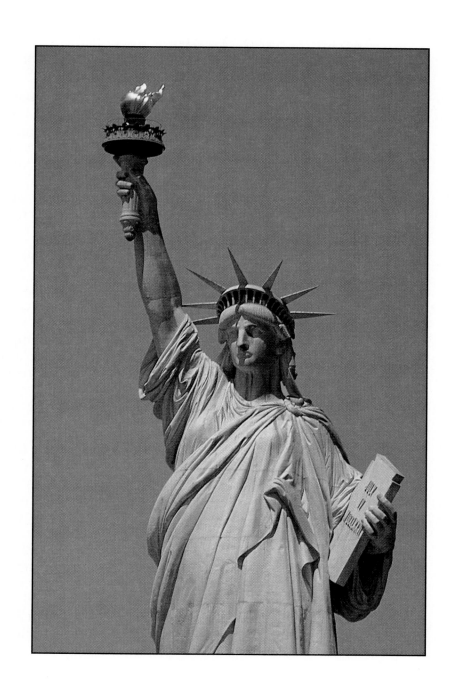

VOCABULARY

The following words or terms will help you to understand this chapter:

Ethics

Assault

Battery

False imprisonment

Invasion of privacy

Confidentiality

Negligence

Slander

Residents' bill of rights

Ombudsmen Committee

Ethics

Ethics are guidelines that are concerned with right or wrong behavior. Personal ethics involve the values we each set for ourselves. These ethics are formed by the moral code of our society and are influenced by our inner feelings. Professional ethics are rules of behavior that apply to members of a profession. Doctors, nurses, and teachers, for example, have developed ethical standards for their professions.

Nursing assistants can develop their own set of ethics, which might include the following:

- Treat each other with respect.
- Treat each resident as an individual.
- Protect the privacy of the resident.
- Protect the resident from harm.
- Avoid the use of drugs or alcohol.
- Be honest and trustworthy.
- Be loyal to your employer and your coworkers.
- Do not do anything illegal.

Legal Responsibilities

There are certain legal responsibilities or laws that all health care workers must obey. Laws are rules of conduct that are decided by the government and are enforced by the courts. The purpose of a law is to protect both the individual and society. It is a crime to break a law, and the person who commits a crime may have to pay a fine, go to jail, or both. Legal problems that you should be aware of as a nursing assistant include the following:

Assault. Assault is a threat to do bodily harm. Any threat of punishment is assault. Using hand gestures, such as shaking a fist at someone, could be considered assault.

Battery. Battery is touching another person's body without permission. Battery is often thought of as hitting someone, but it is not always that violent. Treating a resident roughly or forcing him to do something is a form of battery. Performing a treatment or procedure without the resident's permission is also an example of battery.

False Imprisonment. False imprisonment means to restrain or restrict a person's movements when the person is not in danger of harming himself or herself. A prison is a place where criminals are locked up, and false imprisonment can be compared to locking up a person who has committed no crime. A resident may not be locked in a room or restrained in a chair to prevent wandering. Residents are never restrained for the convenience of the staff.

Invasion of Privacy. Invasion of privacy occurs when either the privacy of the resident's body or the privacy of personal information is not protected. Avoid unnecessary exposure of the resident's body during personal care. Protect the resident's privacy during personal care by closing the door and pulling the curtain. You must knock before entering the resident's room.

Personal information including medical care, must be kept confidential. **Confidentiality** means privacy of resident information. All questions from family or friends concerning medical treatment should be referred to the charge nurse. Do not repeat personal information that the resident has chosen to share with you. Something that is not important to you could be very important to the resident, whose need for privacy may be different from your own.

Negligence. **Negligence** is the failure to give proper care, which results in physical or emotional harm to the resident. You can be negligent when you fail to perform a task. It is also negligent to perform a task incorrectly. Examples of negligence include the following:

- A resident's signal light was on for 20 minutes. The resident got up alone to go to the bathroom, fell, and broke a hip.
- A resident slipped in water that was spilled on the floor, fell, and broke an arm.
- The nursing assistant dropped the resident's dentures (false teeth) and they broke.
- The resident had not been taking fluids. The nursing assistant did not provide fluids or report the problem to the nurse and resident became dehydrated.

Slander. **Slander** is a false statement that damages another person's reputation. If the false statement is written, it is called libel.

You can cause trouble by repeating gossip about a resident or coworker. Avoid this problem by refusing to repeat anything that you are not sure is true.

Legally, you are responsible for your own actions. This means that you can be sued if the resident is harmed because of something you did or something you failed to do. If you are guilty of assault, battery, false imprisonment, invasion of privacy, negligence, slander, or anything else that harms someone, a lawsuit can be brought against you.

The nursing assistant always works under the supervision of a nurse. However, there may be times when you should refuse to follow the nurse's orders. Examples of situations in which you may refuse are included in the following list.

- The nurse asks you to do something that a nursing assistant is not allowed to do. (See Chapter 2.)
- The nurse tells you to do something that would harm the resident.
- The nurse asks you to do something illegal or unethical.

You must *never* ignore the nurse's order. Politely refuse, and be sure the nurse knows

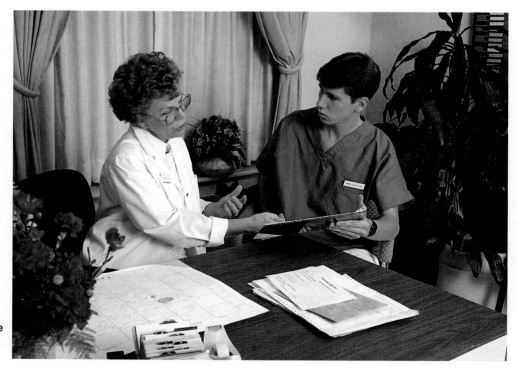

Fig. 3-1
If the nurse's orders are not clear, ask her to explain.

that you are not going to carry out the order. There are special situations when you will need more information before you can carry out the nurse's order. For example,

- The nurse's order is not clear and you are not sure what to do. Tell the nurse that you do not understand and ask for a better explanation. Do not attempt to take any action until you know what you are doing.
- The nurse asks you to do something that you have not been taught to do. Tell the nurse that you do not know how to perform that task and you would like to learn. Make every effort to do those tasks that are required of you, but do not attempt to do anything until you can do it safely.

Wills. A will is a written document that states how a person wants property divided after death. People often write or change their wills when they get sick. You might be asked to witness the signing of a will. Although there is no legal reason why you cannot, it is better if you do not act as a witness. Wills are sometimes contested and you might have to testify in court. Your best response is to tell the person that the nurse will contact the appropriate person.

Residents' Bill of Rights

The **residents' bill of rights** is a list of the rights and freedoms of the residents. It is much like the Bill of Rights of the Constitution of the United States. The Bill of Rights guarantees certain rights to the American people, such as the right of free speech and the right to religious freedom.

To meet federal regulations, long-term care facilities must have written policies to protect the rights of the residents. These must be made available to the resident and the resident's family. Some of the rights are described in the paragraphs that follow. A more complete list of the resident's rights can be found in Fig. 3-2.

The Right to Civil and Religious Liberties. The resident may take part in social, religious, or civic activities and be allowed to vote if able. This includes the right to contact government representatives as desired.

The Right to Complain Without Fear. A resident has the right to make complaints and suggest changes without fear of harm. A resident committee is usually formed to express complaints, concerns, and suggestions for change. This committee represents the resident population. Individuals may express grievances and concerns directly to the administration, at any time.

The Right to Refuse. A resident has the right to refuse medication and treatment. Staff members should explain the importance of following the doctors orders. However, the resident who continues to refuse has a right to do so.

The Right to Be Free from Physical or Chemical Restraints. Restraints can be used only to protect the resident from harm. Restraints require a doctor's order. A violation of this right is considered false imprisonment.

The Right to Be Free from Mental or Physical Abuse. No resident has to endure abuse in any form. Physical abuse is the same as battery, and mental abuse may be assault.

The Right to Personal Privacy and Confidentiality. The resident has the right to personal privacy. This involves providing care in a way that does not expose the body unnecessarily. It also includes privacy of personal belongings. Information about the resident must be kept confidential. It should not be discussed with anyone except those who participate in the resident's care. All records should be handled carefully and not be left where they can be seen by people who are not involved in caregiving. A violation of this right is invasion of privacy.

The Right to Be Treated with Consideration and Respect. The resident must be treated with dignity as an individual. This means that all people are different and should be accepted as such. The resident is to be called by the proper name or the name of choice.

The Right to Personal Belongings. The resident may keep and use personal clothing and other belongings as space permits. Most facilities will encourage residents to bring pictures and mementoes. Sometimes there is room for a piece of furniture, such as a favorite chair or a small table. The things they bring are often the most important and meaningful possessions they own. Their belongings are to be treated with care and respect.

The Right to Privacy for Married Couples. This is a right that assures a husband and wife privacy when a resident's spouse is visiting. It also permits them to share a room when both are residents.

A violation of one of the resident's rights may be illegal, or it may be considered abuse. It is your responsibility to help protect the resident's rights.

Elderly Abuse

Elderly abuse (mistreatment of older people) is a serious problem. Abuse can take place at home or in a health care facility. Most of the time, the person who is abused has physical or mental problems and requires a lot of care. The abuser (the one who mistreats another person) is often the one who provides most of the care. The abuser may be a family member, or it might be a health care worker.

Abuse can be physical, verbal, sexual, or material. Verbal abuse may also be called emotional abuse. Hitting, rough handling, or hurrying the resident are examples of physical abuse. Neglect is also a form of physical abuse. Threats, curses, or anything said that makes the resident feel badly or lowers self-esteem is verbal abuse. Sexual abuse can involve physical contact, gestures, or remarks. Material or financial abuse involves misuse of the resident's money or personal possessions. This can include anything from eating the resident's candy to stealing money.

As a nursing assistant, you may be the first person to discover that a resident is being abused. You might notice that the resident appears to be afraid. Physical abuse

---

RESIDENTS' RIGHTS

A long-term care facility must protect and promote the rights of each resident, including the following:

1. the right to civil and religious liberties
2. the right to file complaints without fear
3. the right to be informed of his/her rights, and the rules of the facility, upon admission
4. the right to inspect his/her records
5. the right to be informed of his/her medical condition and treatment, and to take part in planning the care
6. the right to refuse medication and treatment
7. the right to information from agencies of inspection
8. the right to be informed of responsibility for charges and services
9. the right to manage his/her own financial affairs
10. the right to receive adequate and appropriate health care
11. the right to be free from unnecessary physical restraints and drugs
12. the right to be free from verbal, mental, sexual or physical abuse
13. the right to personal privacy, and confidentiality of information
14. the right to be treated courteously, fairly and with dignity
15. the right to send and promptly receive mail that is unopened
16. the right to have private communication with any person of choice
17. the right to receive visitors at any reasonable hour
18. the right to immediate access to family and friends
19. the right to choose a personal physician
20. the right to have access to private use of a telephone
21. the right to participate in social, religious and group activities of choice
22. the right to retain and use personal possessions and clothing as space permits
23. the right to equal policies and practices regardless of source of payment
24. the right to privacy during visits with a spouse, and to share a room when a married couple resides in the same facility

Fig. 3-2 The resident's bill of rights.

---

can produce fear and anxiety, as well as injuries. Physical or verbal abuse can cause mental or emotional pain and may cause a change in personality. For example, a

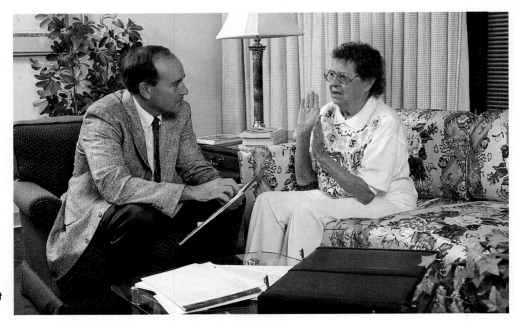

Fig. 3-3
A member of the Ombudsmen Committee will visit the long-term care facility to investigate a complaint of abuse.

friendly, outgoing resident may suddenly become quiet and withdrawn. Any unusual behavior should be reported immediately. Trust your feelings. If something seems to be wrong—it probably is.

What kind of person would hurt an elderly resident? Abusers are often people who are tired and overworked. They lose patience easily and do not handle stress well. They try to hold back their emotions and have difficulty saying what they feel. Many abusers have personal problems that keep them from thinking clearly. Others have been abused themselves.

Protecting the Resident from Abuse.
What can you do about elderly abuse? Begin with yourself, and stay in tune with your feelings. If you find that the complaints and demands of a certain resident annoy you, it is time to withdraw. You may only need to get away for a few minutes to get control of yourself, or you might need to ask the nurse to change your assignment. Be aware of your stress level, and use appropriate coping techniques as needed. There is *never* an excuse for abusing a resident.

The best way to protect a resident is by being observant and reporting anything suspicious. It is your ethical and legal duty to report resident abuse. The first step would be to inform the charge nurse. If that does

not result in immediate action, you must go through the chain of command as far as necessary. If you fail to report abuse, you are just as guilty as the abuser and can be held legally responsible.

Most areas have an abuse hotline that will be listed in the front of the telephone book. Your area might also have an Ombudsmen Committee to whom you may report abuse. The **Ombudsmen Committee** investigates complaints of resident abuse in health care facilities. This committee is composed of concerned citizens who are usually appointed by the governor of the state. The purpose of the Ombudsmen Committee is to protect the residents' rights.

Conclusion

Remember these important points:

1. Ethics are concerned with right or wrong behavior.

2. Personal ethics involve the values we set for ourselves.

3. The resident has the right to refuse medicine or treatment.

4. A nursing assistant should practice total confidentiality.

5. A nursing assistant who fails to give proper care is negligent.

6. You are responsible for your own actions.

7. The purpose of the residents' bill of rights is to protect the resident.

8. Every resident has the right to be treated with consideration and respect.

9. There is never an excuse for abusing a resident.

10. It is your ethical and legal responsibility to report abuse.

11. The purpose of the Ombudsmen Committee is to protect the residents' rights.

Discussion Questions

1. Identify two examples of assault, battery, false imprisonment, invasion of privacy, negligence, and slander.

2. Discuss examples of violations of residents' rights that could be abuse.

3. What would you do if you suspected that a coworker was abusing a resident?

Application Exercise

1. The class will develop a set of ethics for nursing assistants using the following method.

    a. Each student will develop a personal set of ethics.

    b. The students will share individual lists with the other members of the class.

    c. The class will select a set of ethics from the individual lists.

Restorative Care: Promoting Resident Independence

OBJECTIVES

Upon completing this chapter, you will be able to do the following:

1. Explain the meaning of rehabilitation and restorative care.

2. List the members of the rehabilitation team.

3. Describe six rehabilitation departments.

4. Explain the purpose of adaptive equipment and prosthetic devices.

5. Identify the principles of restorative care.

6. Identify six restorative measures and programs.

7. List four guidelines to promote wellness.

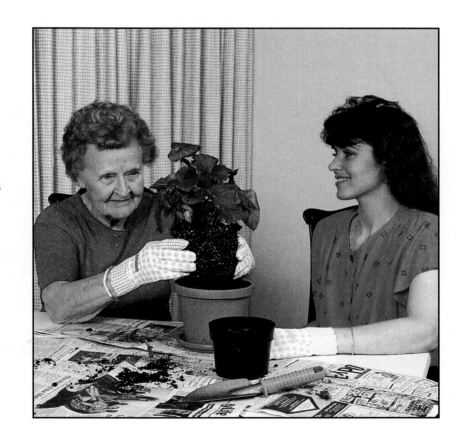

VOCABULARY

The following words or terms will help you to understand this chapter:

Rehabilitation	Reality orientation	Complication
Restorative care	Validation therapy	Ambulate
Independence	Adapt	Health
Mobility	Adaptive equipment	
Prosthesis	Prosthetic device	

Introduction to Rehabilitation and Restorative Care

Restorative care brings rehabilitation into the total care of the resident. All daily activities are carried out with a focus on independence and the quality of the resident's life. Every staff member must be committed to meeting the challenge of assisting the resident, who is struggling to cope with problems. To rise to the call of restorative care, you will be challenged to use enthusiasm, empathy, patience, and all your other emotional strengths. In return, your reward will be the joy and satisfaction of knowing you are making a significant difference in the resident's life.

Rehabilitation is the method that is used to bring the resident back to as nearly normal function as possible. It includes restoring function and preventing further loss. Rehabilitation is concerned with all the resident's needs and problems. It also addresses the resident's feelings and how problems and unmet needs interfere with life. Rehabilitation is one of the best tools available to improve quality of life.

Rehabilitation is needed by any resident who has an impairment or a disability. An impairment is a limitation caused by disease, injury, or a birth defect. A disability is a decrease in the ability to carry out daily activities. For example, a resident who has had a stroke might have an impairment, such as weakness of the right arm and leg. This could lead to a disability, such as difficulty with walking, eating, and self-care.

Rehabilitation would help the resident regain as much function as possible.

Restorative care is the care that is given to assist the resident to attain and maintain the highest level of function and independence. (It is also called rehabilitative care.) All nursing care should be provided in a restorative manner.

Independence means being able to care for yourself and being in control of your life. It allows freedom. The concept of independence is difficult to define because it means different things to different people. To many people, independence means being able to make decisions, while others think independence means bathing, dressing, and feeding themselves.

Of all life's gifts, independence is one of the most treasured. When the need for independence is not met, the resident may become angry, depressed, or demanding. How would you feel if someone else had to help you bathe, dress, and go to the bathroom? What if you lost the freedom to come and go as you please?

The Rehabilitation Team

The rehabilitation team is a group of people who work together to meet the resident's needs. The center of the rehabilitation team is the resident, and the resident's family. Other members of the team include doctors, nurses, nursing assistants, physical therapists, occupational therapists, speech therapists, social workers, activity directors, and members of the clergy. All members of the health care team belong to the rehabilitation team.

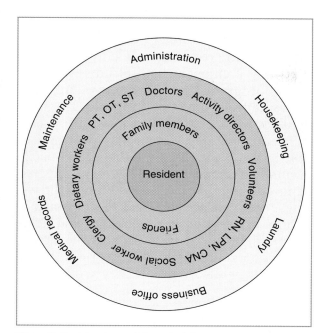

Fig. 4-1 Members of the rehabilitation team.

Rehabilitation Departments

Every department in the long-term care facility might be called a rehabilitation department, since all are concerned with keeping the resident in the best possible health. However, those that provide direct care to the resident have the greatest responsibility.

Nursing Department. The role of the nursing department in rehabilitation and restorative care is introduced in Chapter 1 and continues to be emphasized in every chapter of this textbook. Nurses and nursing assistants must provide restorative nursing care whenever they are working with the residents. Encouragement and praise are the motivating elements of restorative nursing care. The nursing staff must constantly encourage the residents to do as much as possible for themselves. Praise given for even the slightest accomplishment encourages the resident to continue trying. Since nursing assistants provide most of the direct care for the residents, they have many opportunities to use restorative measures. The members of the nursing department extend the efforts of other rehabilitation departments into the daily lives of the residents.

Physical Therapy Department. The physical therapist and physical therapy assistants use special training and equipment to help the resident strengthen muscles and regain physical independence. Responsibilities of the members of the physical therapy department include the following:

- Evaluate muscle strength and **mobility** (ability to move).
- Help the resident to regain muscle strength and mobility.
- Measure, fit, and help the resident to use a **prosthesis** (an artificial body part).
- Teach the use of canes, crutches, and walkers.

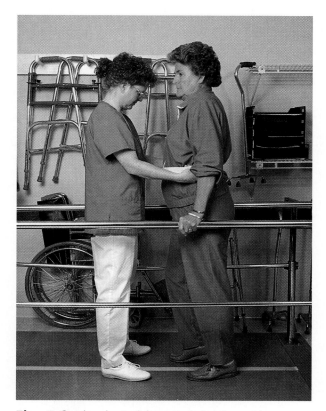

Fig. 4-2 The physical therapist helps the resident to learn to walk again.

Occupational Therapy Department. The primary role of the occupational therapist is to help the resident to perform activities of daily living. This might involve relearning previous skills or developing new ones. New skills might be needed to overcome prob-

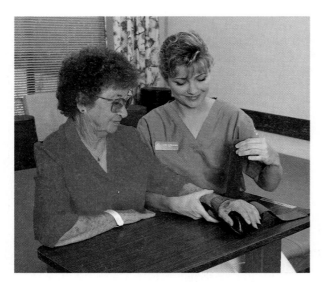

Fig. 4-3 The occupational therapist helps the resident to apply a hand splint.

lems caused by weakness, paralysis or a lack of coordination. The therapist recommends equipment that can help the resident to function with a disability. For example, a resident who has a weak arm might need a splint to keep the hand in a normal position.

Speech Therapy Department. The speech therapist works with the resident who has a communication problem. Speech therapy involves planning and directing the treatment of residents whose ability to speak has been impaired. The therapist also works with residents who have a hearing loss and assists residents with eating and swallowing problems.

Social Services Department. The social worker provides counseling to help the resident and the family adjust to the changes in their lives. Changes in health, independence, and living arrangements are upsetting, not only to the resident, but to the family as well. The social worker helps them to work through their feelings and find ways to cope. Social services also helps the family to work out financial problems and provides information about community resources that are available.

Activities Department. The activity director and activity assistants provide programs that help the residents to socialize, keep busy, and feel worthwhile. They plan daily activities such as exercises, crafts, movies, shopping, and other outside trips. They meet with the residents to identify activities that will be enjoyable and of interest. Many of the programs help to improve the resident's self-esteem. For example, the resident's artwork may be on display or for sale.

The activity department may post notices that indicate the date, weather, and special events that are planned. They help the residents celebrate birthdays and other holidays. These help to provide reality orientation. **Reality orientation** is a technique that helps the resident maintain awareness of person, place, and time. Some elderly residents are confused or disoriented. They may not be aware of where they are, what time of year it is, or even who they are. Another technique for working with confused residents is validation therapy. **Validation therapy** is a technique that creates a climate of acceptance by encouraging the confused resident to explore thoughts. Reality orientation and validation therapy are discussed in more detail in a later chapter.

Other Departments. The responsibility of other departments in rehabilitation is discussed in later chapters. Although each department has specific responsibilities, their activities often overlap.

Adaptive Equipment / Prosthetic Devices

The word **adapt** means to adust or change in order to cope with a situation. **Adaptive equipment** is the equipment that is used to help the resident adjust to a disability and function as independently as possible. A cane is an example of adaptive equipment. A person with a weak leg uses a cane to assist in walking.

A **prosthetic device** replaces or assists a body part to perform its function. A prosthetic device is a type of adaptive equipment. Eyeglasses are an example of a prosthetic device. The sight-impaired person wears glasses to assist the eyes by improving vision.

sive, while others are simple and easy to use. A straw is adaptive equipment when you use it to drink milk out of a carton. It can provide independence for the resident who has difficulty holding a glass. If you shorten the straw by cutting it in half, it may be easier to handle. Can you think of other examples of adaptive equipment that you can make?

Modern technology has led to the development of amazing prosthetic devices. There are artificial hands that can do almost everything a normal hand can do. Prosthetic legs are no longer "peg legs." They look and feel like real limbs. There are disposable contact lenses that can be worn for a week or two, at very little cost.

Wheelchairs, one of the most common pieces of adaptive equipment, come in all shapes and sizes. Some are small and lightweight and easily folded for transporting. Others recline and have headrests. There are electric wheelchairs for ease and convenience. There is also adaptive equipment available for automobiles. These types of equipment increase the mobility of people who might be dependent on others for transportation.

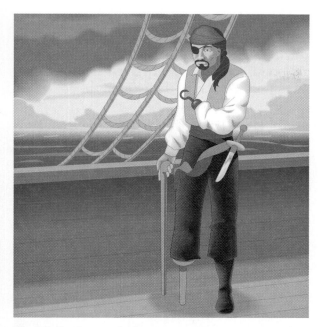

Fig. 4-4 The use of adaptive equipment is not a new idea.

The use of adaptive equipment is not a new idea. In the past, a missing leg was replaced with a wooden peg, and a missing hand with a hook. A straight, strong stick made an effective cane.

There are many types of adaptive equipment. Some are complicated and expen-

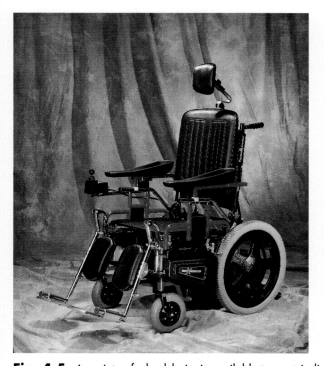
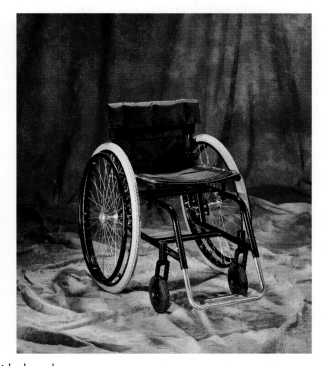

Fig. 4-5 A variety of wheelchairs is available to meet individual needs.

These are only a few examples of adaptive equipment and prosthetic devices. There is equipment designed to meet the needs of each individual restorative program. New equipment is continually being developed. It is the responsibility of the rehabilitation team to be aware of available equipment, and to teach the resident how to use it. The nursing assistant must be familiar with the equipment and encourage the resident to use it.

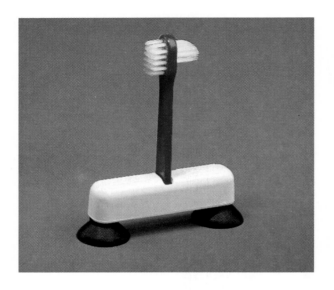

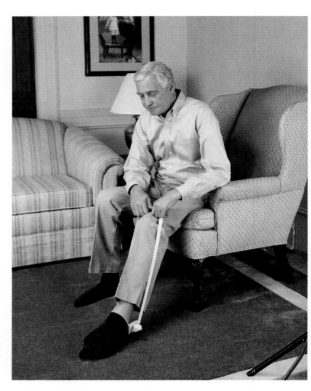

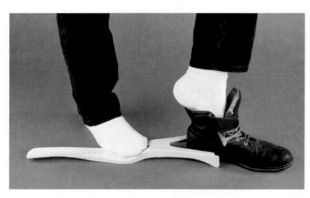

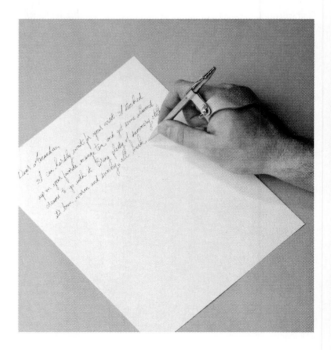

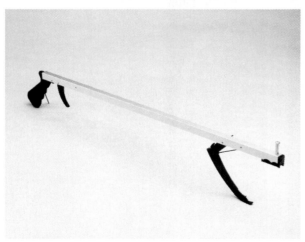

Fig. 4-6 There are many types of adaptive equipment.

Principles of Restorative Care

Restorative care does not "just happen." It requires commitment, thoughtful planning, and an understanding of the rehabilitation process. There are certain principles (basic facts) that will help you to practice restorative care.

RESTORATIVE CARE BASIC PRINCIPLES

- Treat the whole person.
- Start rehabilitation early.
- Stress ability, not disability.
- Encourage activity.
- Maintain a restorative attitude.

Treat the Whole Person. Rehabilitation is directed toward the needs of the "whole person." It is not enough to treat only the physical needs (the needs of the body); a person also has mental, emotional, social, sexual, and spiritual needs. When a person becomes ill, all those needs are affected and must be met in an individual manner. Attitudes, desires, and interests differ, just as body appearance differs. No two people have the same feelings or desires. Therefore, each person must be treated as an individual.

Start Rehabilitation Early. Rehabilitation should begin at the first sign of illness. For the resident who has just entered the long-term care facility, rehabilitation begins on admission. Early treatment prevents complications. A **complication** is an additional problem that results from a disease or other condition. Early treatment also provides a positive approach that is encouraging to the resident. The fact that treatment has begun increases the resident's self-esteem and lessens the chance of depression.

Stress Ability, Not Disability. Restorative care emphasizes what the resident can do, rather than what cannot be done. A person with a disability may be focused on the disability and give up many activities. The fear of failure and embarrassment may cause withdrawal. The resident often tries to meet

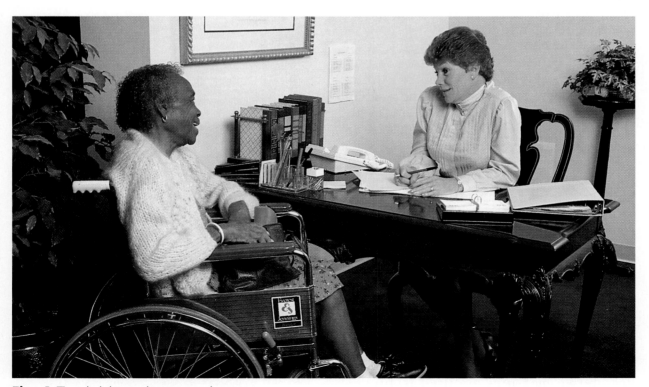

Fig. 4-7 Rehabilitation begins on admission.

your expectations. If you expect the restorative measures to be successful, the resident is likely to be influenced by your attitude. The resident should always be encouraged to be as independent as possible.

Encourage Activity. It is important to encourage the resident to be active. Activity strengthens the mind and the body—inactivity weakens it. Activity improves circulation, digestion, elimination, and mobility. It helps prevent complications, increases mental alertness, and helps prevent depression. The active resident will be more independent, which leads to increased self-esteem and feelings of self-worth. Your praise and encouragement will help the resident to be more active.

Maintain a Restorative Attitude. A restorative attitude includes positive feelings and beliefs. To be successful in providing restorative care, you must believe in its importance, and in the resident's need for this care. You must believe that restorative care will provide a better life for the resident. If you truly believe that a restorative measure will help the resident, it will probably be more successful. If you don't believe that it will work, how are you going to convince the resident to try?

Positive feelings such as empathy, sensitivity, and patience contribute to a restorative attitude. Empathy, the ability to think how you would feel if you were the resident, helps you to understand. Sensitivity means being aware of how the resident feels. Being in tune with the resident's feelings can mean the difference between success and failure. Patience is necessary to prevent frustration, because relearning takes time. Restorative care requires you to make a commitment to continue the care as long as it is needed and to always maintain a positive attitude. The resident could be influenced by your attitude, whatever it may be.

Restorative Measures and Programs

Restorative measures are used to provide resident care in a way that will promote independence. These measures should be used 7 days a week and 24 hours a day, whenever resident care is being provided. Some restorative measures are as follows:

- Understand the resident's abilities and disabilities.
- Be aware of the resident's fears.
- Know what equipment is available.
- Encourage the resident to make decisions.
- Support the family's efforts to help.
- Keep directions simple—one step at a time.
- Be consistent—do a task the same way every time, all the time.
- Arrange furniture and belongings for independence.
- Allow the resident to function independently with as little assistance as possible.
- Allow time—don't rush.
- Allow the resident to struggle—but don't allow frustration.
- Watch for signs of fatigue.
- Never scold or humiliate.
- Praise! Praise! Praise!

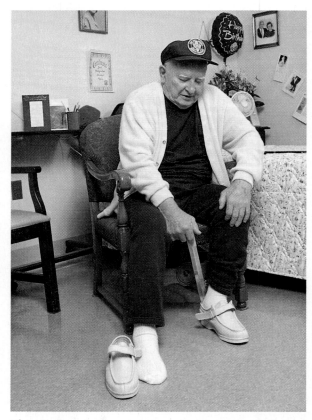

Fig. 4-8 Adaptive equipment promotes independence.

Restorative programs have been developed to meet the needs of residents who have difficulty performing activities of daily living. The purpose of each of these programs is to promote independence and to enable the resident to perform the activities with as little assistance as possible. It is important to remember that a program must be adapted for each individual. The program then becomes a part of the resident's plan of care. All restorative care revolves around this plan.

Personal Hygiene and Grooming Program. This program helps the resident to meet hygiene and grooming needs independently. It includes such activities as bathing, mouth care, hair care, and dressing. These are skills that are needed to help a person stay clean, neat, and healthy. Cleanliness is important to one's well-being and quality of life. Being unable to perform these simple, yet necessary, procedures causes great distress. Personal hygiene and grooming are discussed in more detail in a later chapter.

Restorative Dining Program. The restorative dining program is designed to help residents who are unable to feed themselves. Eating is an enjoyable experience for most people. However, being fed by someone else takes away much of the pleasure. The use of adaptive equipment, learning new skills, and relearning old ones, helps the resident return to independent dining. The restorative dining program is discussed in more detail later.

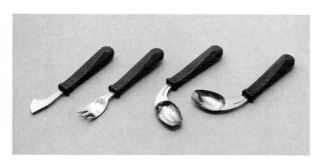

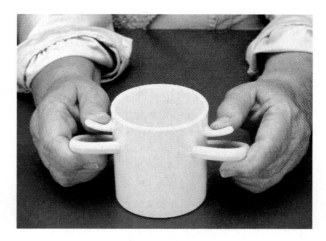

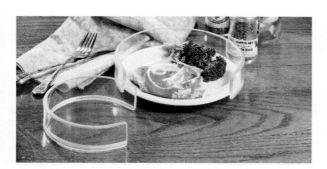

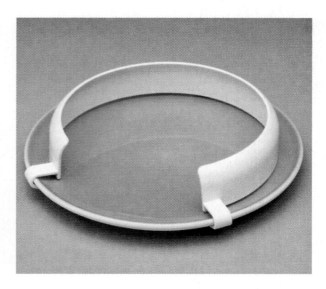

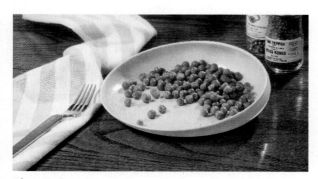

Fig. 4-9 Adaptive equipment for independent dining.

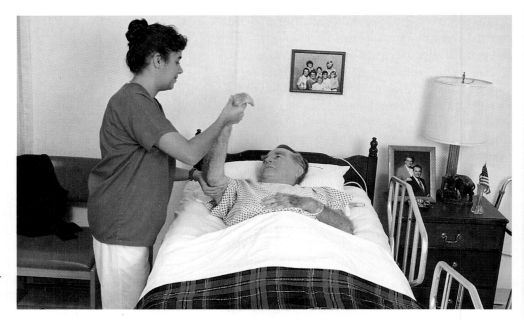

Fig. 4-10
Range-of-motion exercises help to prevent complications.

Bowel and Bladder Program. This program helps residents who are unable to control urine and bowel movements. The loss of the ability to control these body functions can be overwhelming to the resident and his or her family. It can cause physical, emotional, and social problems. The goal of this program is to help the resident regain control of bowel and bladder function. The bowel and bladder program is discussed in more detail later.

Range-of-Motion and Exercise Program. Restorative exercise programs help the resident who has limited mobility. Exercise benefits every system of the body. It keeps a person more alert and oriented. Physical activity promotes a positive emotional outlook, helps reduce stress, improves appetite, and helps the resident sleep more soundly.

Range of motion is a program in which the resident is encouraged to move and exercise. Exercise maintains muscle strength and prevents the joints from getting stiff. If the resident is not able to do the exercises without assistance, you must help. However, encouraging independent exercise will help to regain and maintain function. Range-of-motion and other exercise programs are discussed in more detail later.

Ambulation Program. The word **ambulate** means to walk. The purpose of this program is to increase or maintain the resident's ability to walk. Not being able to get up and go as you wish is very depressing. It is hard to stay emotionally healthy and socially involved if you cannot walk. Ambulation helps keep the resident mobile and independent. The goal is to have the resident walk with as little assistance as possible. The ambulation program is addressed in more detail later.

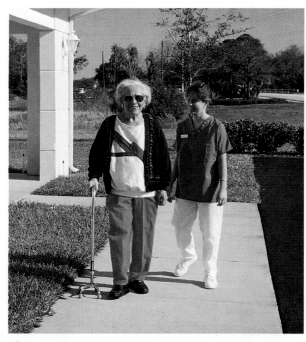

Fig. 4-11 Ambulation helps the resident to maintain independence.

Communicating with the Sight, Hearing, or Speech Impaired. Residents who have an impairment in sight, hearing, or speech will have difficulty communicating. It can be frightening if you cannot see or hear what is happening. Being unable to put fears, needs and concerns into words is very frustrating. There are special techniques to use when working with these individuals. Communicating with the sight-, hearing-, or speech-impaired resident is discussed in more detail later.

Promotion of Wellness

The World Health Organization (WHO) defines health as follows: "**Health** is a state of complete physical, mental, and social well-being, not merely absence of disease and infirmity." Wellness means adapting to change in order to live life to the fullest. Health and wellness are not the same. A person can have an illness and still have wellness. For example, the person with diabetes has an illness that prevents good health. But wellness can be achieved by living the best life that is possible with the disease.

Wellness is physical, mental, emotional, social, and spiritual. It requires a positive attitude, with a high degree of self-esteem and self-respect. The ability to handle stress is important. It is influenced by life-style and environment. Rehabilitation and restorative care help promote wellness. Restorative measures that increase self-esteem and independence also increase wellness. It is your responsibility as a nursing assistant to always be concerned with the wellness of the resident.

GUIDELINES TO PROMOTE WELLNESS

- Remain aware of the resident's health.
- Learn the warning signs of disease.
- Assure personal hygiene.
- Use safety measures.
- Follow infection control policies.
- Assist with nutrition and fluids.
- Encourage rest, relaxation, and sleep.
- Provide continuity of care.

While it is very important that you help the resident to attain wellness, do not forget your own wellness. You can apply to your life many of the measures listed. If you have a positive attitude and are moving toward wellness, you can better assist the resident in that direction.

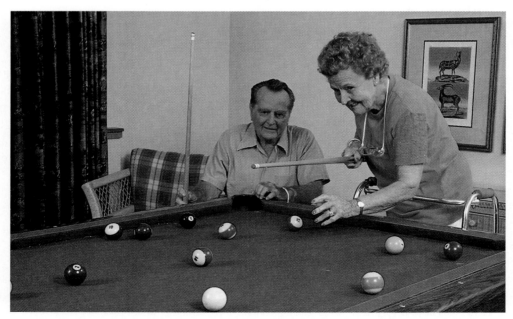

Fig. 4-12
Wellness is living life to the fullest.

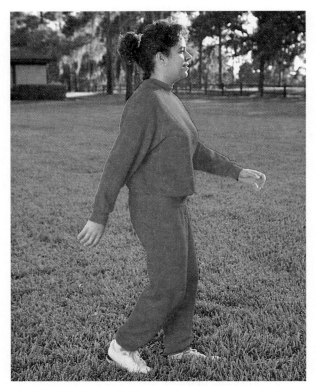

Fig. 4-13 The nursing assistant should also seek wellness.

Conclusion

Remember these important points:

1. Rehabilitation is the method that is used to bring a person back to as nearly normal function as possible.

2. Restorative care assists the resident to maintain normal function and independence.

3. All members of the health care team belong to the rehabilitation team.

4. Encouragement and praise are the motivating elements of restorative care.

5. Physical therapy helps the resident regain muscle strength and mobility.

6. Occupational therapy helps the resident learn to perform the activities of daily living.

7. Rehabilitation is directed toward the needs of the whole person.

8. Rehabilitation should start as early as possible.

9. The resident should be encouraged to function independently with as little assistance as possible.

10. Activity strengthens, inactivity weakens.

11. A restorative attitude includes positive feelings and beliefs.

12. Allow time—don't rush.

13. Restorative care revolves around the resident's plan of care.

14. Wellness means living life to the fullest.

15. Restorative measures that increase the resident's self-esteem increase wellness.

16. Work to achieve wellness in your own life.

Discussion Questions

1. What does independence mean to you?

2. How many decisions did you make today? How important were they?

3. How can you tell that a nursing assistant has a restorative attitude?

4. What fears might the resident have that would interfere with rehabilitation?

5. What is the difference between health and wellness?

Application Exercise

1. The class will visit a long-term care facility. Each student will make a list of the things he or she noticed that would indicate that restorative care was being given. The students will combine their individual observations into one list and discuss the importance of each.

Infection Control

OBJECTIVES

Upon completing this chapter, you will be able to do the following:

1. Explain the purpose of infection control.

2. Explain the difference between pathogens and nonpathogens.

3. List four ways microorganisms are spread.

4. Identify three signs and symptoms of infection.

5. Explain the difference between asepsis and sterilization.

6. Explain the importance of handwashing.

7. List six guidelines for universal precautions.

8. Identify the purpose of isolation.

9. Describe the restorative approach to isolation.

10. Identify the cause, transmission, prevention, legal issues, and behavior changes related to HIV infection.

11. Perform the procedures described in this chapter.

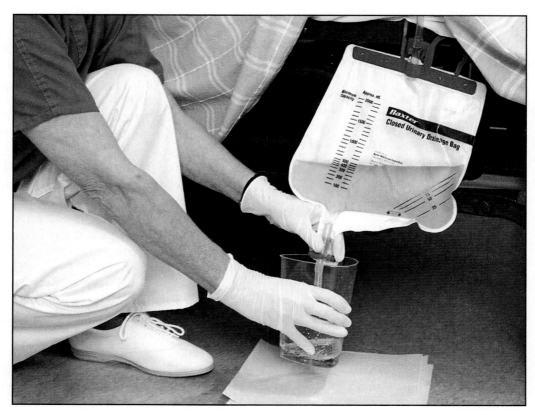

VOCABULARY

The following words or terms will help you to understand this chapter:

Infection	Sterile	Protective (reverse)
Microorganisms	Contaminate	isolation
Nonpathogens	Universal precautions	Biohazardous waste
Pathogens	OSHA (Occupational	Specimen
Normal flora	Safety and Health	HIV (human immunode-
Susceptibility	Administration)	ficiency virus) infection
Asepsis	Isolation	AIDS (acquired immune
Disinfection	Communicable disease	deficiency syndrome)

The Purpose of Infection Control

Infection is a disease condition that occurs when germs enter the body and cause damage. Preventing the spread of infection, and reducing its risk to residents and employees, is an important responsibility of the nursing assistant. Many elderly residents are less able to resist infection because they are weak and frail, or because they have a chronic illness.

Each facility has a committee that writes the facility's infection-control policies and procedures. This committee also keeps a record of infections that occur. It is your responsibility to know the policies and procedures of infection control in your facility. In this chapter, you will learn general infection-control procedures.

The Body's Response to Microorganisms

Microorganisms. Microorganisms are small living things that cannot be seen without the aid of a microscope. "Micro" means small, and "organisms" are living things. Microorganisms are commonly called "germs." They can cause infection and disease by entering the body and damaging cells. We are surrounded by microorganisms. They are always present on skin and in food, air and water (see Fig. 5-1). Some microorganisms are harmful, some are not.

Microorganisms that do not cause an infection are called **nonpathogens**. Some are useful, as for example, in the creation of cheese, yogurt, and alcohol. Even penicillin (a medication) is created by the use of nonpathogens.

Microorganisms that are harmful and cause infection are called **pathogens**. Because they are too small to be seen, it is difficult to remember that pathogens are present. Since the signs of infection do not occur immediately upon contact with pathogens, it is easy to forget how harmful they can be. In other words, "Out of sight, out of mind." The danger of pathogens would be much more real to us if they were large and easy to see.

To stay healthy, the body needs some microorganisms. **Normal flora** are microorganisms that are necessary for good health and are usually found in certain locations. Normal flora exist on the skin to help protect it from infection. The intestine also contains normal flora that help to break down food particles. Normal flora can become harmful and cause infection if they enter another part of the body. For example, the normal flora of the intestine can cause infection if they enter the urinary system or an open wound. The chart in Fig. 5-2 illustrates the relationship between pathogens, nonpathogens, and normal flora.

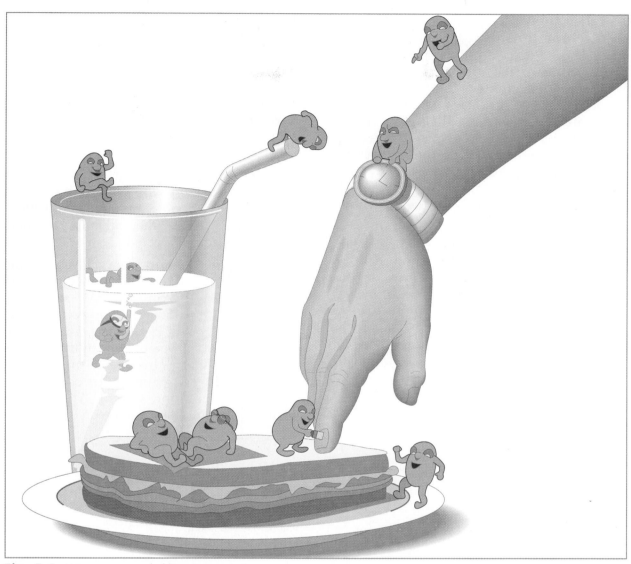

Fig. 5-1 We are surrounded by microorganisms.

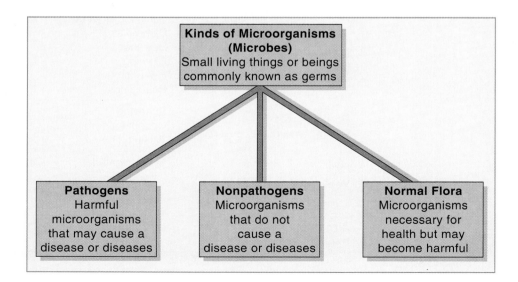

Fig. 5-2
The relationship among pathogens, nonpathogens, and normal flora.

Kinds of Microorganisms (Microbes)
Small living things or beings commonly known as germs

Pathogens
Harmful microorganisms that may cause a disease or diseases

Nonpathogens
Microorganisms that do not cause a disease or diseases

Normal Flora
Microorganisms necessary for health but may become harmful

Conditions That Promote the Growth of Microorganisms. Microorganisms live in humans, other animals, plants, water, food, and dirt. All microorganisms need water and food, and most of them need oxygen. They thrive in a dark, warm (50–110° Fahrenheit), moist area. It is no surprise that humans are so easily infected, because there are many areas of the body that provide excellent conditions for the growth of microorganisms. Think of the body's dark, warm, moist areas that could easily become infected.

Spread of Microorganisms. Microorganisms enter and leave the human body through the nose, mouth, rectum, vagina, and urethra. They also enter and exit by way of the bloodstream, and through broken skin. When a microorganism leaves the body, it can be transmitted to another person. Microorganisms spread in the following ways:

- Direct contact: touching the infected person
- Indirect contact: touching an object that has been in contact with pathogens
- Droplet: inhaling fine drops of moisture caused by talking, sneezing, or coughing
- Airborne: inhaling pathogens that are floating in the air
- Vehicle: entering the body in food, water, blood or medication that contains pathogens

Infection can be spread by a carrier. A carrier is a person who has the pathogen, but has no signs or symptoms of infection. The carrier can give the pathogen to others who may become infected.

The Immune System. The body's immune system attacks invading microorganisms and helps protect against infection. We are always in contact with pathogens. However, because the immune system is working, an infection does not always develop. Poor nutrition, lack of rest, stress, chronic illness, and chemotherapy (a treatment for cancer) can weaken the immune system. A weakened immune system makes a person susceptible

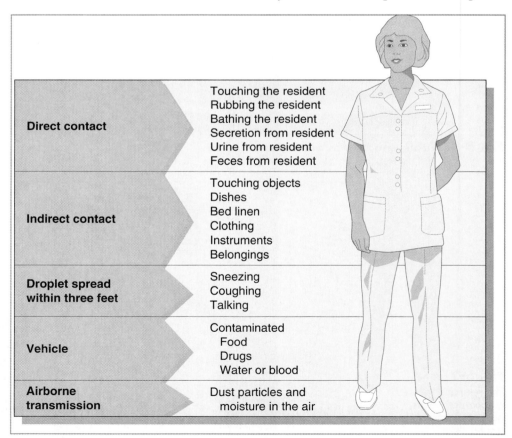

Direct contact	Touching the resident Rubbing the resident Bathing the resident Secretion from resident Urine from resident Feces from resident
Indirect contact	Touching objects Dishes Bed linen Clothing Instruments Belongings
Droplet spread within three feet	Sneezing Coughing Talking
Vehicle	Contaminated Food Drugs Water or blood
Airborne transmission	Dust particles and moisture in the air

Fig. 5-3
Transmission of microorganisms.

to disease. **Susceptibility** means that an individual is more likely to catch a disease.

Signs and Symptoms of Infection

An infection may be a localized infection (located in one part of the body), or it may be a generalized infection (affecting the whole body). Signs and symptoms of localized infection are redness, swelling, heat, drainage, and pain. Signs and symptoms of generalized infection are fever, headache, fatigue, increased pulse and respirations, nausea, and vomiting. The signs of a local infection may also be present with a generalized infection.

It is important to observe for signs and symptoms of infection and report them immediately to the charge nurse. The resident's verbal complaints are as important as the signs that you can see.

Asepsis

Asepsis is the absence of pathogens. When asepsis is practiced, clean procedures are used to prevent the spread of pathogens and lower the risk of infection. If something is clean, it is free of pathogens. **Disinfection** is the use of chemicals to destroy pathogens. These disinfectants include Lysol™, bleach, hydrogen peroxide, alcohol, and Betadine®, among others. Nonpathogens may not be destroyed by disinfection.

An object is **sterile** if it is free of *all* microorganisms. Both pathogens and nonpathogens are destroyed by sterilization. Sterile items will always be in a package that is sealed. If the seal is broken, the item inside is no longer sterile. The difference between clean and sterile may be demonstrated, using gloves as an example. The gloves in an open box are clean, but they are not sterile. Sterile gloves are in a sealed package.

You may see nurses using sterile gloves to perform certain procedures. A sterile proce-

dure requires gloves. Because the hands cannot be sterilized, they must be covered to prevent contaminating the sterile area. To **contaminate** means to dirty or expose to microorganisms. Although you may not perform sterile procedures, you may assist the nurse. Figure 5-4 illustrates the relationship of asepsis, disinfection, sterility, and contamination.

Aseptic Practices. Aseptic practices are used to prevent the spread of pathogens by keeping everything as clean as possible. Everyone should follow aseptic practices at all times. Following are lists of aseptic practices and procedures to be used:

General Infection Control:

- Follow aseptic practices and use gloves when appropriate.
- Wash your hands before handling food, after using the toilet, sneezing, coughing, or blowing your nose and before and after eating.
- Wash fruits and vegetables before preparing or eating them.
- Use individual towels, wash cloths, toothbrushes, drinking glasses, dishes, and other personal items.
- Cover your nose and mouth when coughing, sneezing, or blowing your nose.
- Don't come to work if you have a fever or cold.
- Report all open sores to the charge nurse.
- Dispose of tissues properly.
- Wash dishes with soap and water after each use.

Care of Equipment and Supplies.

- The overbed table is a clean area and must not be used for bedpans, urinals, soiled linen, or other soiled items.
- The stethoscope earpieces and diaphragm should be wiped with alcohol before use.
- Disposable items that are not intended for reuse should be discarded in the dirty utility room immediately after use.
- Personal belongings should be kept in the resident's own area.
- When a mattress is soiled, it should be washed and dried.

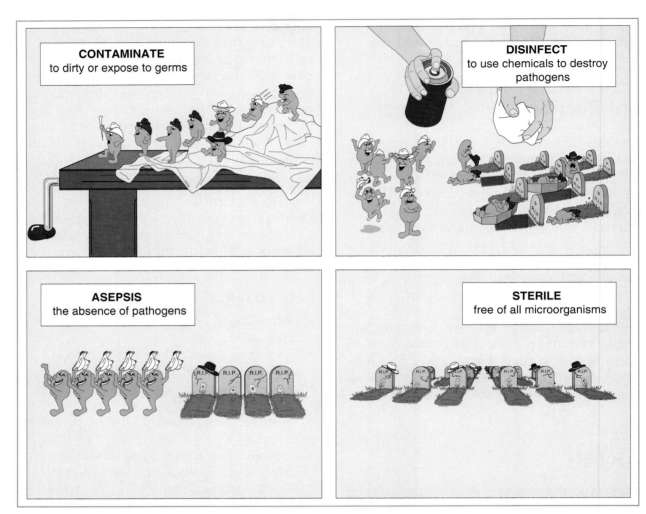

Fig. 5-4 Infection-control terms.

- Urinals and bedpans should be emptied immediately and cleansed and covered after use.
- It is your responsibility to keep brushes and combs clean.
- Personal belongings should not be shared between residents.
- Equipment such as chairs and wheelchairs should be checked daily for cleanliness and wiped off as necessary.
- Utility rooms should be checked and cleaned regularly during each shift.
- All dirty or contaminated items must be taken to the dirty utility room.
- Unused equipment and supplies cannot be taken from one resident's room to another.
- Reusable equipment must be cleaned and disinfected before it is used for another resident.

- Water pitchers and ice scoops must be handled according to facility policy.

Personal Hygiene: Refer to Chapter 2.

Resident Hygiene: Refer to Chapter 19.

Handling Linen: Refer to Chapter 15.

Serving Meals: Refer to Chapter 21.

Handwashing

Handwashing is the most important procedure used to prevent the spread of pathogens and lower the risk of infection. Proper handwashing protects the residents, visitors, yourself, other staff members, and your families.

PROCEDURE

Handwashing

1. Do not touch the sink with your clothes; the sink is considered contaminated.
2. Turn the water on, using a paper towel; adjust the temperature to warm.
3. Wet the hands and forearms thoroughly by holding them under running water. Hold the hands lower than the elbows so that water runs off the fingertips (see Fig. 5-5A).
4. Apply soap to the hands. If bar soap is used, it must be rinsed before and after use.
5. Apply friction to all surfaces of the hands as follows:

   a. Wash the palms and backs.
   b. Interlace the fingers and thumbs. Move the hands back and forth (see Fig. 5-5B).
   c. Wash the wrists and three or four inches above the wrists using rotating movements (see Fig. 5-5C).

6. Rinse well.
7. Steps 4–6 may be repeated as necessary.
8. Dry hands thoroughly, using a separate paper towel for each hand.
9. Use a *dry* paper towel to turn the water off and open the door (see Fig. 5-5D).
10. You may use lotion on your hands to prevent dryness.

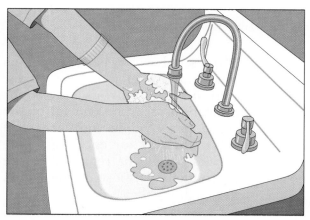

A Hold hands lower than elbows.

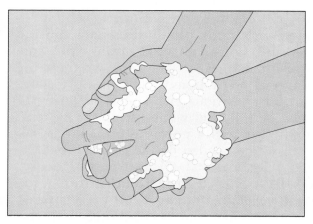

B Interlace fingers and thumbs.

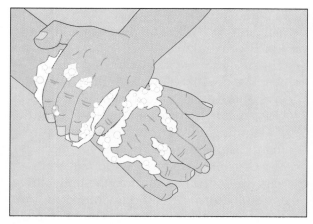

C Wash the wrists with a rotating motion.

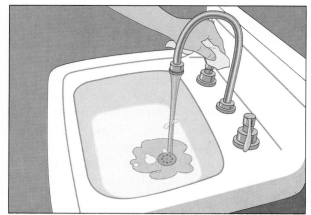

D Turn the water off with a dry paper towel.

Fig. 5-5 Handwashing procedure.

ALWAYS WASH YOUR HANDS

Before eating

After using the bathroom

After coughing or sneezing

After smoking

Before and after giving care to
  each resident

After handling soiled items

Remember: Just because you can't see the pathogens doesn't mean they aren't there!

Universal Precautions

The use of **universal precautions** is a method of infection control in which all human blood and body fluids are considered infectious. Universal means "all," and precautions means "take care", so the term universal precautions simply means to take care in all situations. These precautions must be followed while caring for all residents. The use of universal precautions has been recommended by the Centers for Disease Control (CDC) and mandated by **OSHA (the Occupational Safety and Health Administration)**. OSHA is a governmental agency that is concerned with the safety and health of workers. You will find more detail about OSHA in the following chapter.

Universal precautions include all the rules for asepsis and stresses handwashing as the major method of infection control. It addresses the use of personal protective equipment such as gloves, gowns, face masks, and eye protectors. The most frequently used protection is disposable gloves.

Health care workers should wear gloves anytime there is a possibility of contact with body fluids. Body fluids that are most infectious are blood, semen, vaginal secretions, and any other body fluid that contains visible blood.

Gowns, masks and eye protectors are not often needed in the long-term care facility.

However, your facility must have these types of protection available, should they be needed.

GUIDELINES FOR UNIVERSAL PRECAUTIONS

- Follow standard infection-control practices.
- Wash your hands immediately if they become contaminated with body fluids.
- Do not eat or drink in work areas.
- Clean up spills of body fluids immediately.
- Dispose of sharp objects properly.
- Wear gowns when there is a possibility of body fluids coming into contact with your uniform.
- Wear masks and eye protectors if there is a possibility of body fluids splashing.
- Wear gloves any time you expect to have contact with body fluids.

Use of Gloves. Always wash your hands before applying and after removing gloves. Contamination of your hands may occur during application, use, or removal of the gloves. A clean pair of gloves must be worn for each resident and for each task performed. Gloves should be removed before leaving the resident. Dispose of the gloves according to facility policy.

GUIDELINES FOR REMOVING GLOVES

- The outside surface of gloves should not touch your skin.
- The inside surface is considered "clean."
- Remove the first glove with the gloved fingers of the other hand, by grasping the glove just below the cuff on the outside, and pulling it over your hand, while turning it inside out (see Fig. 5-6A).
- Place the ungloved index and middle fingers inside the cuff of the remaining glove.
- Carefully turn the cuff downward, pulling the glove inside out as you remove it from your hand (see Fig. 5-6B).
- Discard the gloves according to facility policy, and wash your hands.

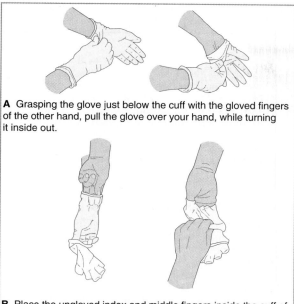

A Grasping the glove just below the cuff with the gloved fingers of the other hand, pull the glove over your hand, while turning it inside out.

B Place the ungloved index and middle fingers inside the cuff of the glove, turning the cuff downward, pulling it inside out, as you remove it from your hand.

Fig. 5-6 Guidelines for removing gloves.

Isolation

Separating a person and using barriers to prevent the spread of pathogens is called **isolation**. Isolation is used when a person has a communicable disease. A **communica-** ble disease is a disease or infection that spreads easily from one person to another.

One practice that is used to prevent the spread of infection from the isolation room is the proper removal of equipment, linen, and trash by double bagging. Double bagging is a procedure in which a contaminated bag of equipment, linen, or trash is placed inside a clean bag for its removal from the room. This is one of the isolation procedures you will learn.

Purpose of Isolation. The usual purpose of isolation is to prevent the spread of pathogens from the isolated person to others. However, a person may also be isolated who is susceptible to infection. **Protective (reverse) isolation** protects the isolated person from pathogens that are present in the normal environment (see Fig. 5-7).

Types of Isolation. Isolation procedures may vary. The correct procedure to be used will depend upon the situation, facility policy and type of infection. Each type of isolation requires that specific precautions be taken (see Fig. 5-8). An isolation sign will be placed on the door of the isolation room to provide information about protection for entering the room.

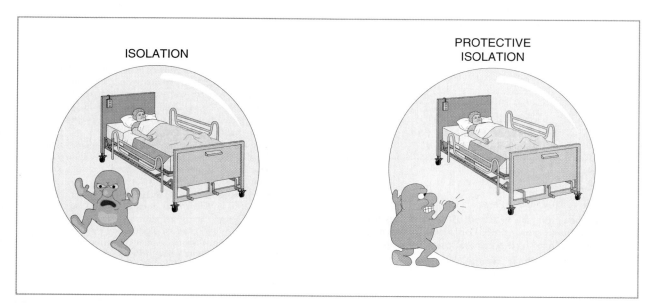

ISOLATION

PROTECTIVE ISOLATION

Fig. 5-7 The difference between regular isolation and protective isolation.

Contact Isolation
Visitors—Report to Nurses' Station
Before Entering Room

1. **Masks** are indicated for those who come close to patient.
2. **Gowns** are indicated if soiling is likely.
3. **Gloves** are indicated for touching infective material.
4. **Hands must be washed after touching the patient or potentially contaminated articles and before taking care of another patient.**
5. **Articles** contaminated with infective material should be discarded or bagged and labeled before being sent for decontamination and reprocessing.

Drainage/Secretion Precautions
Visitors—Report to Nurses' Station
Before Entering Room

1. **Masks** are not indicated.
2. **Gowns** are indicated if soiling is likely.
3. **Gloves** are indicated for touching infective material.
4. **Hands must be washed after touching the patient or potentially contaminated articles and before taking care of another patient.**
5. **Articles** contaminated with infective material should be discarded or bagged and labeled before being sent for decontamination and reprocessing.

Respiratory Isolation
Visitors—Report to Nurses' Station
Before Entering Room

1. **Masks** are indicated for those who come close to patient.
2. **Gowns** are not indicated.
3. **Gloves** are indicated per Universal Precautions (for contact with blood or body fluids).
4. **Hands must be washed after touching the patient or potentially contaminated articles and before taking care of another patient.**
5. **Articles** contaminated with infective material should be discarded or bagged and labeled before being sent for decontamination and reprocessing.

Strict Isolation
Visitors—Report to Nurses' Station
Before Entering Room

1. **Masks** are indicated.
2. **Gowns** are indicated.
3. **Gloves** are indicated.
4. **Hands must be washed after touching the patient or potentially contaminated articles and before taking care of another patient.**
5. **Articles** should be discarded, cleaned, or sent for decontamination and reprocessing.

AFB (Acid Fast Bacillus) Isolation Primarily for Tuberculosis
Visitors—Report to Nurses' Station
Before Entering Room

1. **Masks** are indicated.
2. **Gowns** are indicated only if needed to prevent gross contamination of clothing.
3. **Gloves** are indicated per Universal Precautions (for contact with blood or body fluids).
4. **Hands must be washed after touching the patient or potentially contaminated articles and before taking care of another patient.**
5. **Articles** should be discarded, cleaned, or sent for decontamination and reprocessing.

Enteric Precautions
Visitors—Report to Nurses' Station
Before Entering Room

1. **Masks** are not indicated.
2. **Gowns** are indicated if soiling is likely.
3. **Gloves** are indicated for touching infective material.
4. **Hands must be washed after touching the patient or potentially contaminated articles and before taking care of another patient.**
5. **Articles** contaminated with infective material should be discarded or bagged and labeled before being sent for decontamination and reprocessing.

A private room is indicated for Enteric Precautions if patient hygiene is poor. A patient with poor hygiene does not wash hands after touching infective material, contaminates the environment with infective material, or shares contaminated articles with other patients. In general, patients infected with the same organism may share a room.

Blood/Body Fluid Precautions

1. **Masks** are not indicated unless aerosolization is likely.
2. **Gowns** are indicated if soiling with blood or body fluids is likely.
3. **Gloves** are indicated for touching blood or body fluids.
4. **Hands must be washed after touching the patient or potentially contaminated articles and before taking care of another patient.**
5. **Articles** contaminated with blood or body fluids should be discarded or bagged and labeled before being sent for decontamination and reprocessing.
6. **Care** should be taken to avoid needle-stick injuries. Used needles should not be recapped or bent; they should be placed in a prominently labeled, puncture-resistant container designed specifically for such disposal.
7. **Blood spills** should be cleaned up promptly with a solution of 5.25% sodium hypochlorite diluted 1:10 with water.

A private room is indicated for Blood Body Fluid Precautions if patient hygiene is poor. A patient with poor hygiene does not wash hands after touching infective material, contaminates the environment with infective material, or shares contaminated articles with other patients. In general, patients infected with the same organism may share a room.

Fig. 5-8 Types of isolation.

The type of isolation used, and the precautions necessary, are determined by the following:

- The type of disease being isolated
- The method of transmission of the isolated pathogens
- The way the isolated pathogens enter and leave the body

Contact isolation prevents the spread of pathogens by direct or indirect contact. Severe respiratory infections, scabies, and lice require contact isolation.

- Hands are washed upon entering and leaving the room.
- Masks may be worn.
- Gowns are worn if body contact is likely.
- Gloves are worn if contact with contaminated material or areas is likely.
- Equipment, linen, and trash are double bagged.

Respiratory isolation prevents the spread of airborne pathogens that cause infections such as Staphylococcus aureus pneumonia.

- Hands are washed upon entering and leaving the room.
- Masks are worn.
- Gowns are not necessary.
- Gloves may be worn.

- Equipment, dishes, linen, and trash that have been in contact with secretions are double bagged.

Drainage/secretion precautions are used to prevent the spread of pathogens by direct or indirect contact with the wound or drainage. These pathogens can cause "staph" and "strep" infections of the skin.

- Hands are washed upon entering and leaving the room.
- Masks are not necessary.
- Gowns are worn if body contact with the wound, drainage, or items contaminated with drainage is likely.
- Gloves are worn if direct or indirect contact with the wound, drainage, or body fluids is likely.
- Equipment, linen, and trash that have been in contact with the wound or drainage are double bagged.

Enteric isolation prevents the spread of pathogens by direct or indirect contact with feces. The pathogens are usually spread by contaminated hands. Hepatitis and infectious diarrhea require enteric isolation.

- Hands are washed upon entering and leaving the room.
- Gloves are worn.

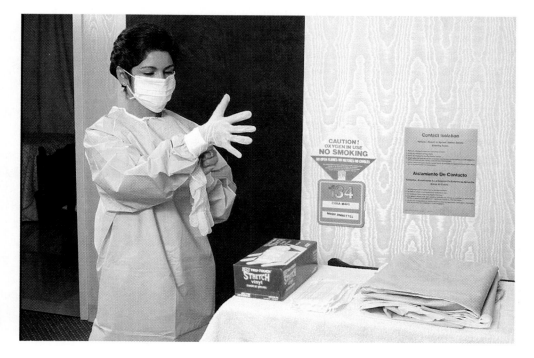

Fig. 5-9
Gloves are put on after the gown, when preparing to enter an isolation room.

- Masks are not necessary.
- Gowns are worn if body contact with the resident, bedpan, toilet, urinal, linen, feces, urine, blood, or other body fluids is likely.
- Equipment, dishes, linen, and trash are double bagged.

Protective or reverse isolation prevents the spread of pathogens to the isolated resident who is highly susceptible. Age, weakness, disease, medications, chemotherapy, stress, burns, and some skin conditions may cause a person to become susceptible. The resident in protective isolation, and items in the room, are considered "clean." All others are "contaminated."

- Hands are washed on entering and leaving the room.
- Masks are worn by all who enter the room.
- Gowns are worn by all who enter the room.
- Gloves are worn for all direct contact with the resident.

To clarify the differences in types of precautions that are used, let us discuss the isolation of a resident with an infected wound. The pathogens causing this infection are present in the drainage or secretions from the wound. Transmission occurs only by direct or indirect contact. The pathogens enter and leave through the open wound.

- A mask is not necessary because the pathogen does *not* enter through the respiratory system.
- Gloves are necessary if you handle contaminated objects or body fluids or you have direct contact with the infected area. The pathogens spread only by direct or indirect contact. They enter and exit the body through the skin.
- Gowns must be worn only if contact with the wound or secretions is likely.
- Articles contaminated with wound secretions or drainage must be double bagged for disposal.
- Handwashing is necessary, as it is for all resident care.

The Isolation Area. To be isolated, a person must be separated from others. Sometimes a special isolation room or a private room is necessary. At other times, a resident may be isolated in a semiprivate room.

The isolation area must contain equipment and supplies that will be required for meeting the needs of the isolated resident. A sink with running water is necessary. The following is a list of other items that are needed:

- A toilet
- Bedpan and urinal
- Toilet paper
- Soap and bath basin
- Water pitcher and glass
- Tissues
- Thermometer and holder
- Equipment for taking vital signs
- Paper towels
- Wastebasket
- Hamper or bag for linen

Storage outside the isolation room will contain masks, gowns, gloves, isolation bags, and isolation tags. All other items necessary for grooming and hygiene can be brought to the room as needed. Before entering an isolation room, plan, organize, and gather equipment and supplies. Make arrangements with a team member for assistance.

PROCEDURE

Putting on a Gown

1. Wash your hands.
2. If you need to wear a mask, put it on first.
3. Let the clean gown unfold without touching any surface.
4. Slide your hands and arms through the sleeves.
5. Tie the neck ties.
6. Overlap the back of the gown.
7. Fasten the waist ties.
8. If gloves are required, put them on last.

Removing a Gown

1. Untie the waist belt or ties.
2. If you are wearing gloves, remove them (see Fig. 5-10A).
3. Wash your hands (see Fig. 5-10B).
4. Untie the neck ties.
5. Pull the sleeve off by grasping each shoulder at the neck line (see Fig. 5-10C).
   a. Do not contaminate your hands by touching the outside of the gown.
   b. Turn the sleeves inside out as you remove them from your arms (see Fig. 5-10D).
6. Holding the gown away from your body by the inside of the shoulder seams, fold it inside out, bringing the shoulders together (see Fig. 5-10E).
7. Roll the gown up with the inside out, and discard (see Fig. 5-10F).
8. Wash your hands (see Fig. 5-10G).
9. If your are wearing a mask, remove it, touching only the strings, and wash your hands (see Fig.5-10H and Fig. 5-10I).

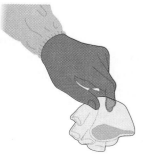

A Remove gloves.

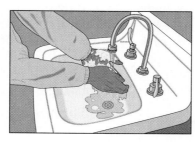

B Wash hands.

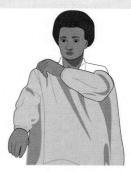

C Grasp each shoulder of gown near neck to remove sleeves.

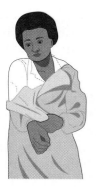

D As you remove sleeves turn them inside out.

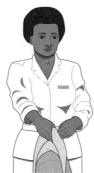

E Fold the gown inside out, holding it away from you.

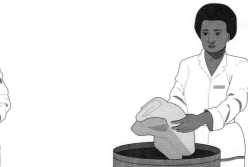

F Roll up the gown and discard it.

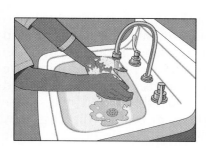

G Wash your hands.

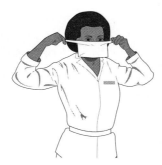

H Remove your mask.

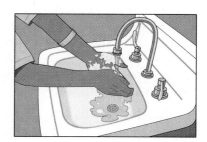

I Wash your hands.

Fig. 5-10 Preparing to leave an isolation room.

PROCEDURE

Putting on a Mask

Put on the mask before putting on the gown or gloves.

1. Wash your hands.
2. Place the upper edge of the mask over the bridge of your nose.
   a. Tie the upper ties.
   b. Place the upper edge under your glasses to prevent fogging.
3. Place the lower edge of the mask under your chin.
   a. Tie the lower ties at the nape of your neck.
4. If the mask has a metal strip in the upper edge, form it to your nose. A good fit prevents microorganisms from entering behind the mask.
5. If the mask becomes damp, it must be changed. It should not be worn more than 20–30 minutes.

PROCEDURE

Removing a Mask

1. Gloves must be removed before removing the mask.
2. Wash your hands. Microorganisms can be spread to your head and neck from your hands or from the gloves.
3. Untie and discard the mask by touching only the strings. Each mask should be worn only one time.
4. Wash your hands after removing the mask.

Isolation Procedures. To care for the isolated resident you must be able to follow isolation procedures and guidelines as listed:

- Handwashing
- Putting on and removing gloves, gown, and mask
- Removing contaminated linen, equipment, and trash
- Serving meals and disposing of food and dishes
- Taking vital signs
- Collecting specimens

Double Bagging. Double bagging is an isolation procedure in which two bags are used to prevent the spread of pathogens. It is used to remove items from the isolation room. Everything in the isolation room is contaminated. This procedure prevents the spread of pathogens to other persons and to other areas of the facility.

Items to Be Double Bagged: Soiled linen and trash are usually double bagged and removed from the isolation room at the end of each shift. Any other items that are to be removed from the room must also be double bagged.

Supplies for Double Bagging: The exact procedure and supplies that are used for double bagging will differ from one facility to another. In some facilities the linen is first placed in a special bag called a "soap bag." A soap bag melts or dissolves in water. The linen is removed from the hamper and placed into the soap bag, while you are inside the isolation room.

Soap bags allow the laundry personnel to empty the linen into the washer without touching it. If a soap bag is used, you should try to place wet linen into it in a way that will not soak the bag. Too much wetness will dissolve the bag before it gets to the washer. A plastic isolation bag will be used if a soap bag is not available.

Red bags are usually used as a second outer bag. Red makes it very obvious that the contents are contaminated items. Isolation tags or labels may be used on the red bags. A biohazard label indicates that the contents are infectious. **Biohazardous waste** is waste matter that has been contaminated with blood or body fluids and may cause infection. Methods of sealing the bags may differ. Often the bags are simply tied at the top to seal them.

Many facilities have contracts for special services to dispose of biohazardous waste.

PROCEDURE

Double Bagging

Before this procedure you must perform the following basic steps: collect the equipment, wash your hands, and explain the procedure.

Follow universal precautions and wear gloves when appropriate.

1. Before entering the room, arrange for a team member to stay outside the door to help you.
2. While you are inside the room and before your help arrives, place items that are to be removed from the isolation room into an isolation bag (see Fig. 5-11A). Seal the contaminated isolation bag by tying it. Prevent drafts that may carry pathogens from the bag into your face.
3. The team member outside the door will hold a clean red isolation bag wide open by making a folded cuff (about 8 inches wide) over the hands (see Fig. 5-11B).
4. Carefully place the contaminated bag inside the clean bag that is being held at the door. You must stay inside. Do not touch your team member or the outside of the clean bag (see Fig. 5-11C).
5. Your team member will tie the outer bag, being careful not to create a draft from it (see Fig. 5-11D). The team member will label and dispose of it properly.

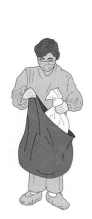 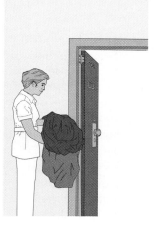 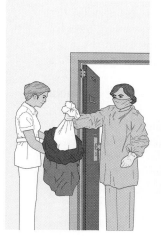 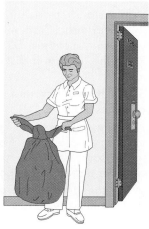

A Before help arrives, bag the items to be removed.

B Hold the red bag open by making a folded cuff over your hands.

C Do not touch your assistant or the outside of the red bag.

D Tie the bag without creating a draft.

Fig. 5-11 Removing items from an isolation room.

In this case, special containers are provided. These containers and their contents stay in the room until a pickup is scheduled. You may not be responsible for removing these from the room. Keep the containers covered and place only the correct items into them.

Serving a Meal in an Isolation Room.
Most facilities use disposable dishes for meals served in isolation rooms. When serving a tray to the resident in isolation, you should transfer the food to a tray that stays in the isolation room. Do not contaminate the clean tray.

Encourage the resident to do as much as possible. Take time to talk to the resident, and do not hurry. Mealtime is a good time for communication and observation. Be sure to record the amount eaten.

PROCEDURE

Serving a Meal Tray in an Isolation Room

Before this procedure, you must perform the following basic steps: collect the equipment, wash your hands, identify the resident, and explain the procedure.

Follow universal precautions and wear gloves when appropriate.

1. Ask a team member to help you. The person will stand outside the door.
2. Put on the appropriate isolation clothing, and enter the isolation room.
3. Wipe the tray that has been left in the room with a damp paper towel, and take it to the door.
4. While standing inside the room, take the food and dishes from the tray being held by your team member. Do not touch the tray. Place the food and dishes on the resident's tray.
5. Serve the resident and assist with the meal as necessary.
6. After the resident has eaten, flush uneaten food down the toilet. Place bones or seeds in the trash, not in the toilet. Discard the disposable dishes in the room.
7. Wipe the tray with a damp paper towel, and put it away.
8. Remove the isolation clothing, using the proper procedure.
9. Wash your hands.

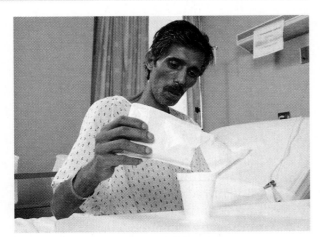

Fig. 5-12 Disposable food containers may be used in isolation.

Taking Vital Signs in the Isolation Room. The equipment needed to take vital signs may be kept at the bedside when the resident is in isolation. The following items will be needed: a glass thermometer (in a container of disinfectant solution that must be changed daily), a stethoscope, a blood pressure cuff, a pencil, and pad of paper.

PROCEDURE

Taking Vital Signs in an Isolation Room

Before this procedure, you must perform the following basic steps: collect the equipment, wash your hands, identify the resident, explain the procedure, and provide privacy.

Follow universal precautions and wear gloves when appropriate.

1. Put on the correct isolation clothing.
2. If a gown and gloves are required, you may need to remove your watch first. It will be placed on a clean paper towel, so that you will be able to see it while taking the pulse and respirations.
3. Measure the vital signs by the usual procedure.
4. Write the vital sign measurements on a piece of paper, so you will be able to remember them.
5. Remove the isolation garments and wash your hands, in the proper order.
6. Pick up the watch.
7. Look at the vital signs measurements that you have written. Leave the pencil and paper in the isolation room.
8. Record the vital signs immediately.

Collecting a Specimen in the Isolation Room. A specimen is a sample of material from a person's body. Because of the possibility of differences in collection procedures, you must be aware of the procedure used in your facility. There is a basic procedure for collecting a specimen from an isolated resident. The exact procedure for each type of specimen can be found in a later chapter.

PROCEDURE

Collecting a Specimen in an Isolation Room

Before this procedure, you must perform the following basic steps: collect the equipment, wash your hands, identify the resident, explain the procedure, and provide privacy.

Follow universal precautions and wear gloves when necessary.

1. Collect the specimen container, label, a bag (to place the specimen in), and any other supplies or equipment that will be needed.
   a. On the outside of the bag, write the kind of specimen that you are going to obtain, the resident's name and room number, date of collection, and the word "isolation." A biohazard label indicates infectious contents.
   b. Label the container as you did the bag.

2. Leave the bag outside the room.
3. Put on the appropriate isolation clothing.
4. Place the specimen container and the lid, with the inside facing up, on a clean paper towel in the resident's room.
5. Collect the specimen.
6. Transfer the specimen to the container and replace the lid, touching only the outside of the container and lid.
7. Remove the isolation clothing by using the proper procedure.
8. Take the specimen from the room and place it in the bag. Some specimens may need to be double bagged.
9. Wash your hands.
10. Take the specimen to the proper area.
11. Tell the nurse that you have collected the specimen.

Using a Restorative Approach to Isolation Care

Encourage the independence of the isolated resident by using restorative measures. While coping with the emotional experiences of isolation, the resident may become depressed and less motivated. Encouraging self-care may require additional time and effort. Using a restorative approach is important in meeting both the resident's emotional and physical needs.

Isolation greatly affects the resident's emotional well-being. Can you remember the last time you chose to be alone? to isolate yourself? It probably felt good because you needed to be alone—it was your choice. How would you feel if you were forced to stay away from others whom you wanted to be near? if no one could hug you? if no one could touch you without wearing gloves? Would you be bored if you were not allowed to leave a small room?

The resident who has been placed in isolation may be experiencing many feelings. Being isolated can cause feelings of rejection and fear. The resident might feel "dirty," and self-esteem may be affected. The resident might resent being confined and wish visitors and staff members could stay longer.

It is challenging to meet the emotional needs of the isolated resident. Your attitude, comfort, and confidence are important. You must use your communication skills to encourage self-esteem and to promote emotional well-being. The resident who is isolated from others may be more dependent upon you to fulfill emotional needs. The resident may need to express fears and concerns. You should encourage this type of communication. If you feel that more reassurance or information is needed, ask the nurse to talk to the resident.

To reassure the resident, you must first be aware of your own feelings about isolation. Fear of becoming infected, pressure for time, or being unfamiliar with isolation procedures may interfere with your emotional support of the resident. If you have fears, you should discuss them with the charge nurse. You may need to remind yourself and the resident *that it is the pathogens that are being isolated and not the person.*

You will feel more confident about your own safety if you understand isolation procedures and perform them properly. If you are unfamiliar with a procedure, ask the charge nurse for supervision. You must maintain the resident's safety by keeping the call signal in reach and answering it promptly. Be sure that the resident understands the necessary precautions. Your thorough observation and reporting continue to be very important safety factors.

The resident's family will also need extra care and consideration. Family members play a very important role in meeting the emotional needs of the isolated resident. They may need explanations and assistance in carrying out their responsibilities.

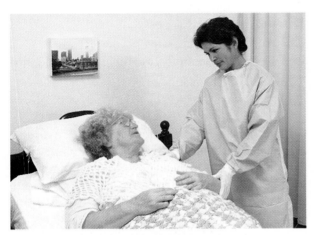

Fig. 5-13 Remind yourself and the resident that it is the pathogens that are being isolated and not the resident.

HIV Infection (AIDS) and Other Bloodborne Diseases

Definition. HIV (human immunodeficiency virus) infection is a disease that destroys the immune system and leaves the body unable to fight the pathogens that cause other infections. AIDS (acquired immune deficiency syndrome) is the term used to describe the final stage of HIV infection. The immune system is the body's defense system. The term "immune deficient" means that the immune system does not have enough cells to defend the body. Although the disease was originally called "AIDS", "HIV infection" is the correct term to use when describing this condition.

History. AIDS was first reported in the United States in 1981, in New York City and San Francisco. Cases now have been diagnosed throughout the world, and the numbers are increasing rapidly. Although the first cases involved mostly homosexual men, it is *not* a "gay disease." Anyone who participates in risky sexual behavior or shares needles when using illegal drugs can get HIV.

Cause. AIDS is caused by the HIV virus, which enters the bloodstream where it continues to live and reproduce. Once a person is infected with HIV, he or she is contagious and can transmit the disease to someone else.

Signs and Symptoms. Persons who are infected with HIV may have no symptoms for an extended period of time. They may not be sick, and may not even realize that they are infected. The virus can have a long incubation period, but most people who are infected with HIV develop AIDS within a few years.

People with an HIV infection eventually develop many severe symptoms. These symptoms include fatigue, diarrhea, weight loss, fever, night sweats, and loss of appetite. AIDS patients are very ill. The diarrhea is endless, vomiting goes on for days, and fever leaves them drenched in sweat. Opportunistic diseases like thrush (an infection of the mouth and throat) may develop because the immune system has weakened. Most HIV patients die of either a rare form of pneumonia or of cancer. It is a terrible, painful way to die.

Transmission. HIV is transmitted by

- Sexual activity
- Injectable drug users sharing contaminated needles and syringes
- Transmission to babies from HIV infected mothers
- Transfusion of blood contaminated by the HIV

Risk Groups. A risk group includes people who are susceptible to a disease. Because of the way HIV is spread, we can identify those who are more likely to catch it. The following is a list of risk groups for HIV:

- Men who have sex with men
- Injectable drug users
- Sexual partners of persons infected with HIV
- Babies born to HIV-infected mothers
- People who receive blood transfusions
- Hemophiliacs

The first two groups are at highest risk. Since 1985 all blood collected for transfusions is tested for evidence of the virus. If the blood tests positive for HIV, it is discarded. This practice has reduced the risk to hemophiliacs and others who have blood transfusions or blood products.

How Contagious Is HIV? It is not easy to get HIV. The virus is not airborne and cannot live long outside the human body. The virus must enter the bloodstream. Every exposure does *not* result in infection. There is no evidence that HIV is spread in any of the following ways:

- Casual contact
- Sharing equipment
- Using rest rooms
- Working together
- Eating together
- Coughing or sneezing

Prevention. Since HIV is transmitted primarily by sexual contact, some changes in behavior must be made to stop its rapid spread. People must remain aware of the danger of some homosexual practices and of having multiple anonymous sex partners. The practice of "safer sex" with the use of condoms also helps to prevent the spread of HIV.

The second most common way that HIV is spread is by sharing needles and syringes that are contaminated. The best way to stop this type of transmission is to avoid the illegal use of drugs, particularly those that are injected into the body. Realizing that all drug users may not quit, some states are furnishing clean needles and syringes to addicts to prevent sharing.

Correct infection-control practices, especially handwashing, are very important.

Always use universal precautions when there is a possibility of contact with any body fluid. The use of protective barriers like gloves, gowns, and masks, in performing resident care, depends on many factors. Refer to the guidelines for universal precautions given earlier in this chapter. If you are not sure of precautions to be taken, check with the nurse.

Needles should be disposed of promptly and never bent, broken, or recapped. Needle sticks are a major source of infection in health care. Although nursing assistants don't give shots, you may handle needles and syringes. For example, a urine specimen is collected from a urinary drainage system by needle and syringe. That is a procedure that you may be asked to do. As soon as you are through using the needle and syringe, or any sharp object, dispose of it in a puncture-proof container (see Fig. 5-14).

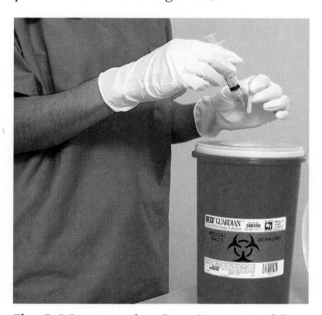

Fig. 5-14 Dispose of needles and syringes carefully.

Disinfection. The AIDS virus is easily killed by chemicals that are commonly found in the facility. These chemicals include alcohol, Lysol®, peroxide, and any other approved germicide. Bleach, the most commonly available disinfectant, will kill the virus, even in a diluted solution. Mix one part bleach with ten parts of water, and make a new solution every 24 hours.

Aseptic techniques currently required in health care facilities are sufficient to prevent the spread of HIV and other diseases. Dietary, laundry, housekeeping, and maintenance already have policies and procedures that, when followed, will destroy HIV.

Education. One of the ways to stop the spread of HIV is through education. Health care facilities are required to provide inservice education about HIV, so be sure to attend. Much information is available in newspapers and magazines, and on television. Question information that you are not sure about, as some things you hear or read may not be true. Information changes continually. It is your responsibility, as a member of the health care team, to stay informed with current information about HIV.

Testing. There are tests to find out if a person has developed antibodies to the virus. An antibody is a substance that is produced by the immune system when a foreign body (a virus, for example) invades the body. However, it takes several weeks after infection for the antibodies to develop. There is a period of time when a person who is infected might test negative. During that time, the infected person could infect someone else. If no antibodies develop within five or six months after an exposure to HIV, the exposed person probably has not been infected and will not develop AIDS. *Every person who is exposed to HIV does not get AIDS.*

Treatment of HIV. At the present time, HIV is considered a terminal illness because it has no cure. The first drug approved by the Food and Drug Administration was AZT. Other drugs now available to treat HIV are limited, and all have severe side effects. The person with AIDS, who has pneumonia or cancer, will receive treatment for those diseases. Millions of dollars are being spent on research to develop a vaccine and new medications for treatment of HIV.

Emotional Response to HIV. The person with HIV will need your help in dealing with many emotions, such as anger, fear, depression, anxiety, or guilt. All these feelings are a normal response to a terminal illness. The loss of job, friends, family, and self-control can damage self-esteem. Experiencing so many losses within a short period of time can be overwhelming.

Your attitude toward HIV will affect your response to the resident with HIV. Develop a supportive, nonjudgmental attitude. Tact, sensitivity, and empathy are necessary. The resident with HIV is entitled to the same loving care you give to the other residents.

Legal Issues. Laws have been passed concerning HIV. They cover reporting, education, testing, confidentiality, and discrimination. Laws vary between states and are constantly changing. It is your responsibility to keep up with current legal issues in your area.

Hepatitis

Hepatitis is a disease that affects the liver and causes the skin to look yellow. You may have heard this called "yellow jaundice" or "yellow John." The two most common types of hepatitis are hepatitis A and hepatitis B. Both are contagious.

Hepatitis A is caused by a virus. It is usually spread through contaminated food or water. Persons who have hepatitis A will be in isolation. Hepatitis B is caused by a virus called HBV. It is spread in the same way that HIV is spread, through sexual contact and blood. The hepatitis virus is able to live outside the body longer than the HIV virus, and it is more difficult to kill. You must also protect yourself from HBV by using universal precautions.

As in HIV, HBV can infect people who do not get the disease but are carriers. They can give the disease to someone else. Precautions to prevent the spread of HBV are the same as those for HIV.

There is a vaccine available to prevent hepatitis B. OSHA regulations mandate that this vaccine be offered at no cost to health care workers who might be exposed to infectious material. The vaccine provides immunity to hepatitis B and has few side effects or reactions.

MRSA

MRSA (methicillin-resistant Staphylococcus aureus) is a disease caused by a pathogen that is resistant to many antibiotics. MRSA exists in warm, moist areas like the nose and mouth. It may also be found in urine, stool, or wound drainage. It affects people whose resistance is low. Because the elderly are more susceptible to disease, MRSA may occur in the long-term care facility.

The signs and symptoms of MRSA are similar to those of other infections and might include redness, fever, and drainage. It is a highly contagious disease and spreads rapidly. Once MRSA occurs in a facility, it is difficult to prevent it's spread.

The most frequent transmission of MRSA is on the hands of health care workers. Poor handwashing practices cause the worker to carry the pathogens from an infected resident to others. The health care worker who is infected may also infect others. Prevention measures for MRSA include universal precautions and aseptic technique. The most important measure is handwashing.

Conclusion

Remember these important points:

1. Preventing the spread of infection is the responsibility of all employees.

2. Pathogens are microorganisms that cause infection.

3. Normal flora are microorganisms that live in certain areas of the body, but can cause infection if they leave their usual location.

4. All microorganisms prefer darkness, warmth, moisture, and food. Most need oxygen.

5. Pathogens spread from one person to another by direct contact, indirect contact, air, and vehicle.

6. It is important to observe and recognize the signs of infection and report them immediately.

7. Aseptic practices that prevent the spread of pathogens include handwashing, disinfection, sterilization, and universal precautions.

8. Handwashing is the most important procedure that is used to prevent the spread of infection.

9. Universal precautions should be followed while caring for all residents.

10. Gloves should be worn when you are in contact with blood, semen, vaginal secretions, or any body fluid. Always wash your hands before and after using gloves.

11. The usual purpose of isolation is to prevent the spread of pathogens from the isolated person to others.

12. Protective isolation protects the isolated person from pathogens that are present in the environment.

13. The type of isolation is determined by the type of infection, method of transmission, and the way the pathogen enters and leaves the body.

14. Everything in the isolation room is contaminated and must be disinfected or double bagged before being removed from the room.

15. Encourage the isolated resident's independence by using restorative measures.

16. Isolation has a major effect on the resident's emotional well-being.

17. Your attitude toward infection will affect your response to the isolated resident. Be aware of your own feelings about isolation.

18. Remind yourself and the resident that it is the pathogens that are being isolated, not the resident.

19. It is your responsibility to provide extra care and consideration to the families of isolated residents.

20. The risk of HIV infection or hepatitis in the workplace is very low if basic infection-control practices and universal precautions are followed.

Discussion Questions

1. *How are microorganisms spread from one person to another? Be sure to discuss all methods of transmission.*

2. *What is the difference between asepsis and sterilization?*

3. *Discuss aseptic practices that are used in resident care.*

4. *How do your feelings about infection affect your response to the resident in isolation?*

5. *How would you feel about caring for a resident with HIV infection?*

Application Exercise

1. The instructor will divide the class into groups and assign each group a different type of isolation. Each group will prepare a report. The report will include

a. Method of transmission

b. Protection required and why it is necessary

c. List of necessary supplies

A representative of each group will deliver the report to the class, allowing time for questions and discussions.

Safety in the Long-Term Care Facility

OBJECTIVES

Upon completing this chapter, you will be able to do the following:

1. List four reasons why elderly residents have accidents.

2. Identify three common accidents that happen to the elderly.

3. List six safety measures to prevent accidents.

4. List ten guidelines for using body mechanics.

5. Explain the role of OSHA in safety.

6. Explain the purpose of an incident report.

7. Describe the effects of restraints on the residents.

8. Identify six substitutes for restraints.

9. List six guidelines to be followed when applying restraints.

10. List six rules of fire prevention.

11. Explain the purpose of a disaster plan.

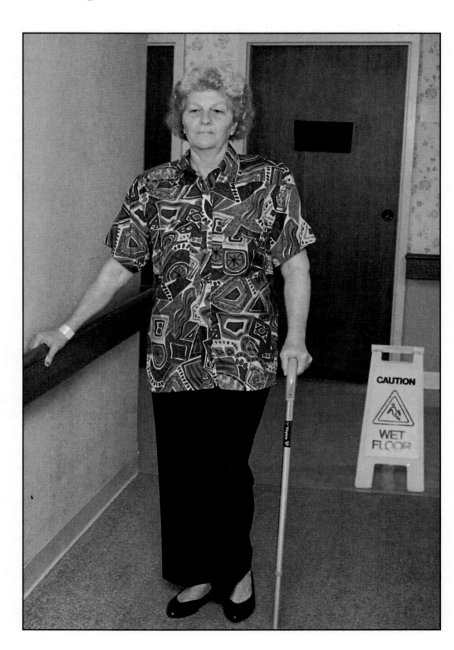

VOCABULARY

The following words or terms will help you to understand this chapter:

Toxic	OSHA (Occupational	Incident report
Suffocation	Safety and Health	Restraint
Body mechanics	Administration)	

Safety Concerns of the Elderly

Elderly people have more accidents than any other age group, except children. Reasons for this include physical changes of aging, disease process, mental disorders, life changes, and medications.

Physical Changes of Aging. The physical changes of aging often increase the risk of an accident. Slower blood circulation may cause a person to be weak or dizzy. Physical changes may result in limitation of mobility, as muscles weaken and joints stiffen. Because the elderly cannot move quickly, they are often unable to get out of the way of danger. Balance and coordination might be affected. They are less able to protect themselves in falls, and when the elderly person falls, brittle bones may break.

Many older people have some loss of vision and hearing. They may not be able to hear or see warnings of danger. Because the sense of touch and the awareness of pain are decreased, the older person may get burned. Slowed reflexes can prevent the resident from reacting quickly in an emergency.

Disease Process. There are many diseases that place the elderly resident at risk for accidents. For example, many geriatric residents suffer from arthritis, a joint disease that interferes with movement. This can lead to loss of balance and falls. The desire for independence may cause the resident to attempt to do things that are unsafe.

A stroke may result in paralysis, poor balance, and poor coordination. Paralyzed residents are more at risk for accidents because of their decreased ability to protect themselves. A stroke may affect the ability to speak or to think clearly. This impairment also increases the risk of an accident.

Mental Impairment. Diseases like Alzheimer's or chronic brain syndrome can cause the elderly resident to be confused. Confusion and disorientation are major causes of accidents. Confused people can accidentally injure themselves or others. Unconscious residents are even more at risk because they are totally dependent on others for their safety. Any decrease in awareness creates a hazard.

Life Changes and Losses. Leaving home and being admitted to a long-term care facility requires a major adjustment. The resident may be upset about leaving home and belongings. The environment has changed drastically and everything is unfamiliar. The resident may wake up at night and be unable to find the bathroom. An accident might occur because furniture isn't arranged the way it was at home.

While some people adjust quickly to the change, others do not. Many become depressed, which makes them less concerned for their safety. The elderly person may have lost a spouse, a home, and friends. Loss of health or even loss of life no longer seem important.

Medications. As people age, they react differently to medications. Medications may have a stronger effect, and the effects may last longer. The need for several medications increases the risk of drug interaction. Some medication causes confusion or drowsiness. Have you ever taken a medication that made you drowsy or sleepy? A confused or drowsy resident is at great risk.

Types of Accidents

An accident may be caused by carelessness or negligence. Some examples include

- Failure to identify the resident
- Not answering the signal light promptly
- Incorrect moving and lifting
- Failure to lock brakes on equipment wheels
- Lack of knowledge about using equipment
- Failure to clean up spills
- Failure to place signal light in reach

Some types of accidents involving the elderly include

- Falls
- Burns
- Poisoning
- Suffocation

Falls. A fall is the most frequent accident in the long-term care facility. The most common cause of falls is wet, slippery floors. Water, or any other liquid spilled on the floor, creates a hazard for everyone. The resident with poor vision and unsteady gait is more likely to slip on wet floors. Picture the confused resident coming down the hall, totally unaware that directly ahead is a puddle of water. The result will likely be a fall. The following list includes other factors that can cause a fall:

- Improper footwear
- Loose rugs or a hole in the carpet
- Poor lighting
- Clutter
- Staff carelessness or negligence

Burns. Burns are often caused by careless smokers. The resident who smokes may drop hot ashes or a lit cigarette. Hot water and other liquids may also cause burns. Extra precautions are necessary when performing any procedure involving heat or cold. A decreased sensitivity to heat can result in a burn. Burns can be caused by negligence.

Poisoning. Residents who have poor vision or are confused may pick up a toxic substance and eat or drink it. **Toxic** means poisonous. Cleaning solutions and disinfectants are examples of toxic substances.

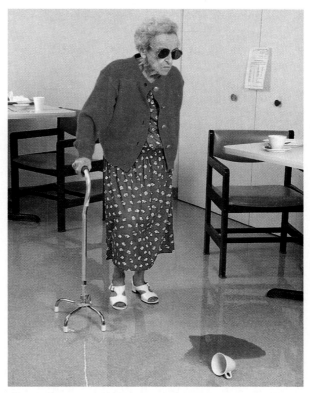

Fig. 6-1 The confused or vision-impaired resident may not be aware of spills.

Suffocation. **Suffocation** means the interruption of respiration, preventing the intake of oxygen. Some causes of suffocation include choking, drowning, smoke inhalation, and electrical shock. Suffocation leads to death.

Safety Measures to Prevent Accidents

The purpose of safety control in the long-term care facility is to prevent accidents. The following is a list of safety measures:

- Correctly identify the resident.
- Keep the signal light in reach.
- Clean up spills immediately.
- Use safety equipment such as a gait belt or hydraulic lift.
- Encourage the resident to use safety bars and rails.
- Make sure the resident is wearing proper footwear.
- Raise side rails when appropriate.

- Follow aseptic practices to prevent the spread of infection.
- Lock wheels on beds, chairs, and other equipment.
- Provide adequate lighting.
- Report faulty equipment and other safety hazards.
- Return beds to the lowest position and fold bed cranks out of the way.
- Keep hallways and rooms free of clutter.
- Understand and use correct procedures.
- Get help when necessary.
- Use proper body mechanics.

Correct Identification. Correct identification of the resident is a very important safety measure. The safest way to identify the resident is by checking the identification bracelet. Never rely on calling the resident by name because the wrong person may answer. Have you ever had someone mispronounce your name or call you by the wrong name? Did you answer them anyway? If you did, was it because you were confused or hard of hearing? Probably not—you were just being polite. The resident may respond in the same way.

You cannot depend on checking the room number or the name on the bed. Residents sometimes enter the wrong room and occasionally get into the wrong bed. Always check the I.D. bracelet. It doesn't matter how well you perform a procedure if you don't have the right resident.

Using the Call Signal. The call signal (also referred to as a call bell or signal light) should be placed where the resident can reach it. If the resident is in bed, the signal can be fastened to the pillow. When the resident is up in a chair, it should be within reach. A confused resident who is out of the room in a wheelchair should be within sight of staff members. Check to be sure the call signal is working and that the resident knows how to use it. Answer all call signals promptly. A serious accident can happen because a resident does not get help when it is needed. A fall may occur if the resident attempts to go to the bathroom without assistance. Even if a resident is confused, the call signal must be in reach at all times.

Cleaning Up Wet Floors and Spills. Cleaning up spills is everyone's responsibility. The person who sees the spill first should take action to prevent an accident. If you are unable to clean it up yourself, tell someone else immediately. Observe "wet floor" signs, and remind residents and visitors to avoid those areas.

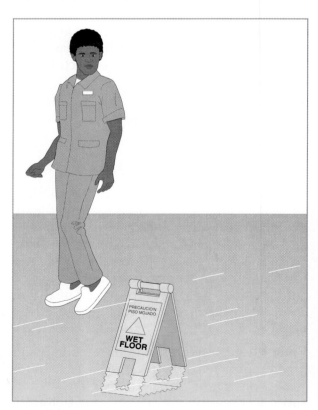

Fig. 6-3 Obey "Wet Floor" signs.

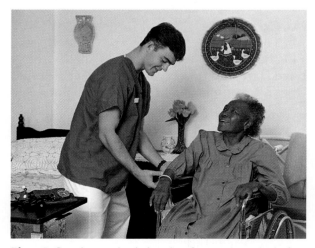

Fig. 6-2 Always check the identification bracelet before you perform resident care.

Wearing Proper Footwear. The resident should wear nonskid shoes when out of bed or walking. Check to be sure that shoes fit properly and are in good repair. Tie shoestrings and fasten buckles as needed. Bedroom slippers should not be worn unless they provide support and have nonskid soles. The resident should not attempt to walk in stocking feet. "Scuffs" or any footwear with an open heel are unsafe. The safest shoe for the elderly person is one that has nonskid soles and a closed heel and toe. This is also the safest type of shoe for you to wear to work.

Body Mechanics

Body mechanics refers to the use of the body to produce motion. Correct body mechanics means using the body in a careful and efficient manner. The three most important reasons for using correct body mechanics are

- To protect the resident from injury
- To protect you from injury
- To save energy and prevent fatigue

GUIDELINES FOR USING CORRECT BODY MECHANICS

- Maintain a wide base of support by standing with your feet 8–12 inches apart for balance.
- Bend at your knees, not at your waist.
- Keep your back straight.
- Use the large muscles of your legs and arms. The strongest muscles are in your thighs and the weakest are in your back.
- Stand close to the object or the person you are working with. Hold the object you are lifting close to your body.
- Turn your whole body at once, don't twist.
- Use smooth, coordinated movements.
- Push or pull an object rather than lift it.
- Use correct posture (head up, chin and stomach tucked in).
- Keep beds and other surfaces at the proper working height, when possible.
- Plan ahead and get help if needed.

Use correct body mechanics all the time, not just at work. Consider the guidelines you have just read, and how you could use them while sitting, standing, walking, working, lifting, or moving objects. To prevent fatigue and back strain, change position frequently, stretch and relax occasionally, and use correct body mechanics.

OSHA (The Occupational Safety and Health Administration)

OSHA (Occupational Safety and Health Administration) is a government agency that is concerned with the health and safety of workers. These concerns include infection-control practices and other safety issues. Regulations are in effect concerning bloodborne pathogens, such as HIV and hepatitis B. Rules specify the type of protective supplies, equipment, and techniques to be used in the health care facility.

Hazard Communication Standard. OSHA's hazard communication standard states that you have the right to know what hazards you may be exposed to at work. This standard also requires that you protect yourself against possible hazards. All hazardous material must be labeled. The employer must provide information and training to help you understand labels and safe procedures.

Incident Reports

An incident is an event that occurs that is not a part of the routine care of the resident or a part of the regular routine of the facility. An accident is one type of incident. An error in performing resident care is another type. An **incident report** provides written documentation of an incident. It includes information such as the persons involved, the date, time and location of the incident, witnesses, and injuries, if any. See Fig. 6-5 for a sample incident report.

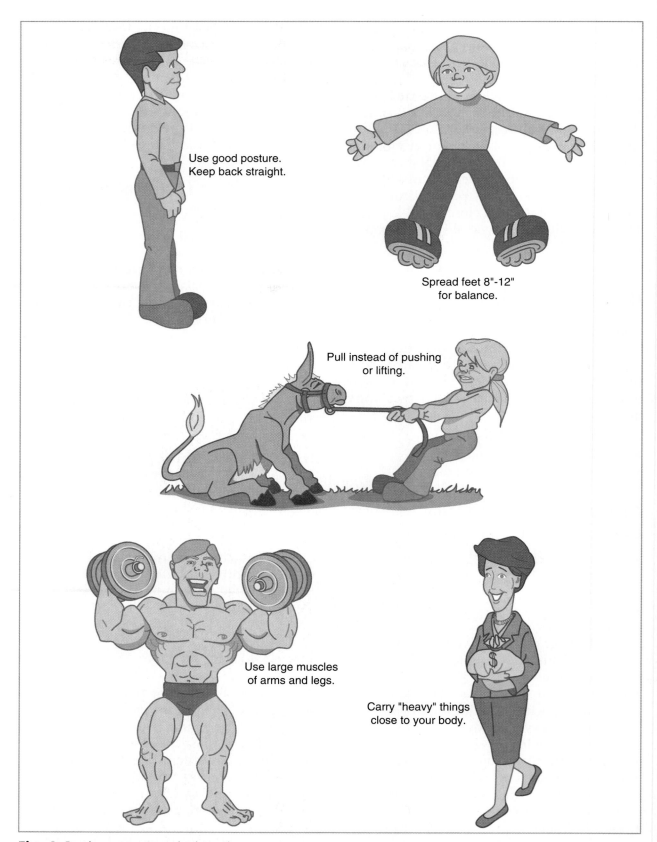

Fig. 6-4 Always use correct body mechanics.

ACCIDENT/INCIDENT REPORT

1. Patient ☒   Visitor ❑   Employee ❑   Other ❑

2. Date of this report <u>12/25</u> 19 <u>98</u>   Date of incident _____ <u>12/25/98</u> _____

3. Name _____ <u>Johnson, Henry A.</u> _____ Age <u>79</u> Sex <u>Male</u> Marital Status ____
   Department _____ Position _____

4. Location incident occurred at _____ <u>Room 407</u> _____ Time <u>1:00</u> a.m.
                                                                                              p.m.

5. Reported to _____ Patient seen by Dr. <u>Ralph A. Jones</u> _____
   _____ Time _____ a.m.   _____ Time <u>1:05</u> a.m.
                                   p.m.   p.m.

6. Statement of doctor or resident (diagnosis, parts of body affected and treatment)
   _____ <u>Patient examined—no injuries sustained—left elbow slightly abraded.</u> _____
   _____
   _____
   _____ Attending Physician _____ M.D.

7. Describe incident and how accident occurred. (Statement of nurse or person in charge.)
   <u>Patient found on floor—stated he attempted to get out of bed, slipped</u>
   <u>and fell to floor. Slight abrasion of left elbow. No property damaged.</u>
   Signed _____ Title _____

8. Witness's name _____ <u>Fred R. Smith</u> _____ Address <u>33 Yale St., New Brunswick, N.J.</u>
   Witness's name _____ Address _____

9. Name of machine involved _____

10. Kind of work performed by machine _____

11. Part of machine causing injury _____

12. Any protective device on machine _____

13. Action taken to prevent recurrence _____
    _____
    _____ Signed _____ Title _____

14. Did employee lose time?   Yes ❑   No ❑   If yes, give last day worked   mo   day   yr
                                                                                          __   __   __
    If unable to rusume work, give probable date of return   mo   day   yr   if already returned   mo   day   yr
                                                              __   __   __   __   __   __

15. If patient accident, signed _____ Date _____
                          Ass't. Adm. Nursing Service
    Reported to administration on _____ at _____ a.m. Signed _____ Adm.
                                                      p.m.

Department director must complete necessary information in duplicate. Duplicate must be forwarded immediately to chairperson of the safety committee.

Reviewed by safety committee on _____ Signed _____ Chairperson.

(FILL OUT IN DUPLICATE)

Fig. 6-5 An example of an incident report.

An incident report must be written any time you are involved in an accident, witness an incident, or make an error that could result in an injury. Some examples of incidents that would require an incident report include

- You fall or injure yourself.
- You perform a procedure on the wrong resident.
- A resident falls or is injured.
- A visitor falls or is injured.

Write the incident report immediately. The sooner you get the information down on paper, the less likely you will be to forget something. The report should be accurate and specific. Include only the facts—what you saw, not what you think may have happened. Use quotes to describe what someone tells you. Try to remember, as closely as you can, what was said. Study the following situation to see how to make a correct incident report.

You walk into Mrs. Day's room and find her sitting on the floor. She has a small bump on the left side of her forehead. She tells you, "I fell and bumped my head."

What should you write on the incident report? You should *not* write that she fell and bumped her head, because you don't know that for a fact. She may have bumped her head on the door and then sat down on the floor. You should chart, "Mrs. Smith found sitting on the floor in her room. She has a small bump on the left side of her forehead. She says she fell and bumped her head." This is called objective reporting.

An incident report should be written, even if there are no obvious injuries or the person involved thinks they are not hurt. If an injury develops later, as a result of the incident, all the facts will be available. Always write the incident report before you leave the facility. If you are not sure how to fill out an incident report, ask the charge nurse to help you.

An incident report protects you, the resident, visitors, and the facility. Incident reports are also used to identify and resolve safety problems.

Restraints

A **restraint** is a device that is used to restrict a person's freedom of movement. A restraint may be used only for the safety of the resident, *never* for the convenience of the staff.

Legal Issues. There are federal and state laws regarding the use of restraints. Restraining a resident unnecessarily is false imprisonment. It is also abuse and a violation of the resident's rights. A restraint requires a doctor's order.

Effects of Restraints. Being restrained affects the resident physically and emotionally. Physical effects can include skin breakdown, constipation, pneumonia, blood clots, muscle weakness, and loss of mobility. Emotional effects can be just as severe and include loss of dignity, independence, and control. These losses lead to a loss of self-esteem. Confusion, disorientation, anxiety, frustration, and anger can also result. There is a decrease in both communication and social activity.

Most people don't like to have their movements restricted. It causes them to become upset and angry. If the resident is already angry or combative, a restraint will only increase the anger. Your goal should be to calm the resident down.

Residents who suffer from chronic wandering, such as those with Alzheimer's disease, should not be restrained, except in extreme situations. Always try to encourage independence. It is important to protect the resident without damaging self-esteem.

Using Restraints. A resident might need to be temporarily restrained if he or she

- Has a history of severe falls
- Needs postural support in a chair
- Might experience self-injury or injure others
- Might interfere with treatment (remove tubes or dressings)

Substitutes for Restraints. A restraint should always be the last resort, used only after other methods have failed to protect the resident. Try one of the following methods or others you may know about before restraining the resident. As a substitute for restraints, you may do the following:

- Interrupt behavior that might lead to the need for restraints.
- Use music to calm the resident.
- Use TV and radio for diversion.
- Encourage activities as an outlet for energy.
- Closely observe confused residents.
- Allow residents to walk in safe areas.
- Encourage family participation.
- Use pillows, padding, and other equipment for support.

The facility may use bed alarms, door alarms, and arm band alarms to signal the location of the confused resident. Always respond immediately to the sound of an alarm.

Types of Restraints. There are many types of restraints designed to protect the resident in different situations (see Fig. 6-6). The doctor decides which type of restraint, for what length of time, and in what circumstance it may be used. Some types of restraints commonly used in long-term care include

- Soft belt restraint: A soft belt restraint is used to prevent the resident from falling out of a wheelchair or bed (see Fig. 6-6A). It is applied over the clothing and around the waist and fastened to the bed or chair. Some styles may look like a car seat belt and may fasten the same way.
- Safety vest: A safety vest is also used to prevent the resident from falling from a chair or bed (see Fig. 6-6B). It provides more support than a belt. It is a sleeveless, cloth vest that is applied over clothing and tied to the chair or bed frame. The safety vest must always cross in the front to prevent the resident from being injured. It should also be kept clean and free of wrinkles.
- Wrist restraint (limb holder): The wrist restraint is used to prevent the resident from removing dressings or pulling out tubes that are a part of the treatment. This type of restraint is a cloth band that is sometimes padded with fleece or some other soft material (see Fig. 6-6C). It is

applied around the wrist and secured to the bed or chair. It must not be applied over jewelry or the identification bracelet. Since it is applied over a bony area, it must be well padded to prevent skin breakdown. A wrist restraint must be checked every 15 minutes to be sure that it is not interfering with circulation. Signs of circulation problems include cold, pale, or bluish skin; absence of a pulse or complaints of pain; numbness; or tingling. If any of these occur, loosen the restraint and report to the nurse immediately.

- Mitt restraint: A mitt restraint looks like a big mitten without a thumb (see Fig. 6-6D). It is used for the same purpose as the wrist restraint. The mitt restraint is the better choice of the two. It restricts finger movement, without preventing movement of the hand or arm.
- Safety bars: Safety bar kits can be applied to wheelchairs to help prevent the resident from falling (see Fig. 6-6E). They are less restricting than soft belts.

GUIDELINES FOR APPLYING A RESTRAINT

- A restraint requires a doctor's order.
- Use only when necessary, never for convenience.
- Use restorative techniques first (activities or recreation).
- Use the least restrictive device when possible (a belt instead of a vest, a mitt instead of a wrist restraint).
- A geri-chair (geriatric chair) is considered a restraint, if the lap table is in place.
- Explain what you are doing and why you are doing it.
- Use the correct size and type of restraint.
- Apply the restraint properly.
- Tie a knot that can quickly be released (half-bow).
- Do not tie the restraint too tightly. You should be able to insert four fingers under the waist of the vest restraint and two fingers under the wrist restraint.
- Tie the restraint to the part of the bed frame that does not move, never to the side rail.
- Never use a sheet as a restraint.

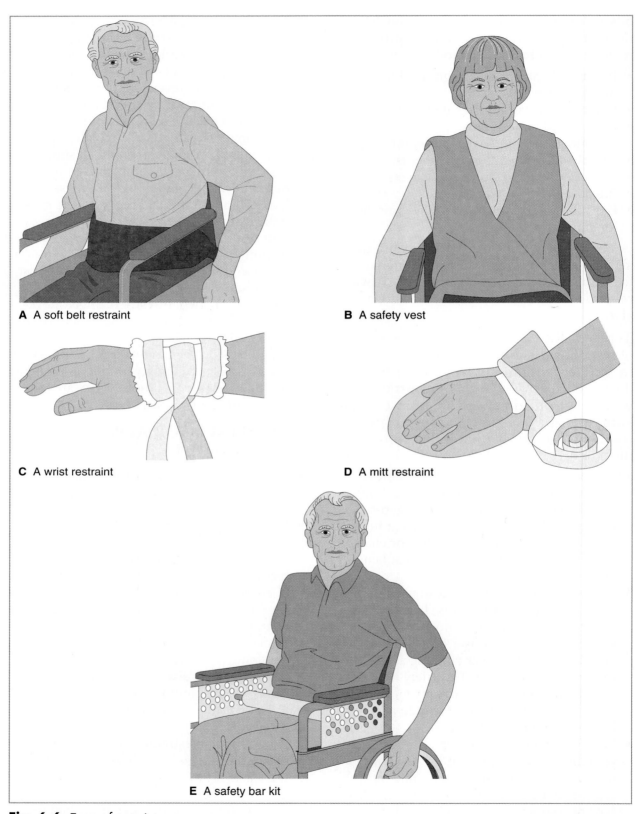

A A soft belt restraint

B A safety vest

C A wrist restraint

D A mitt restraint

E A safety bar kit

Fig. 6-6 Types of restraints.

- Do not restrain a resident to the toilet or a bedside commode.
- Allow as much movement as possible.
- Pad bony areas.
- Protect the resident's rights.

GUIDELINES TO FOLLOW AFTER RESTRAINTS HAVE BEEN APPLIED

- When a resident is restrained, you will be responsible for meeting basic needs.
- Visually check the resident's safety every 30 minutes.
- Remove the restraint every two hours, provide exercise and skin care, and reposition. Offer toileting and fluids at this time.
- Observe for complications such as skin irritation, injury, circulatory impairment, or increased anxiety.
- Observe for comfort and alignment.
- Reassure frequently.
- Check wrist restraints every 15 minutes.
- Keep the signal light within reach.
- Make sure the restraint is clean and undamaged.
- Document the type of restraint and the time of application.

Fire Safety

Fire safety focuses on the prevention of fires. It also includes information on how fires start and the correct response to a fire. Health care facilities are built with safety features to prevent fires and to reduce the need for evacuation. These safety features include fire exits, closed stairwells, smoke detectors, sprinkler systems, and automatic fire door closers.

Elements of a Fire. The three elements needed for a fire are fuel, oxygen, and a spark. Draperies, linens, clothing, wood, or any material that will burn provide fuel. Since there is fuel almost everywhere, and oxygen is found naturally in the air, all that is needed for a fire is a spark.

Causes of Fires. Careless smoking causes more fires than any other factor. Fire is often the result of improper disposal of matches or cigarette butts. Sometimes a smoldering cigarette is left on a surface and forgotten by the smoker. Many health care facilities do not allow smoking in the building. Not only does this reduce pollution from tobacco smoke, it also lessens the chance of a fire.

Defective electrical equipment can cause fires. Frayed wires, overloaded circuits, and ungrounded plugs are dangerous. Electrical appliances that are used improperly, or are in need of repair, are another hazard.

Other factors that contribute to fires include improper trash disposal, cooking materials, flammable liquids, and oxygen equipment.

Sometimes the resident will need more oxygen than is present in the air. This oxygen is usually provided by tank, wall outlet, or a concentrator. Because oxygen will explode and burn, special rules apply when it is used.

GUIDELINES FOR FIRE SAFETY WHEN OXYGEN IS BEING USED

- Place "No Smoking" signs outside the door and over the bed.
- Remove radios, televisions, and electric razors from the area.
- Use cotton blankets, not wool or synthetic fabrics.
- Remove smoking materials from the room.
- Remind residents and visitors not to smoke in the room.

Fire Prevention. The prevention of fire is the responsibility of everyone. Rules of fire prevention include

- Obey "No Smoking" signs.
- Smoke only in designated areas.
- Extinguish smoking materials carefully.
- Dispose of waste material correctly.
- Store flammable liquids properly.
- Check electrical equipment and report any hazards.
- Observe all the rules for oxygen safety.

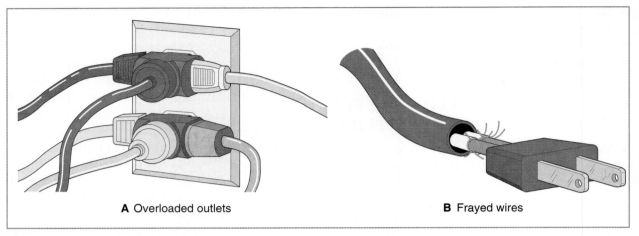

A Overloaded outlets   **B** Frayed wires

Fig. 6-7 Report defective electrical equipment immediately.

Fire Emergency Rules. If a fire occurs, it is important that you stay calm and do not panic, run, or scream. Reassure residents and visitors. The first step in the event of fire is to remove residents who are in immediate danger. The fire should be contained by closing doors. Halls are cleared of people and equipment to allow easy access by the fire department. Each facility has a policy and procedure for fire, and it is your responsibility to know the correct procedure to follow. One system that is used in many public buildings is the RACE system (see Fig. 6-8)

A smoldering fire is very dangerous. In a fire, more people die from smoke inhalation than from the fire itself. Smoke can kill even if there is no flame. If you are in a room that is smoke filled, drop to your knees on the floor, cover your mouth and nose, and crawl to an exit. There is less smoke just above floor level, because smoke rises.

Fire Extinguishers. There are several kinds of fire extinguishers. Your facility will provide inservice classes to show you which type to use in any situation. These classes are often taught by the local fire department. When you are using a fire extinguisher, you should point the nozzle toward the base of the fire.

Fire Drills. Your facility will have regular fire drills in which everyone participates. It is your responsibility to know the fire emergency plan for your facility. You must be able to respond quickly and correctly.

Disaster Planning

A disaster is an event that may cause injury or death to a large number of people. It may also cause great property damage. Some examples of disasters include explosions, bomb threats, fires, transportation accidents, earthquakes, floods, hurricanes, tornadoes, or other severe weather conditions.

Every health care facility must have a disaster plan that describes the role of all employees. The plan includes policies and procedures for the protection of the residents and the staff. There are also procedures for handling large numbers of people and providing medical care for the wounded.

In a long-term care facility, an interruption in water or electrical supply is addressed in the disaster plan. A failure in the facility's heating or cooling system may also be included.

Disaster safety drills are held on a regular basis in a health care facility. They may be combined with a community disaster drill. In this way, the authorities can evaluate the ability of the entire community to deal with an emergency.

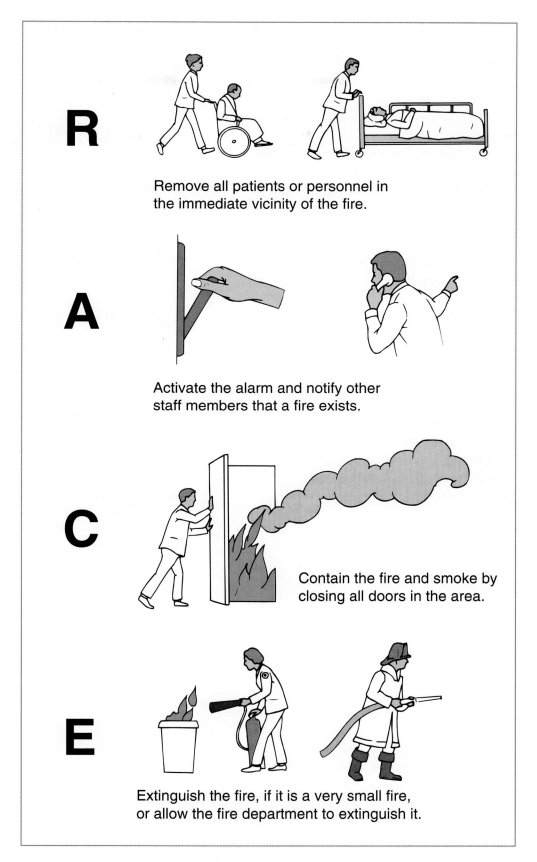

R Remove all patients or personnel in the immediate vicinity of the fire.

A Activate the alarm and notify other staff members that a fire exists.

C Contain the fire and smoke by closing all doors in the area.

E Extinguish the fire, if it is a very small fire, or allow the fire department to extinguish it.

Fig. 6-8
The RACE system.

Conclusion

Remember these important points:

1. Elderly people and children have the most accidents.

2. Any decrease in awareness creates a safety hazard.

3. The most common accident in a long-term health care facility is a fall.

4. Staff carelessness or negligence can result in an accident.

5. The safest way to identify the resident is by checking the identification bracelet.

6. Always use correct body mechanics.

7. OSHA regulations help protect the safety of workers.

8. An incident report protects you, the resident, visitors, and the facility.

9. A restraint may be used only to protect the resident.

10. Try restorative techniques before using a restraint.

11. When a resident is restrained, you are responsible for all basic needs.

12. Restraints must be removed every two hours.

13. Fire prevention is everybody's responsibility.

14. In case of fire, remove the residents who are in immediate danger first.

15. A disaster plan describes the role of the employees in an emergency.

Discussion Questions

1. *Why do elderly people have more accidents?*

2. *What might happen if you fail to write an incident report?*

3. *How would you feel if you were restrained?*

4. *Have you ever taken part in a disaster drill? If so, what observations did you make?*

Application Exercise

1. Members of the class will place their chairs in a circle. They will select a leader whose chair will be placed in the center of the circle. All the students, except the leader, will restrain one another to a chair. They will remain in restraints for 15 minutes. During this time, the leader will record their reactions to being restrained. The leader will share the list with the class, and they will discuss what they have learned from the experience.

First Aid and Emergency Care

OBJECTIVES

Upon completing this chapter, you will be able to do the following:

1. Identify eight general rules to be followed in emergencies.

2. List four life-threatening conditions.

3. Explain how to recognize and prevent shock.

4. Describe the emergency care for airway obstructions, hemorrhage, and seizures.

5. Demonstrate the procedures for the Heimlich maneuver and one-rescuer CPR.

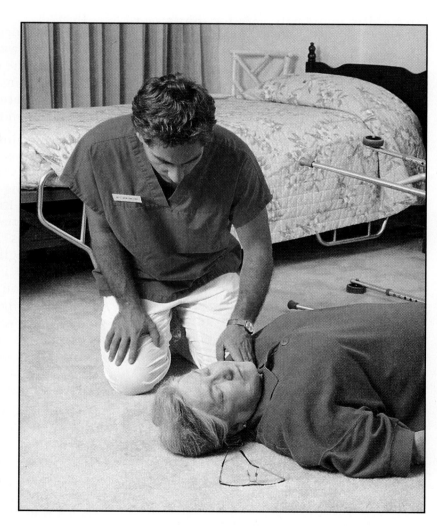

VOCABULARY

The following words or terms will help you to understand this chapter:

First aid	Cardiac arrest	Aspirate
Pulse	Respiratory arrest	Heimlich maneuver
Respirations	Hemorrhage	Cyanosis
Trauma	Cardiopulmonary	Sternum
Assess	resuscitation (CPR)	Seizure

Introduction to First Aid

First aid is immediate care for injuries or sudden illness that is given to prevent further injuries and save lives. Although you may be the first to discover a life-threatening emergency in the facility, it is your responsibility to notify the nurse. When a nurse is present you will provide emergency care as directed.

You will best be prepared for handling emergencies if you complete a course of first aid, which is offered by the American Red Cross. You may also prepare yourself for cardiac and respiratory emergencies by taking a CPR course that is offered by the American Heart Association or the American Red Cross. This chapter will discuss emergency care for situations that might occur in a long-term care facility.

You should also be familiar with the facility's disaster plan. Follow the general rules for emergencies. These rules will be helpful, although you may not know specific care to be given in each type of emergency. Don't forget to complete an incident report. Incident reports are discussed in Chapter 6.

General Rules for Emergencies

Some general rules that must be followed in every emergency situation follow:

- Stay calm and reassure the resident.
- Know your limitations.
- Do not move the injured resident.
- Be sure the environment is safe.

- Observe for life-threatening conditions.
- Call for help. Stay with the resident, if possible.
- Prevent shock by keeping the resident lying down and warm.
- Reassure the resident frequently.
- Monitor consciousness, **pulse** (heartbeat), and **respirations** (breathing).
- Keep bystanders away.

Staying calm helps you to function well. The victim may develop shock as a result of **trauma** (physical or emotional injury or upset). Staying calm will help reduce the victim's anxiety. Knowing what you cannot do is just as important as knowing what you can do for victims. This prevents further injury.

Before beginning first aid, be sure the environment is safe. Look for hazards that may harm you or the victim. Avoid moving the resident because movement may cause additional injuries. Movement can be especially dangerous if head, neck, or spinal injuries are present. Remember that if you are in the facility, you must call for the nurse and work under his or her direction.

Observing for Life-Threatening Conditions. Life-threatening emergencies must be treated first. When injury or sudden illness has occurred, you must first **assess** (check or evaluate) the resident's condition to determine if it is life threatening. Some situations that threaten life are **cardiac arrest** (the absence of heartbeats), **respiratory arrest** (absence of breathing), drowning, smoke inhalation, electric shock, **hemorrhage** (severe bleeding), and stroke.

The heart, lungs, and brain are all dependent upon each other for survival. If any one fails, they all fail. Every cell of the body, including the cells of the heart, must have a constant flow of oxygenated blood to continue functioning. If breathing or heart action stops, the oxygenated blood will not be available to cells. If cells are deprived of oxygen for four to six minutes they begin to die. Death of brain and heart cells could make recovery impossible.

You must determine if life is threatened by checking for responsiveness, breathing, and pulse. If these are absent, immediate steps must be taken. The procedure for emergency care to restore heart and lung function is called **cardiopulmonary resuscitation (CPR)**. CPR is described later in this chapter.

Calling for Help (Activating the EMS System). When beginning care for life-threatening conditions, the Emergency Medical Services (EMS) must be called. The nurse will either call EMS or designate someone else to do so. Information to be given should include location (with the name of the nearest cross street), the nature of the injuries, number of victims, and emergency care that is being given. Always wait to hang up after the operator disconnects. To notify EMS, you must dial 911 or call the operator, fire department, or police.

Recognizing and Preventing Shock. In any emergency situation, shock may result from a drop in blood pressure. This may happen because of loss of blood or physical injury. Shock may also occur as a result of extreme emotional upset. If the blood pressure drops too low, the vital organs will not receive oxygenated blood and death will result.

Attempt to prevent shock in all emergency situations. The signs and symptoms of shock include

- Rapid pulse and respirations
- A blue color of the skin, especially at the lips and nails
- Cool, damp skin
- Perspiration
- Thirst
- Dilated pupils
- Nausea and vomiting

Keeping the victim calm and reassured helps to prevent shock. It is also important to keep the victim lying flat and warm (see Fig. 7-1A). The feet may be elevated if there is no evidence of leg injury, head injury, or breathing difficulties. If there is vomiting or bleeding at the mouth, you must prevent *aspiration* (choking or inhalation of food or fluid) by positioning the resident on the side (see Fig. 7-1B). If the resident is hemorrhaging, the bleeding must be stopped.

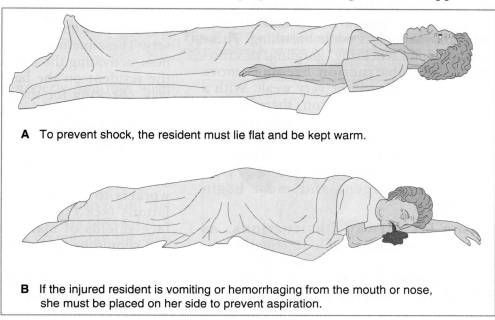

A To prevent shock, the resident must lie flat and be kept warm.

B If the injured resident is vomiting or hemorrhaging from the mouth or nose, she must be placed on her side to prevent aspiration.

Fig. 7-1
Positioning the shock victim.

- Lean toward the victim's head to give ventilations. Do not move your knees back and forth between ventilations and compressions (see Fig. 7-9).
- Continue cycles of 15 compressions and 2 ventilations for four cycles or one full minute. Check for recovery of the pulse. If the pulse is present, resume rescue breathing and continue to monitor pulse. If the pulse is not present, resume CPR.

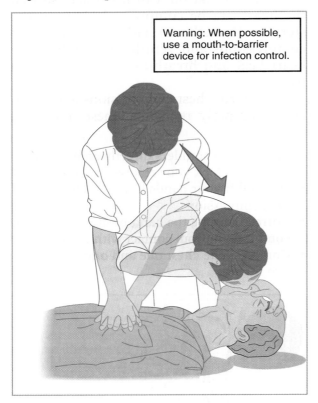

Warning: When possible, use a mouth-to-barrier device for infection control.

Fig. 7-9 Lean toward the victim's head to give ventilations. Do not move your knees between ventilations and compressions.

Emergency Care for Hemorrhage

If the victim is hemorrhaging, direct pressure must be placed upon the wound until bleeding stops (see Fig. 7-10). Follow universal precautions regarding contact with blood. Pressure is applied by holding a sterile pad over the injury. If a sterile pad is not available, a clean dressing or piece of cloth may be used. If the dressing becomes saturated, add additional pads as needed. Do not

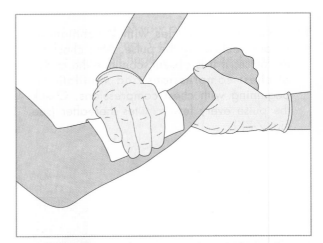

Fig. 7-10 Direct pressure is used to stop hemorrhage.

remove the original dressing. Maintain pressure over the wound while adding the pads. While maintaining direct pressure over the wound, pressure may also be applied with the fingers to the pressure points of the artery supplying blood to the area of the injury. Some pressure points are shown in Fig. 7-11.

Emergency Care for Seizures

A **seizure** (convulsion) is a sudden spasm of muscles that is caused by abnormal brain activity. Tremors may also occur. The intensity, length, and extent of the seizure may vary. Loss of consciousness occurs.

The most important first aid given for seizures is the prevention of injuries. Call for a nurse. Clothing should be loosened. The resident who is in bed must be kept from falling. A resident who is standing or sitting should be lowered to the floor. The resident must be protected from striking objects that might cause injury during the seizure. Never attempt to hold down or restrain the resident. Stay with the resident and notice how long the seizure lasts.

Learning first aid procedures will help you to protect your family and friends, as well as the residents in your care. If an injury or sudden illness occurs while you are at work, you should stay with the resident and call the nurse who will direct further care.

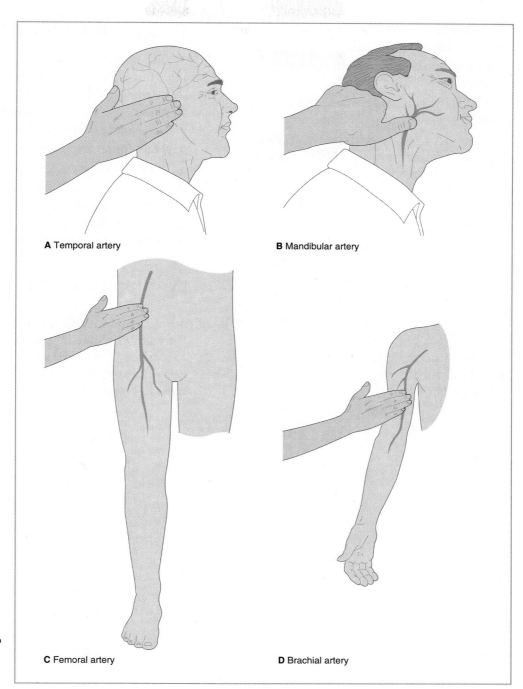

A Temporal artery

B Mandibular artery

C Femoral artery

D Brachial artery

Fig. 7-11
Pressure points may be used, in addition to the use of direct pressure, to stop hemorrhage.

Conclusion

Remember these important points:

1. First aid is the immediate care that is given for injury or sudden illness.

2. The American Red Cross and the American Heart Association offer courses to prepare for emergencies.

3. Staying calm helps you to function well.

4. Avoid moving the resident.

5. Life-threatening emergencies must be treated first.

6. Dial 911 or call the fire or police departments for help.

7. Keeping the victim flat and warm helps to prevent shock.

8. Severe respiratory distress is a life-threatening condition.

9. Grabbing the throat with the hands is the universal signal for choking.

10. The Heimlich maneuver is the first aid for a complete airway obstruction.

11. The unconscious victim with an airway obstruction must have the airway opened and be checked for respirations before abdominal thrusts are given.

12. Rescue breathing is given for a victim who is not breathing but has a pulse.

13. CPR replaces lung and heart function when respiratory and cardiac arrest have occurred.

14. Pressure is used to stop hemorrhage.

15. The first aid for seizures is the prevention of injuries.

16. If an injury or sudden illness occur you should call for the nurse and follow instructions.

Discussion Questions

1. Discuss situations that could be life-threatening. How would you determine if there is a life-threatening condition?

2. When should EMS be called and what information should be given?

3. What causes shock and why is it dangerous?

4. What are some causes of airway obstruction?

5. How do you decide when it is necessary to use the Heimlich maneuver?

6. How does the rescuer know that chest compressions are necessary for the unconscious person?

Application Exercise

1. Each student will watch a television program or movie in which emergency scenes take place. The student will observe for correctness of first aid care that is provided. The class as a group will discuss their observations.

Communicating in the Long-Term Care Facility

OBJECTIVES

Upon completing this chapter, you will be able to do the following:

1. Explain the importance of communication in the long-term care facility.

2. List three effects of communication as a restorative measure.

3. Give two examples each of verbal and nonverbal communication.

4. Demonstrate listening skills.

5. List six barriers to communication.

6. List four guidelines each for communicating with vision-, hearing-, and speech-impaired residents.

7. Describe the nursing assistant's role in communicating with the resident's family and friends.

8. List four observations that should be made of the elderly resident.

9. Explain the nursing assistant's role in reporting resident information.

10. Identify four guidelines that are to be followed when recording information about the resident.

11. Explain the purpose and use of the resident's care plan.

12. List five guidelines for answering the telephone in the long-term care facility.

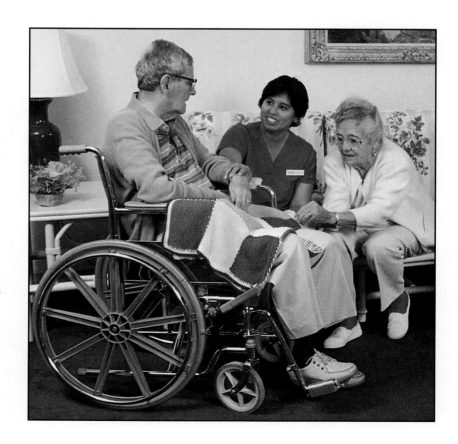

VOCABULARY

The following words or terms will help you to understand this chapter:

Communication
Verbal communication
Nonverbal communication
Listening
Communication barriers
Communication impairments
Aphasia

Report
Observation
Symptom
Objective reporting
Recording
Charting
Care plan

The Importance of Communication

Communication is the sharing of information (a message). The person who is receiving the information must understand what the speaker (or sender) means (see Fig. 8-1). Communication is a lifelong process involving a message, a sender, and a receiver. The newborn baby enters this world communicating with a cry and a dying person continues to hear until death occurs.

In the health care facility, communication flows through the doctors, the staff members, the residents, and the residents' family members. Staff members must communicate to provide resident care that is efficient and helpful. For example, if a resident is having chest pain, failure to communicate could be life threatening.

Communication assures that the residents receive the care that is needed. The dietary department must know about diet changes, and the laundry must know when the nursing unit is in need of additional linen. When

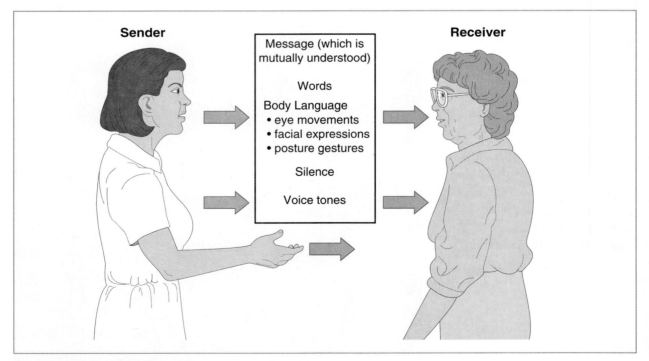

Fig. 8-1 The communication process.

an employee is too ill to come to work, the supervisor is notified so that arrangements can be made for another employee to work. If the doctor has ordered "Nothing by mouth after midnight," the staff must have this information. Failure to communicate any of this information successfully could cause significant problems.

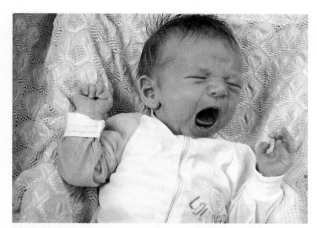
Fig. 8-2 Communication begins at birth and continues through death.

Communication as a Restorative Measure

Communication is an important part of providing restorative care for the residents of the long-term care facility. Everyone, even a person who likes being alone, needs contact with others. This is impossible without communication. Have you ever been in a room full of people and felt alone? Communication was the missing "bridge" between you and the crowd. Residents need this communication "bridge" to others. It is necessary for physical and emotional health. Some residents have no family or visitors and must depend upon the staff and volunteers for much of their communication.

You will find many opportunities to talk with the residents while you are providing care. Ask them questions about their interests, families, and histories. Because many are no longer able to function as totally independent individuals, their self-image, and sense of individuality may be threat-

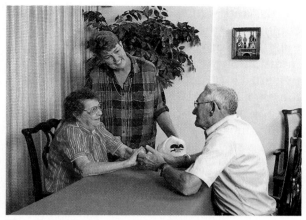
Fig. 8-3 Communication is a bridge.

ened. Talking about themselves, and topics that are important to them, helps residents to stay in touch with their identities and encourages self-esteem. Communication also helps the confused resident to stay in touch with reality. During your conversations with residents, it is helpful to frequently mention dates, time, places and the identity of individuals. It is also important to call the resident by name.

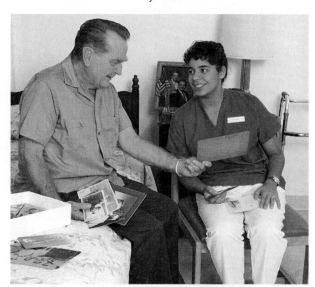
Fig. 8-4 Encourage the resident to talk about himself.

Forms of Communication

Verbal and Nonverbal Communication. **Verbal communication** is the use of words to share information. This form of communication includes spoken words, written words, and sign language. Another type of communication is called nonverbal communication. **Nonverbal communication** shares information without the use of words. These two forms of communication may be used together or separately.

Look at the following list of nonverbal communications and recall the last time you were given a message with one of them.

- Body language—includes facial expressions (smiles, frowns, and eye movements), posture, body position, hand gestures, and other body movements
- Touch (patting, hugging)
- Silence (can be pleasant or uncomfortable)
- Odor (body odor or perfume)
- Listening (shows you care)

Nonverbal communication often reflects a person's true feelings when verbal communication may not. Although loudness and tone of voice affect the verbal message, they are not verbal communication. For example, a pleasant or angry tone of voice adds information. Voice tone may change the message being spoken. Does it always sound like a person is having a good morning when he says, "Good morning?"

The nonverbal message may disagree with the words that are spoken. People often think about their verbal communication. Nonverbal communication is usually not planned, and it is more difficult to control. For better understanding, it is important to be aware of nonverbal communication. Your words, body language, and voice tones

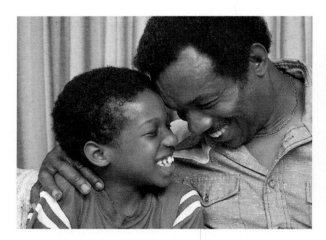

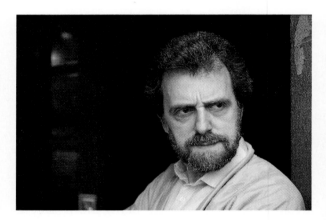

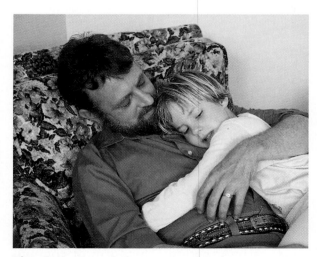

Fig. 8-5 Nonverbal communication relates a message without the use of words.

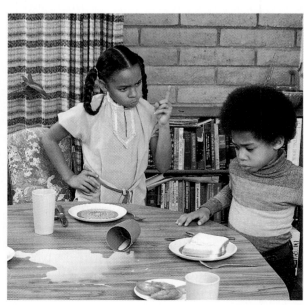

should agree so that you don't send confusing messages.

Listening. One form of nonverbal communication is listening. **Listening** is giving your attention to what you are hearing, while you think about its meaning. The quality of care that is given can be affected by your ability to listen. The health and safety of the resident depend upon your ability to understand orders and directions.

It is important to listen to pleasant conversation as well as to the resident's verbal complaints. It reassures the resident to know that you care enough to take the time to listen. Your listening helps maintain the resident's sense of worth and self-image.

You can become a good listener by developing the following skills:

- Keep eye contact with the speaker.
- Stop other activities while you are listening.
- Ask questions occasionally.
- Be sincere; don't just pretend to listen.

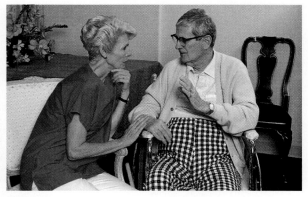

Fig. 8-6 Listening is giving attention to what you are hearing.

Have you ever recognized that someone was not truly listening, although he or she appeared to be doing so? If you have ever been ignored, think about the feelings and thoughts that you experienced afterward.

Communication Barriers

The quality of relationships between people depends upon the quality of the communi-

cation between them. Communication does not occur if the message is misunderstood, or if it is not received. Problems that interfere with communication are called **communication barriers**.

There are many barriers to communication, some of which are listed here:

- Different language levels (using medical terms with the public)
- Words with more than one meaning (sick, crazy)
- Different languages (Spanish, English, German, etc.)
- Speaking too fast
- Failure to listen
- Feelings (anger, defensiveness, embarrassment)
- Daydreaming
- Distractions (bright light, noise, odors)
- Being unable to ask questions
- Illness
- Loss of hearing, vision, or speech

Communicating with the resident who speaks a different language requires special skills. Using and observing body language and hand gestures often are the primary methods. Being able to point to or draw pictures is sometimes helpful. Listen carefully for poorly pronounced words. It is important to consider cultural differences. Because of these differences, the resident's reactions may be misunderstood. The best communication plan would include the help of a person who speaks the resident's native language.

Many barriers can be avoided if you will learn to communicate clearly and skillfully. Both the speaker and receiver should make sure the message is understood. One way to do this is to ask questions or to repeat what has been said. The sender may correct any misunderstanding. Be aware of signs of misunderstanding, such as frowns or doubtful expressions.

Communication Impairments

A resident may have a **communication impairment**. This means that the resident

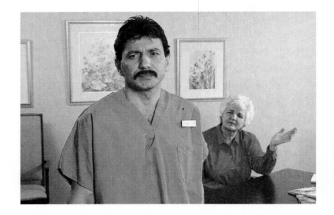
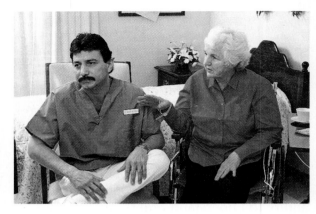
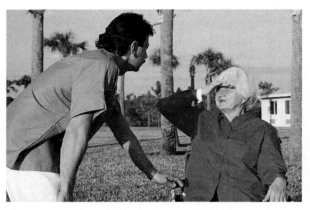
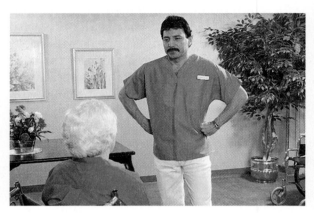

Fig. 8-7 Can you identify the barriers to communication in each photograph?

has difficulty communicating because of one or more disabilities. These impairments or disabilities may include problems with vision, hearing, speech, sense of touch, or movement. All these are important to successful communication.

The Blind or Vision-Impaired Resident. A person with a vision impairment may not be totally blind. Those who have vision impairments are more dependent upon the use of their other senses to maintain contact with their world. Touch and hearing are very important communication methods for the blind or sight-impaired resident.

GUIDELINES FOR COMMUNICATING WITH THE VISION-IMPAIRED RESIDENT

- Speak to announce your presence.
- Gently touch the resident after you have verbally announced your presence.
- Allow the resident to touch and handle unfamiliar objects.

- Encourage the resident to express feelings.
- Provide a predictable schedule to help the resident feel a sense of security and control.
- Provide good lighting and avoid glare.
- Face the person you are talking to.
- Explain everything that you are going to do.
- Be sure the resident's eyeglasses are clean.
- Describe surroundings, when appropriate to do so.
- Describe the location of personal items.
- Describe the location of food at mealtime.
- Describe the new location of furniture, if it must be moved.
- Allow the resident to take your arm while walking.
- Provide large-print reading material and a magnifying glass for reading.
- Provide tapes and talking books.
- Do not leave the resident in the room alone for long periods of time.
- Stimulate the senses by encouraging the resident to smell and touch objects.

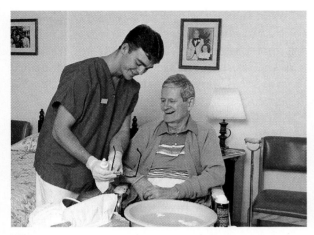

Fig. 8-8 Be sure the resident wears clean eyeglasses.

The Deaf or Hearing-Impaired Resident.

The hearing-impaired resident is also more dependent upon the other senses for communication. It is very important to emphasize the use of sight and touch in communicating with this resident.

GUIDELINES FOR COMMUNICATING WITH THE HEARING-IMPAIRED RESIDENT

- Approach the hearing-impaired resident so that you can be seen.
- Touch the resident gently after you are seen.
- Speak into the better ear, if possible.
- Writing notes is helpful.
- Provide good lighting and avoid glare.
- Be sure the resident wears a hearing aid, if required. Check the batteries.
- Face the resident to whom you are speaking. Because the resident may depend on lip reading, provide the opportunity to see your face and lips clearly.
- Do not exaggerate lip movements.
- Provide a predictable schedule to help the resident feel a sense of control and security.
- Carefully explain everything, one step at a time.
- Speak slowly and clearly. Do not shout.
- Do not leave the resident alone for long periods of time.
- Stimulate the senses of vision, touch, and smell.
- Use written messages, if necessary.

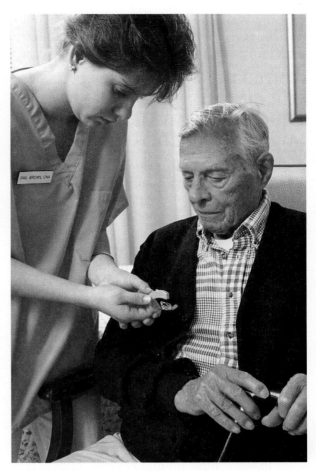

Fig. 8-9 Be sure the resident's hearing aid is working properly.

The Aphasic or Speech-Impaired Resident.

Aphasia is the loss of ability to express oneself through the use of speech, writing, and/or gestures. The most common cause of aphasia is brain damage. Some chronic diseases can also cause aphasia. This impairment can take many forms.

- The aphasic resident may not be able to understand what is said.
- Aphasia may allow the resident to understand what is said, while interfering with the ability to communicate accurately.
- The aphasic resident may speak with a normal rhythm, but without the use of meaningful words.
- Aphasia may involve the loss of control of the muscles needed for speech.
- Aphasia may leave the muscle control intact, but the memory of how to form words is lost.

Some residents are not confused but may not be able to speak clearly and correctly. Others may be confused.

GUIDELINES FOR COMMUNICATING WITH THE SPEECH-IMPAIRED (APHASIC) RESIDENT

- Remember that the resident hears and responds emotionally, although speech is not possible.
- Treat the resident as an adult.
- Speak in a normal voice.
- Don't speak or fill in words for the aphasic resident. Help only if the resident is overly tense or under pressure.
- Allow time for response (at least 10–30 seconds).
- Do not correct or criticize. Repeat what is said so that the resident may hear errors.
- Don't talk about aphasic residents as if they were not there.
- Maintain a relaxed atmosphere.
- Ask questions that can be answered with simple words.
- Use key words. If you want the resident to go to the dining room, say "eat."
- Encourage drawing or writing if the resident is able.

- Stand where the resident can see you when you are talking.
- Don't assume that the resident understands.
- If the resident has difficulty understanding you, speak slowly in short, simple sentences.
- Continue to regard the resident as a communicating person.
- Be sensitive to the resident's emotions.

Be patient with anyone who has a communication impairment and develop empathy. Think about how you might feel if you could not see, hear, or speak! The world would be a lonely place if you lost your ability to communicate.

Communicating with the Resident's Family and Friends

You will be an important link between the facility and the resident's visitors. You may be the staff member that the resident's family and friends see first, or most often. Their opinion of the facility will often be affected by their impression of you. They will be reassured if they believe that you care about the residents, and if you are helpful to them

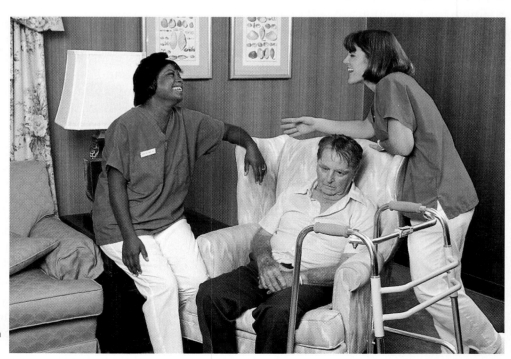

Fig. 8-10
Include the resident in your conversation when he is present.

in regard to their concerns and needs. Often family members experience anxiety about the resident and his care. If they trust you, their nervousness will be relieved.

A visitor needs to be listened to when angry or upset. Knowing that someone cares enough to listen to a problem is often the key to solving it and calming the anger or concern. Do not become defensive. Remind yourself that listening is the key to helping another person deal with problems. Mentally separate yourself from blame, while you attentively listen to what is being said. Even if the problem is not related to you, listen carefully. Show concern and take the visitor to the nurse, who will continue to assist. Think of how you would feel if you were very upset about something and the person that you turned to seemed unconcerned. You would probably become more upset.

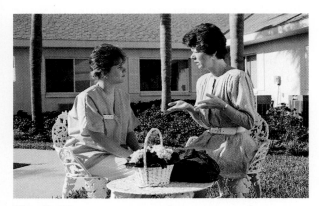

Fig. 8-11 It is important to be concerned when someone is upset.

No matter who you are communicating with, be pleasant, polite, and considerate. Be aware of your body language. A successful relationship depends upon the quality of communication that takes place within it. Communication skills can be learned and are worth every effort to do so.

Observation, Reporting, and Recording

Observation, reporting, and recording are methods of communication that are used by the health care team. Every shift begins with a report. A **report** is the communication of resident information and assignments to those who are coming on duty. Each resident is discussed briefly. The nurse may give this information to the nursing assistants after receiving a report from the nurse that is going off duty. The nurse may include the information on each assignment sheet. The report may be given orally, in writing, or by tape recording. Sometimes resident information is communicated at a nursing report that takes place with all nursing team members present.

The nursing assistant must receive information about the residents that includes the care that is to be provided and changes that have taken place. Remember that you are responsible for providing the correct care for your residents. If you have any questions or doubts about your assignment, you must ask for additional information and make sure you clearly understand. Be familiar with the resident's care plan.

Observation. **Observation** means using the senses of sight, smell, hearing, and touch to gather information. The nursing assistant's observation will be very important to the safety and well-being of the resident. The person who notices early changes in the resident's condition is often the nursing assistant. Some problems become worse very quickly, and early detection may prevent them from becoming life threatening.

Using all your senses to recognize change is a skill. As you learn about the elderly resident, the changes that take place with aging, and what is normal for the resident, you will have a better understanding of which observations are important. Figure 8-12 lists some general observations that should be made. Sometimes the changes that occur in the resident's body, behavior, or mood may be very slight and difficult to observe.

Bath time is an excellent time to communicate, and to perform a thorough observation. Not only is it a time to observe the entire skin and body, but it is usually the longest period of time that is spent with the resident. This extra time allows you to use your listening skills to hear complaints and

MAKING OBSERVATIONS USING THE SENSES

VISUAL OBSERVATIONS are made by the use of sight. These include:

Resident Activities such as: eating, drinking, walking, dressing, socializing, and toileting
Body Posture and Movement
The Shape and Form of Body Parts
Skin: color, perspiration, injuries, and swelling
Breathing: depth and difficulty
Bowel Movement: consistency, color, amount, frequency, and control
Urine: consistency, color, amount, frequency, and control
Vomitus: consistency, color, amount, and frequency
Drainage: color, consistency, and amount
Bleeding
Facial Expressions
Unusual Actions
Safety Hazards

AUDITORY OBSERVATIONS are made by the use of hearing. These include:

Body Sounds such as: breathing sounds, coughing, cracking, and popping of joints or bones, and bowel sounds
Verbal Complaints
Speech Problems
Confused Speech

TACTILE OBSERVATIONS are made by the use of touch. These include:

Skin: temperature and texture
Pulses
Response to Touch

OLFACTORY OBSERVATIONS are made by smelling. These include:

Odors of: drainage, vomitus, urine, bowel movement, mouth and breath, and poor hygiene
Any Unusual Odor

Fig. 8-12 Using the senses to make general observations of the resident.

comments. Asking questions may also give you information about how the resident is thinking and feeling. The resident may be experiencing something that cannot be seen or observed by others. An evidence of disease that cannot be observed is called a **symptom**. Headaches, nausea, and pain are symptoms.

As you gain experience, your observation skills will improve. In addition to observa-

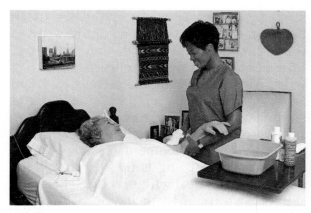

Fig. 8-13 Communicating during the bath provides an excellent opportunity to observe thoroughly.

tions about the resident's condition, you must also be observant of safety hazards in the long-term care facility.

Reporting. Reporting is communicating information to another person. You must always report your observations to your charge nurse. Changes in the resident must be reported immediately so that measures can be taken to prevent a more serious problem. The nurse may have to call the doctor or take some other action.

It is important that you report facts without influencing them with your own ideas and judgment. This reporting of specific factual information is called **objective reporting**. If your statements are not strictly facts, if they are vague or are influenced by your own opinions, they may not be correct. Some examples of objective reporting are as follows:

Vague Reporting	Objective Reporting
The injury is small.	The injury is the size of a dime.
Mr. Smith is combative.	Mr. Smith shoved Mr. Jay.
Mrs. Jones is crying with pain.	Mrs. Jones is crying and says her chest has been hurting for 10 minutes.
Mr. Dye has been in the bathroom for a long time.	Mr. Dye has been in the bathroom for 30 minutes.
Ms. Seth ate well.	Ms. Seth ate all of her lunch except the bread.

Be objective as you report information. Organize your thoughts, use familiar words, be brief, and report only the facts. Do not use words that have more than one meaning, such as the word "sick." It would be better to say that the resident "complained of nausea and is vomiting" than to use the less specific term "sick." The resident may offer the most accurate description of symptoms being experienced. Use the same words as the resident when reporting complaints.

Sometimes you may not be able to be specific about the change that you have observed. You may just "sense" that something is wrong or different about your resident. It is important to report this to the nurse and continue to observe closely.

Nothing is too small or unimportant to report to the nurse. Have you heard the phrase, "An ounce of prevention is worth a pound of cure?" It would be better to report more than is necessary than to report too little, or too late. You have a responsibility to prevent problems by thorough observation and prompt reporting.

Recording. Writing information about the resident is called **recording**. The purpose of recording is to create a permanent communication of care given, and other resident information. This information can be reviewed to determine if the resident is improving, remaining stable or getting worse. Information to be recorded includes observations, treatments provided, and the resident's response to treatments. Activities, events, and checklists of items such as clothing are also recorded.

GUIDELINES TO FOLLOW WHEN RECORDING INFORMATION ABOUT THE RESIDENT

- Make entries throughout the shift, when care is provided.
- Entries must be in order of occurrence, and they must include the date and time.
- Never record on a page that does not contain information identifying the resident. The resident's name, room number, doctor's name, date of admission, and birthdate may be included.
- Be specific and use objective observations.
- Never omit information or leave blanks, empty spaces, or lines. Omissions in the record indicate failure to provide care.
- Never chart for another team member.
- Always include your signature and title as required by facility policy (for example, Maria Gonzalez, C.N.A.).
- Use correct grammar and spelling.
- Write with nonerasable ink, in the color that is required for your shift.
- Correct an error by drawing a single line through it, writing "error," and signing your name and title. Chart the correct entry, and sign it. Never erase, use correction fluid, or remove errors from sight (see Fig. 8-14).
- Learn and use symbols, abbreviations, and initials that are allowed by your facility.
- Maintain the confidentiality of resident information.
- If the resident or a visitor asks to see the chart, politely refer them to the nurse.

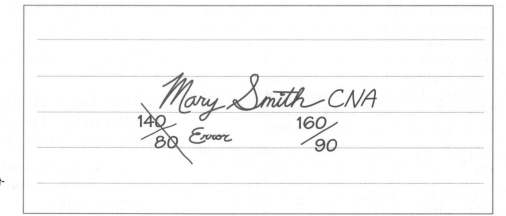

Fig. 8-14
Errors are corrected by drawing a single line through the error and writing the word "error" with your name and title.

Medical Records and Care Plans

Recording of information into the resident's medical record (chart) is called **charting**. This is a form of documentation that allows information to be communicated to other shifts. It preserves important information for future reading. The chart is a legal document and can be used in court. Not all facilities allow nursing assistants to read or record in the resident's chart. Check your facility's policy regarding the use of the medical record.

The doctor uses the chart to review the resident's progress, record observations, plan further treatment, and communicate new orders. The resident's plan of treatment and care depends upon the information that the nursing assistant and other health team members have recorded. Accuracy is very important.

Each section in the medical record has a specific purpose. Some of the forms that might be included are

- Admission sheet
- Nurses notes
- Doctors' notes and orders
- Resident history and physical examination
- Lab and X-ray reports
- Flow sheets
- Care plan
- Kardex

Flow Sheets. There may be a variety of titles and forms for flow sheets. These may also be called graphic sheets, ADL sheets, or daily records. A flow sheet is a brief way to record information about residents. See Fig. 8-15 for a sample of this form. Observations, measurements, care, treatments, and activities are usually recorded on the flow sheet. A flow sheet may be specifically for ADLs. Some facilities provide a separate form for recording specific restorative efforts or rehabilitation programs that are provided by the RNA (restorative nursing assistant).

Care Plan. The **care plan** is a plan of care for the resident. Problems, needs, or concerns of the resident and actions that will be taken by staff members are listed. All departments are involved in creating and following the plan. Meetings are held regularly with representatives from all departments for the sole purpose of reviewing, evaluating, and revising the plan of care for each resident.

Nursing assistants can be very helpful with suggestions for care planning. You may be asked to attend and participate in the care plan meeting. By reporting your observations to the charge nurse, you are contributing to care planning. You may be the source of information regarding new problems, needs, or concerns of the resident. These will be entered into the care plan.

The nursing assistant should read the resident's care plan to be familiar with it. Many of the actions to be taken are the responsibility of the nursing assistant. If your resident has achieved a goal, or is failing to meet one, it is important that this information be reported to the nurse. It will affect the care plan.

The Kardex. A card file consisting of the care plans of all residents is called a kardex. Sometimes a kardex is kept separate from, and in addition to, the care plans. It is used to summarize information, special needs and care to be given. The kardex can be used for quickly getting information about each resident.

Using the Telephone

Nursing assistants are not allowed to answer the telephone in many facilities. Check the policies of your facility regarding telephone use. If you are responsible for telephone communication in your facility, you become someone's link to the facility. The impression you make will help form an impression of the facility.

GUIDELINES TO FOLLOW WHEN ANSWERING THE TELEPHONE IN THE LONG-TERM CARE FACILITY

- Speak slowly and clearly.
- Always answer by stating your work area, name, and title.

ACTIVITIES OF DAILY LIVING CHECKLIST

Self — Done by resident
Assist — Resident assisted by nursing staff
Total — Done by nursing staff
✔ — Check procedure performed
Include time if appropriate

DATE															
DIET	B'fast	Dinner	Supper	B'fast	Dinner	Supper	B'fast	Dinner	Supper	B'fast	Dinner	Supper	B'fast	Dinner	Supper
Ate all food served															
Ate approx. 1/2 food served															
Refused to eat															
PROCEDURE	11-7	7-3	3-11	11-7	7-3	3-11	11-7	7-3	3-11	11-7	7-3	3-11	11-7	7-3	3-11
A.M. or H.S. Care															
Oral hygiene															
Bath-Bed bath complete															
Bed bath partial															
Shower															
Tub															
Self care															
Back care															
Bed made															
ELIMINATION															
Bowel movement															
Involuntary B.M.															
Voided															
Incontinent															
Foley catheter															
Sitz bath @															
ACTIVITY															
Bed rest complete															
Dangle															
Bed rest–B.R.P.															
Up in chair															
Up in room															
Walk in hall															
Ambulatory															
POSITION CHANGED															
Flat in bed															
Semi-Fowler's															
Deep breathe, cough															
Range of motion															
Turn from side to side															
Side rails–Up															
Down															
Fresh water @															
SIGNATURE & TITLE															

Fig. 8-15 A flow sheet provides a brief way to record information about the resident.

- Be polite and helpful.
- If you must transfer the caller to another extension, watch to be sure it is answered.
- Write messages and include
  - Date and time
  - Person being called
  - Message
  - Caller's name
  - Your name

Using Computers

Computers are being used as a method of communication in many health care facilities. A computer is used to store information that can be easily recovered. It is an efficient, fast, and accurate method of communication and recording. Mistakes are less likely to be made when information is computed.

There are many ways to use computers in the long-term care facility. Information can be exchanged between departments and facilities. Resident records, inventory of supplies, and billing information can be stored in the computer. The computer may print your assignment, if information about the residents has been entered. Body functions or vital signs may be measured by a computer. An alarm notifies the staff of changes. This improves the safety of the residents and makes it easier to provide quality care.

Using a computer may frustrate you, because you think you know nothing about it. You may already be using one without realizing it. When a bank card is used to obtain cash, a computer is used. Most late-model cars are equipped with computers. Paychecks are often printed by a computer, which has determined the amount you are to be paid. If you have the opportunity to learn to use a computer, it will add to your job qualifications.

Conclusion

Remember these important points:

1. Communication is the sharing of information and is an important part of providing quality care.

2. For communication to take place, there must be a sender, a receiver, and a message.

3. A restorative approach must be taken when communicating with the resident of the long-term care facility.

4. Encouraging the resident to talk about topics of interest, helps to maintain and/or restore a sense of self-worth.

5. A skillful communicator avoids using conflicting verbal and nonverbal messages.

6. Listening is giving your attention to what you are hearing, while thinking about its meaning.

7. Listening to the resident provides reassurance and helps to maintain a sense of worth and self-esteem.

8. Barriers that interfere with communication should be identified and avoided.

9. Communicating with the resident who has a communication impairment requires special techniques.

10. The nursing assistant has a responsibility to communicate with the resident's family and friends.

11. The quality of relationships depends upon the quality of the communication that takes place within them.

12. Communication with the health care team is done by observing, reporting, and recording.

13. Observation is using your senses to gather information.

14. Never erase, use correction fluid, or cover up an error on a chart.

15. A care plan is a plan of care that lists problems, needs, and concerns of the resident.

16. Nursing assistants can provide valuable assistance in care planning.

Discussion Questions

1. Discuss how poor communication could decrease the quality of resident care in the long-term care facility.

2. Identify some barriers to communication that you have experienced.

3. Make a list of questions that you might ask an elderly person. These questions should be

aimed at encouraging the elderly person's sense of identity and self-worth.

4. Discuss communication impairments and methods to be used with each impairment.

5. How would you respond if an angry family member began to complain to you about the care that her mother received during another shift?

Application Exercises

1. As a homework assignment, students will observe elderly individuals in a public place.

> a. Each student will record a list of observations of physical appearance and behavior.

> b. Each student will verbally report these observations to the class.

> c. The instructor will evaluate the students' observations, verbal reports and recording.

2. The instructor will provide a sample of an incomplete care plan for the class. Random areas of the care plan will be blank.

> a. The class will divide into groups.

> b. Each group will discuss the problems, concerns or needs, steps to be taken, and goals that are missing.

> c. When the groups have completed the activity, they will share their ideas with the class.

Using the Language of Medicine

OBJECTIVES

Upon completing this chapter, you will be able to do the following:

1. Define and give examples of a word root, a prefix, and a suffix.

2. Define medical terms by dividing them into their elements.

3. Identify abbreviations commonly used in the long-term care facility.

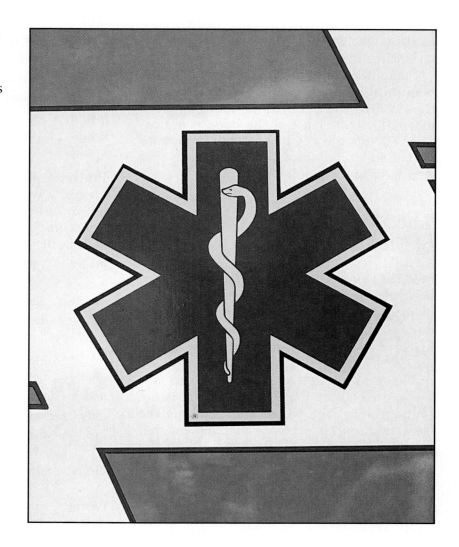

VOCABULARY

The following words or terms will help you to understand this chapter:

Glossary	Root	Prefix	Suffix	Abbreviation

Introduction to Medical Terminology

The medical field has a language of its own, one that the nursing assistant must be able to understand to perform safely. Medical terms may refer to body parts, measurements, orders, activities, treatments, diagnoses, time, or place. Some terms are general and can be used in any health care facility, while others are specific to long-term care.

There is a list of vocabulary words at the beginning of each chapter. Knowledge of those words will help you to understand the material. At the back of the book is a glossary. The **glossary** is like a small dictionary that includes definitions of many words that are found in this book.

The Word Elements of Medical Terms

Medical words are usually a combination of word elements or parts. There are thousands of medical terms, so you cannot expect to memorize all of them. However, you can learn to identify the elements that define words.

Three elements of medical terms are roots, prefixes, and suffixes. The **root** is the foundation of the word, and contains the basic meaning. A **prefix** is the element that is at the beginning of a word. A **suffix** is the element that is at the end of a word. Words can be formed by adding a prefix or a suffix to a root. For example, the root "cardi" means heart, and the suffix "ology" means study of, so the medical term "cardiology" means study of the heart. You will need to learn some commonly used roots, prefixes, and suffixes to understand medical terms.

Root. The root forms the basic meaning of a word. Word roots are the building blocks of medical terminology. A word root can be combined with a prefix, a suffix, or another root to form a medical term. Sometimes the letter "o" or "i" is added to the root to make the word easier to pronounce. Roots commonly used in the long-term care facility include

Root	Meaning	Root	Meaning
arthr(o)	joint	*neur(o)*	nerve
cardi(o)	heart	*oste(o)*	bone
col(o)	colon	*psych(o)*	mind
derma	skin	*pulmo*	lung
gastr(o)	stomach	*septic*	infection
glyc(o)	sugar	*thoraco*	chest
hema	blood	*trache(o)*	trachea
my(o)	muscle	*ven(o)*	vein

Prefix. A prefix is always found at the beginning of a word. A prefix cannot stand alone, but must be combined with another element to become a word. Some prefixes commonly used in the long-term care facility include

Prefix	Meaning	Prefix	Meaning
a, an	without, not	hyper	high, above normal
ab	away from	*hypo*	low, below normal
ad	toward	*micro*	small
ante	before	*non*	not
anti	against	*per*	by, through
auto	self	*poly*	many
bi	double, two	*post*	after, behind
brady	slow	*pre*	before, in front
circum	around	*retro*	backward
dys	difficult, abnormal	*semi*	half
epi	on, over	*sub*	under
hemi	half	*tachy*	fast, rapid

Suffix. A suffix is always placed at the end of a word. A suffix must be combined with another element to become a word. Suffixes commonly used in the long-term care facility include

Suffix	Meaning	Suffix	Meaning
algia	pain	*pathy*	disease
ectomy	surgical removal	*phasia*	speaking
emia	blood	*phobia*	fear
gram	record	*plegia*	paralysis
itis	inflammation of	*pnea*	to breathe
meter	measuring instrument	*scope*	examining instrument
ology	study of	*therapy*	treatment
ostomy	surgical opening	*uria*	condition of urine

Combining Word Parts. Medical terms can be formed by several different combinations of word parts. For example, a word might contain a prefix and a root, a root and a suffix, a prefix and a suffix, or two roots. The following list shows some common medical terms that have been divided into their elements.

WORD COMBINATIONS

Medical Term	Prefix	Root	Suffix
antiseptic	*anti*	*septic*	
arthritis		*arthr*	*itis*
colostomy		*colo*	*stomy*
dyspnea	*dys*	*pnea*	
hypoglycemia	*hypo*	*glyc*	*emia*
hemiplegia	*hemi*	*plegia*	

Abbreviations

An **abbreviation** is a shortened form of a word or phrase. It is developed by leaving out or substituting letters. The purpose of an abbreviation is to save time and space. Abbreviations are an important part of the health care system. Learning some commonly used abbreviations will help you to understand and communicate clearly. Some will be obvious to you, while others will have to be memorized. The following chart includes some suggestions that will help you to learn the meaning of abbreviations.

Clues to Help Understand Abbreviations

An abbreviation may

- Use the first letter of each word (VS = vital signs).
- Use the first and last letter of the word (ht = height).
- Use three or four letters of a word (amb = ambulate).
- Use a chemical symbol that includes a numeral (O_2 = oxygen; H_2O = water).

Remember that
The letter "q" usually means "every" (qd = every day).

or

it may indicate four (qid = four times a day).
The letter "h" usually means hour (qh = every hour).

It helps to
Associate ac with am (ac = *before* meals, am = *before* noon and pc with pm (pc = *after* meals, pm = *after* noon).
Think of bid, tid, and qid as 2 *in* a day, 3 *in* a day, and 4 *in* a day.

The following list contains only a few of the thousands of abbreviations that exist. All facilities do not use the same abbreviations. It is your responsibility to find out which ones are acceptable in your facility. Anytime you are not sure how to abbreviate a word or a phrase, you should write it out in full.

Abbreviation	Meaning
ac	before meals
ADLs	activities of daily living
ad lib	as desired
am	morning

Abbreviation	Meaning (cont.)
amb	ambulate
amt	amount
bid	twice a day
BM	bowel movement
BP	blood pressure
BR	bedrest/bathroom
BRP	bathroom privileges
BSC	bedside commode
$\bar{c}$	with
CA	cancer
cc	cubic centimeter
C.N.A.	certified nursing assistant
c/o	complains of
CPR	cardiopulmonary resuscitation
CVA	cerebrovascular accident/stroke
dc	discontinue/discharge
D.O.N.	director of nurses
GI	gastrointestinal
GU	genitourinary
H_2O	water
HOH	hard of hearing
hr, h	hour
HS	hour of sleep/bedtime
ht	height
I&O	intake and output
IV	intravenous
liq	liquid
L.P.N.	licensed practical nurse
L.V.N.	licensed vocational nurse
LTC	long-term care
meds	medications
ml	milliliter
NPO	nothing by mouth
O_2	oxygen
OOB	out of bed
OT	occupational therapy
oz	ounce
p	after
pc	after meals
pm	afternoon

Abbreviation	Meaning (cont.)
po	by mouth
prn	when necessary/as needed
pt	patient
PT	physical therapy
q	every
qam	every morning
qd	every day
qh	every hour
q2h, q3h, q4h, etc.	every 2 hours, every 3 hours, every 4 hours
qhs	every night at bedtime
qid	four times a day
qod	every other day
qs	quantity sufficient/enough
R.N.	registered nurse
ROM	range of motion
$\bar{s}$	without
S&A	sugar and acetone test
SOB	shortness of breath
stat	at once/immediately
tid	three times a day
TLC	tender loving care
TPR	temperature, pulse, and respirations
VS	vital signs
w/c	wheelchair
wt	weight

Conclusion

Remember these important points:

1. You must be able to understand medical terminology to perform safely.

2. Most medical terms are a combination of roots, prefixes, and suffixes.

3. Separating a word into its elements may help you understand its meaning.

4. An abbreviation is a shortened form of a word or a phrase.

5. It is your responsibility to know which abbreviations are acceptable in your facility.

6. If you are not sure of an abbreviation, you should write it out in full.

Discussion Questions

1. How can you use the information in this chapter to help you understand the care you will provide?

2. What could happen if you used terms or abbreviations that were not accepted at your facility?

3. Discuss methods, other than those listed in the text, that will help to identify abbreviations.

Application Exercise

1. The class will work as a group to develop flash cards of commonly used abbreviations. The cards will be placed in a central study area.

The Resident

OBJECTIVES

Upon completing this chapter, you will be able to do the following:

1. Define and give an example of three types of illnesses.

2. List three factors that affect aging.

3. Identify four common beliefs about aging that are not true.

4. Describe the geriatric resident.

5. Describe the developmentally disabled resident.

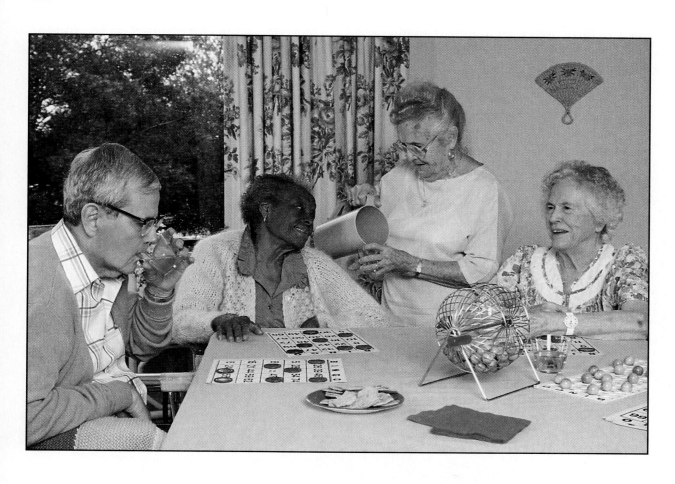

VOCABULARY

The following words or terms will help you to understand this chapter:

Developmentally
  disabled
Acute illness

Chronic illness
Complications
Terminal illness

Hospice
Environment
Pollution

Geriatric resident
Disoriented

It is difficult to identify "typical" residents of long-term care facilities because they represent assorted age groups and cultures. However, most of the residents are elderly. Their numbers include more women than men. The majority are physically or mentally impaired, and they suffer from a wide variety of illnesses. Heart disease, strokes, respiratory disorders, and diabetes are the most common. Many residents have mental or emotional problems.

Some of the residents are developmentally disabled. A **developmentally disabled** person is someone who has not developed normally, due to a birth defect, an injury, or an illness.

Many long-term care residents have difficulty performing activities of daily living (ADLs). A person with this problem needs help with bathing, dressing, toileting, and other daily needs. People often enter a long-term care facility because they can no longer care for themselves at home.

Types of Illnesses

Generally, illnesses are divided into three categories (acute, chronic, and terminal). These are classified according to onset, length, and expected outcome of the illness. Some health care facilities specialize in one type of illness.

An **acute illness** is an illness that begins suddenly and is short term. This type of illness is usually severe, but can often be successfully treated and cured. Hospitals treat these illnesses. In fact, we sometimes use the term "acute care facility" in referring to a hospital. Appendicitis is an example of an acute illness. The person with this condition may suddenly become very ill, be rushed to a hospital, have surgery, and return home, all within a period of a few days. The best response to an acute illness is to seek medical assistance immediately.

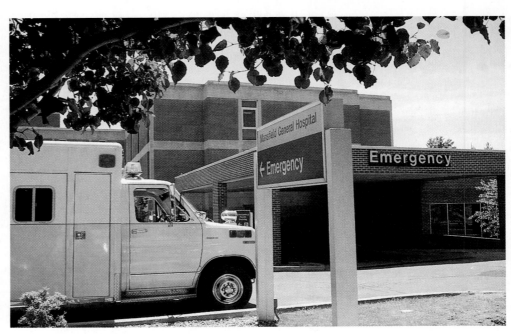

Fig. 10-1
An acute illness is often treated in a hospital.

A **chronic illness** is an illness that usually begins slowly and lasts for a long time. The person who has a chronic illness may not be sick continuously. Although most chronic illnesses are not curable, they can be controlled by treatment. In fact, correct treatment and care are necessary to prevent complications. **Complications** are additional problems that can occur as a result of a disease or other condition.

Diabetes is an example of a chronic illness. Many of the residents of long-term care facilities suffer from one or more chronic illnesses. The appropriate response to chronic illness is to seek treatment and prevent complications from occurring.

A **terminal illness** is an illness that is expected to end in death. There is very little hope of recovery. Many diseases become terminal when treatment is not successful. **Hospice** is a program that provides care for the terminally ill and their families. Although hospice specializes in the treatment of terminally ill patients, such patients are also cared for in other facilities. The key to caring for a person who has a terminal illness is to provide comfort for the resident and support to the family. Hospice is described in more detail in Chapter 25.

All three types of illness can be found in a long-term care facility. A chronic illness may get worse, until the person needs more care than is possible at home. Any resident might suffer an acute illness. The illness would be treated in the facility if possible, or the resident would be transferred to a hospital until the acute episode was brought under control. A resident's disease might become terminal, or the resident might be admitted with a terminal illness. Sometimes hospice patients are admitted to a long-term care facility.

The Process of Aging

Aging is not a sudden event that begins at a particular age. It begins at birth and continues until death. In the 1950s, Erik Erikson, a psychologist, proposed the theory that specific developmental tasks must be accomplished as an individual passes through certain stages of life. The accomplishment of these tasks allows a person to remain emotionally healthy.

The major developmental task of the elderly is to find meaning in life's experiences. This involves remembering, discussing, and perhaps writing about past events. This "life review" helps the individual let go of the past and adjust to the present. It raises self-esteem and gives life more quality. An experience of my own might help you understand this concept.

Each time I visited a certain long-term care facility to teach an inservice, one of the residents would come by to talk to me. First, she would tell me that she used to be a teacher, and then she would proceed to share her teaching experiences with me. Although I heard the same story over and over again, I never failed to delight at the change that would come over her. She would enter the classroom in a wheelchair, her shoulders slumped and her eyes downcast. After sharing her experiences with me, she would leave smiling, with straightened shoulders and sparkling eyes. Why? Because she had reaffirmed her self-worth. She was no longer "just a resident." She was a retired teacher. By reliving her past, she once again experienced her value as an individual. Life review is a valuable tool the elderly frequently use to help complete the developmental tasks of that age group.

All people do not age at the same rate. Some appear old in middle age, while others seem to age very slowly. You may know an elderly person who is healthy, happy, and mentally alert. Aging is greatly influenced by one's state of mind. The person who feels old will often look, feel, and act old. It would seem obvious, then, that the solution to aging would be to "think young." Unfortunately, life is not that simple.

Many factors, such as heredity, environment, lifestyle, physical health, and mental health affect aging. Heredity refers to all the characteristics that a person inherits from parents and other ancestors. One of those characteristics is life span or length of life. In some families, many members live to be very old.

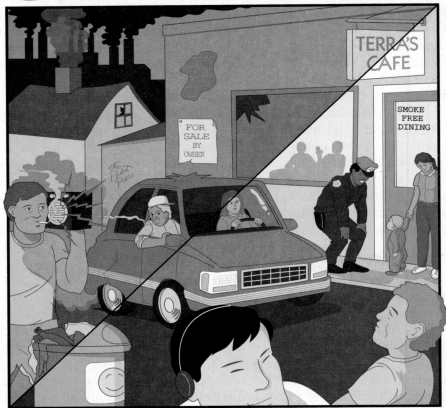

Fig. 10-2
Protecting the environment is everybody's responsibility.

Environment is also important. **Environment** means all the conditions and influences around us. That includes air, water, and noise level in the home, neighborhood, and workplace. **Pollution** occurs when we contaminate the environment with such things as trash and cigarette smoke. Automobiles, hairspray, insecticides, and garbage contribute to pollution. The prevention of pollution is necessary today, and will continue to be a major issue in the future. People live longer in an environment that is clean, quiet, and less polluted.

Lifestyle directly affects how long and how well a person will live. Smoking and the abuse of alcohol and other drugs shorten life. A person's social, emotional or sexual activities may contribute to a destructive lifestyle. Many people have too much stress in their lives, or are not able to cope well with stress. The inability to handle stress can literally "worry a person to

death." Good nutrition, adequate sleep, and regular exercise contribute to a healthy lifestyle. Developing this type of lifestyle helps to lengthen the life span.

People who are in good health usually do not age as quickly. They are able to be more active and involved in meaningful activities. This allows them to feel useful and independent. Those who have either physical or mental health problems often do not feel well enough to remain active. Although the discovery of new medicines and treatments has extended life, many diseases still have no cure.

False Beliefs About Aging. There are some common beliefs about the elderly that are not true. Some of these false beliefs are as follows:

Age 65 Is Old: Although there was a time when this was so, it is no longer true. People are living longer today. The average life span in the United States increased from 65 to 75 between 1940 and 1986. This increase is expected to continue into the future. Many people live into their nineties, and a growing number are past 100. There are a lot of people over 65 who are still working and leading productive lives. They are involved in civic and community affairs. They do not consider themselves old, nor does society.

The Elderly See Themselves as Sick and Helpless: The few who do are often expressing negative feelings they have had for years. The majority of elderly people see themselves as physically healthy, mentally alert, and independent. You often hear the remark, "I'm in pretty good shape for my age." Most people speak with pride of the way that they have weathered the years.

All Old People Are Confused: Confusion is the result of an injury or a disease process and does not necessarily happen as we grow older. Scientists once thought that people became less mentally alert as they aged, because cells in the brain died faster than new cells could replace them. They believed that a decrease in mental ability was a normal change of aging. However, recent studies have shown that the human mind slows down more from lack of use than from a reduction in brain cells.

Most of the Elderly Live in Nursing Homes: Actually, the opposite is true. In the United States, only 5 percent of the elderly live in nursing homes. Most of them live at home with family or friends, and many still live in their own homes. Those who need assistance usually receive it from family members or government programs.

Having purpose, being useful, and being independent delay the aging process. People who have a purpose in life are still setting goals. They are making plans for the future. They have a reason for living as they look forward to what tomorrow might bring. We all have a need to be useful. People who age early often complain that "Nobody needs me, I'm just in the way." Being useful means that what you are doing is worthwhile. This increases feelings of self-worth.

Independence also helps to keep us young. The ability to take care of oneself, and to make choices and decisions, is important. Even a slight amount of independence helps. The person who is able to do only a little will feel better than the person who is totally dependent. A more positive self-image will usually result in a more youthful appearance.

It is important to remember that aging is a normal process. It is not a disease. However, there are some changes of aging that may affect the ability to maintain complete independence. These changes are described in the next chapter.

The Geriatric Resident

A **geriatric resident** is an elderly person who lives in a long-term care facility. The majority of geriatric residents are women. Most are widowed. Some have outlived all their immediate family members, and there is no one to care for them. Many require care that can no longer be provided at home.

The personalities of geriatric residents are as varied as those of people in any other age group. Think about the personalities of the members of your class. Are they all the same? The individual elderly residents are no more alike than are the individual members of your class. The basic personality that a person has developed over the years does not change with age. However, certain characteristics of the personality often get stronger and are more noticeable. A pleasant, happy, young person usually becomes a pleasant, happy, older person, and the older person who is hard to get along with now probably was disagreeable earlier in life.

Geriatric residents may have many health problems. Some are caused by body changes that take place. All the body systems slow down as a person gets older. Response and coordination decrease. Stiff joints and weak muscles make it difficult to get around. Bones become brittle. Vision and hearing loss may occur. These changes place the elderly person at greater risk of injury from

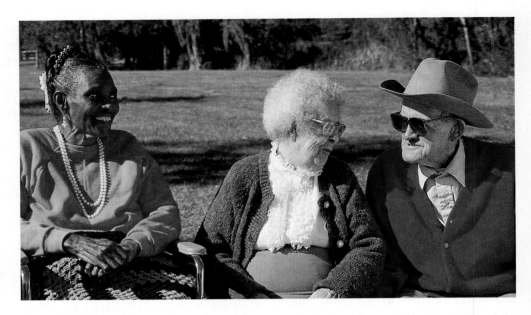

Fig. 10-3
The nursing assistant helps to care for the geriatric resident.

falls and other accidents. The body does not heal as quickly as a person gets older, and rehabilitation may take a long time. Some geriatric residents are confused and disoriented. **Disoriented** means confused as to person, place, or time. The disoriented resident may not even be aware of his own identity. Confused residents have a communication problem because they cannot always follow directions or understand what is being said to them. They have difficulty keeping facts straight. Many geriatric residents are neither confused nor disoriented.

It is important that you develop an understanding of geriatric residents and their problems. They are often frail and are likely to catch a disease if they are exposed to one. Protection of their health and safety is your main concern. Use empathy and care for the geriatric residents as though they were elderly members of your own family.

The Developmentally Disabled Resident

The person who is developmentally disabled has a chronic condition that limits normal function. Many are unable to live independently or take care of themselves. They may have trouble communicating, and learning ability may be reduced.

Some of the developmentally disabled are mentally retarded. Mental retardation occurs early in life, sometimes before birth. These people may have low intellectual and learning skills. The degree of retardation may range from mild to very severe.

The developmentally disabled person may have a disease that causes difficulty in controlling muscle activity. These people are often in wheelchairs. Developmental disability may also be caused by an injury to the brain. Some of these residents may be paralyzed or unconscious.

The needs of the developmentally disabled resident may vary from supervised self-care to total care. It is important that each be treated as an individual with dignity and respect. There are only a small number of developmentally disabled residents in long-term care because most are cared for at home or in special learning centers.

Conclusion

Remember these important points:

1. Most of the residents of a long-term care facility are elderly.

2. The three types of illnesses are acute, chronic, and terminal.

3. Physical health, mental health, heredity, environment, and lifestyle are factors that affect aging.

4. It is everybody's responsibility to prevent pollution of the environment.

5. Confusion is not a normal change of aging.

6. Being useful, having purpose, and being independent delay the aging process.

7. A geriatric resident is an elderly person who lives in a long-term care facility.

8. Geriatric residents have many health problems.

9. Your main concern with geriatric residents is to protect their health and safety.

10. It is important to treat the developmentally disabled person as an individual, with dignity and respect.

Discussion Questions

1. What is the difference between an acute and a chronic illness?

2. Do you feel younger or older than you really are? Why?

3. What can you do to prevent environmental pollution?

Application Exercise

1. The class will go to a long-term care facility. The instructor will assign each student to a resident for a one-hour visit. After returning to the classroom the class will share their experiences and discuss the following observations.

a. Describe your resident.

b. Identify health problems that you observed.

c. Did you have trouble communicating with your resident?

d. How did the resident respond to your attention?

Body Structure and Function: Changes of Aging

OBJECTIVES

Upon completing this chapter, you will be able to do the following:

1. Describe the structure and function of cells, tissues, organs, and systems.

2. Identify two changes of aging in each system of the body.

3. Identify and describe the special senses of the body.

4. Describe the relationships of all the body systems.

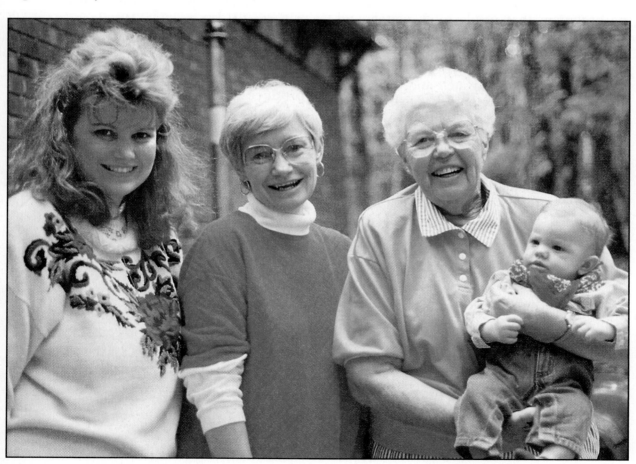

VOCABULARY

The following words or terms will help you to understand this chapter:

Body structure
Anatomy
Function
Physiology
Cell

Tissue
Mucous
  membranes
Organ

System
Appendage
Respiration
Diastole

Systole
Peristalsis
Feces
Metabolism

Basic Body Structure

The human body is composed of many parts that work together in an amazing way. The term **body structure** refers to how the body parts are arranged. **Anatomy** is the study of body structure. The term **function** means purpose or specific action. **Physiology** is the study of body function.

Cells. The smallest unit, the basic building block of the body, is the **cell**. A cell is a living organism that needs food, water, and oxygen. The two basic parts of a cell are the membrane and protoplasm (see Fig. 11-1). The membrane is the outer, protective covering. It permits food, water, and oxygen to enter and allows waste products to exit. Protoplasm is the material inside the cell. It contains cytoplasm and a nucleus that directs and controls the cell. Cell activities are carried out from the cytoplasm.

Cells are so small they can only be seen through a microscope. The human body contains millions of cells that differ in size, shape, and function. For example, skin cells overlap, like the shingles on a roof, to form a protective barrier. Most cells do not work alone, but combine with other cells that are alike in size, shape, and function.

Tissues. A **tissue** is a group of cells that work together to perform a certain function. Tissues can be divided into five different types:

- Blood and lymph
- Epithelial
- Nerve
- Connective
- Muscle

Mucous membranes are thin sheets of tissue that line certain parts of the body. They produce mucus, a thick, sticky fluid that lubricates and protects the membranes. Your mouth and nose are two of the body parts that are lined with mucous membranes.

Organs. An **organ** is a group of tissues that work together to perform a certain function. Organs are located in compartments of the

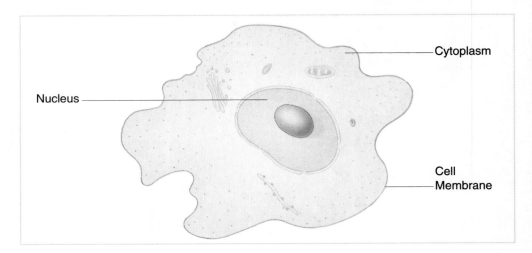

Fig 11-1
Structure of the cell.

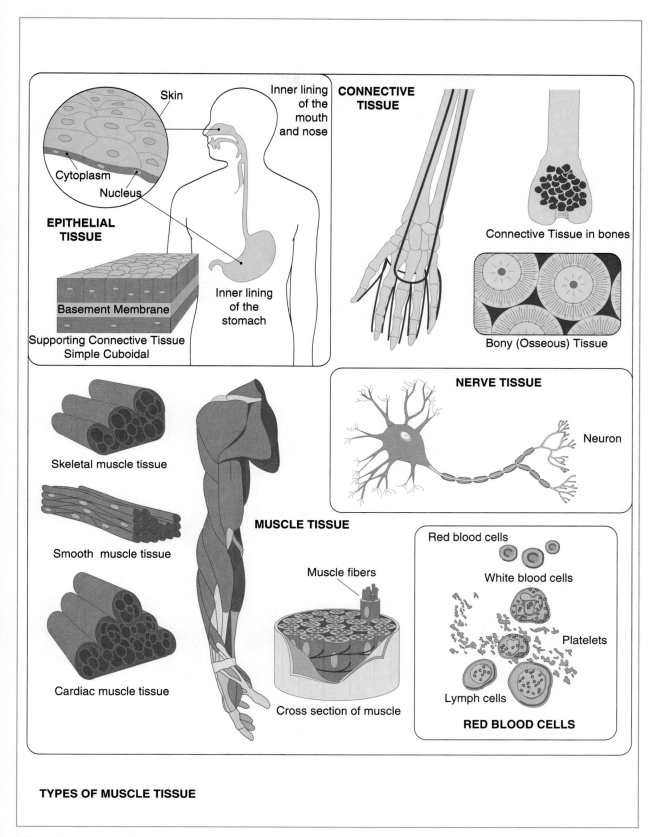

TYPES OF MUSCLE TISSUE

Fig. 11-2 Types of body tissues.

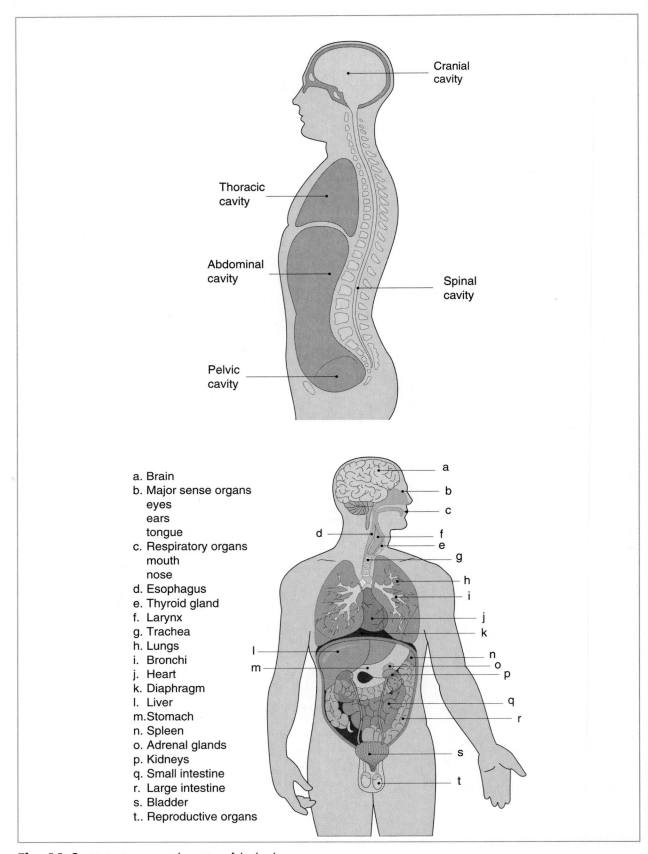

a. Brain
b. Major sense organs
   eyes
   ears
   tongue
c. Respiratory organs
   mouth
   nose
d. Esophagus
e. Thyroid gland
f. Larynx
g. Trachea
h. Lungs
i. Bronchi
j. Heart
k. Diaphragm
l. Liver
m. Stomach
n. Spleen
o. Adrenal glands
p. Kidneys
q. Small intestine
r. Large intestine
s. Bladder
t. Reproductive organs

Fig. 11-3 Major organs and cavities of the body.

body called cavities. See Fig. 11-3 for the location of some major organs and cavities of the body.

Systems. A group of organs that work together to perform a function is called a **system**. The systems of the body include

- Integumentary system
- Urinary system
- Musculoskeletal system
- Nervous system
- Respiratory system
- Endocrine system
- Circulatory system
- Reproductive system
- Digestive system

The human body is a combination of all these systems. You might compare the construction of the body to the construction of a concrete block house. A block is the basic building unit of the house, just as a cell is the basic building unit of the body. Walls are groups of blocks, rooms are groups of walls, and living areas are groups of rooms. All together they create a house. Tissues, organs, and systems are grouped together in a similar way to form the body. See Fig. 11-4 for a better understanding of this comparison.

No system of the body works independently; therefore, a change in one system will affect the others. Although you will study the systems separately, remember that a healthy body requires the combined func-

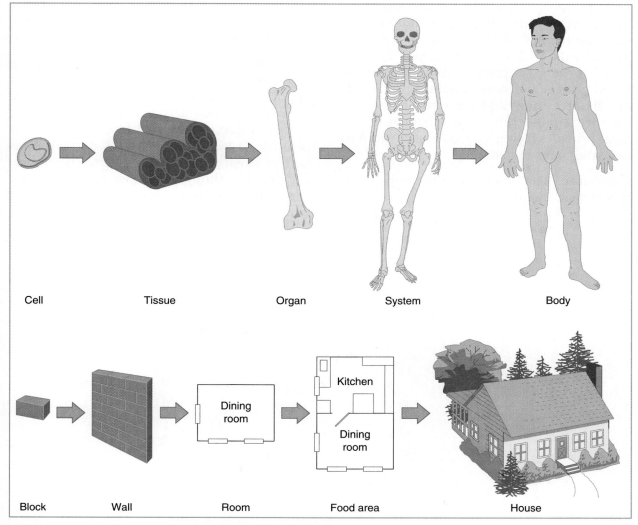

| Cell | Tissue | Organ | System | Body |

| Block | Wall | Room | Food area | House |

Fig. 11-4 Man is built of cells similar to the way in which a house is built of blocks.

tion of all systems. In this chapter, basic information concerning structure, function, and the effects of aging is presented. For more detailed structural information, refer to the physiology and anatomy insert. A summary of the changes of aging is shown in Fig. 11-18 on page 140.

The Integumentary System

Structure. The integumentary system is composed of the skin and its appendages. An **appendage** is an extension of a body part. Appendages of the skin include fingernails, toenails, hair, sweat glands, and oil glands.

There are three layers of skin: the epidermis, the dermis, and the subcutaneous fat layer (see Fig. 11-5). The epidermis is the outer layer of skin. It is very thin and contains the pigment that determines skin color. The dermis, which is often called the "true skin," is the inner layer of skin that contains blood vessels and nerve endings. Cells flake off the epidermis and are replaced by new ones from the dermis. The subcutaneous fat layer provides a shock absorbing cushion for insulation and protection.

Function. The functions of the integumentary system include the following:

- Protection
- Regulation of the body temperature
- Elimination
- Lubrication
- Awareness of environment
- Storage of nutrients

The skin's protective covering helps prevent injury to the internal parts of the body and forms a barrier against germs. The skin protects water balance by preventing too much moisture from leaving the body. It helps to maintain normal body temperature by controlling the flow of blood near the surface, and by the process of perspiration. Perspiration also helps eliminate waste products through pores in the skin. Oil glands provide lubrication to keep the skin and hair soft. Nerve endings in the skin allow a person to feel sensations such as heat and cold or those that bring pleasure. Some fats and vitamins are stored in the skin.

Changes of Aging. The first signs of aging are often seen in the integumentary system. Hair thins and loses its color or turns gray. Brown spots, sometimes called liver spots, may develop. As the skin loses elasticity (its ability to stretch), wrinkles appear. Less active sweat and oil glands cause the skin to be dry. The skin gets thinner and more fragile, which means it is easily damaged.

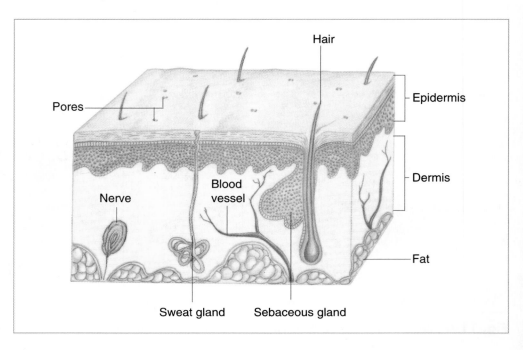

Fig. 11-5
The layers of the skin.

The fatty layer that provides padding between the skin and bones gets thinner, leaving the skin with less protection and less insulation. Because there is less insulation, the elderly often complain of feeling cold.

A decrease of sensitivity in nerve endings causes the elderly person to be less able to identify sensations. The sense of touch may not be dependable.

Fingernails and toenails become thick, hard, and yellowed. Torn cuticles and ingrown nails can occur. The nails may become diseased because they are hard to clean.

Changes of aging in the integumentary system leave the elderly person less protected from the environment.

The Musculoskeletal System

Structure. The musculoskeletal system is composed of bones, joints, and muscles. Although bones are hard and rigid, they are made of living cells that grow and harden slowly. The human skeleton contains 206 bones. The four most common types of bones are long bones, short bones, flat bones, and irregular bones (see Fig. 11-6).

Joints connect the bones and are composed of ligaments, tendons, bursa, and cartilage. Ligaments connect bone to bone, while tendons connect muscle to bone. Bursa are small sacs of fluid that lubricate and prevent friction in the joint. Cartilage provides padding between bones. There are several types of joints that allow a variety of movements (see Fig. 11-7).

There are three types of muscles: voluntary, involuntary, and cardiac. Voluntary muscles are muscles that are controlled by will. For example, you can move the muscles in your arms or legs by thinking about doing so. Involuntary muscles work automatically, without conscious thought. These muscles help you to breathe and digest food. Cardiac muscle is a special type of involuntary muscle that controls the heartbeat.

Muscles work together in groups. Some muscles, like those in your upper arm, work in pairs. A muscle in the front of the arm contracts (shortens), while the one in the back relaxes (lengthens). This allows you to bend your arm (see Fig. 11-8). Working muscles use food for energy and produce body heat.

Functions. The functions of the musculoskeletal system include the following:

- Produce movement
- Protect vital organs

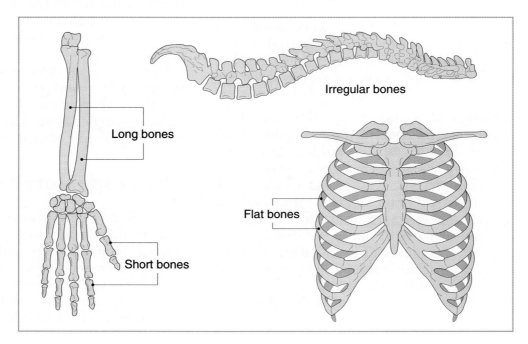

Fig. 11-6
Types of bones.

Long bones

Irregular bones

Flat bones

Short bones

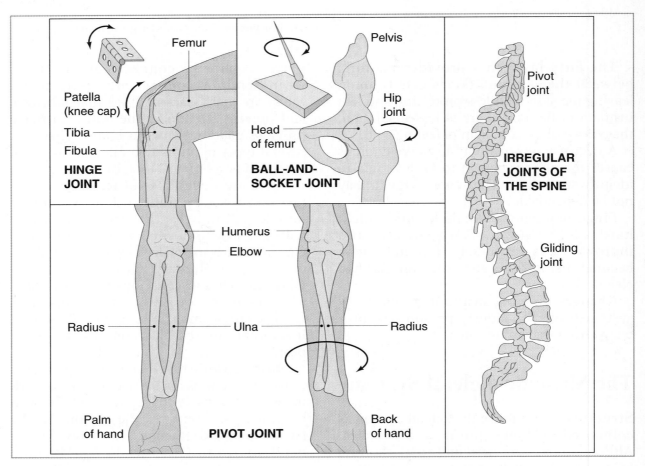

Fig. 11-7 Types of joints.

- Provide support and framework for the body
- Produce blood cells
- Produce body heat
- Store minerals

Muscles and bones must work together to move the body. The musculoskeletal system must work with other body systems to allow you to accomplish even a small movement such as lifting one finger.

Changes of Aging. As a person gets older, many changes occur in the musculoskeletal system. Muscles weaken and lose their tone. This weakness affects many parts of the body. For example, a decrease in heart function or breathing difficulties may be the result of weak muscles. Strength and endurance decrease, while body movement slows.

Joints become stiff as cartilage deteriorates and tissue hardens. This can make movement difficult, which may lead to decreased activity and further loss of muscle tone.

Bones become porous and brittle. Because they are not as hard as they once were, bones are easily broken. Some older people lose calcium, making the bones even more fragile. Changes in the spinal column (the bony structure that protects the spinal cord) can result in stooped posture and a loss of height.

Changes of aging in the musculoskeletal system may interfere with the ability of elderly people to care for themselves and remain independent. These changes also place the resident at increased risk of injury.

The Respiratory System

Structure. Structures of the respiratory system include the nose, pharynx, larynx, trachea, bronchi, lungs, and alveoli (see Fig. 11-9). Air enters the body through the nose and pharynx. The pharynx (throat) is a passageway for both air and food. The larynx ("voice box") contains the vocal cords and

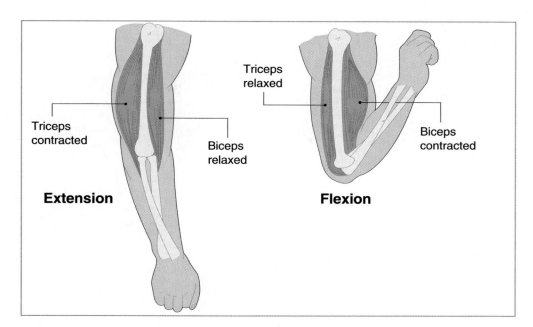

Triceps
contracted

Biceps
relaxed

Extension

Triceps
relaxed

Biceps
contracted

Flexion

Fig. 11-8
Coordination of
muscles.

is located at the opening to the trachea (windpipe). After leaving the pharynx, air enters the trachea and flows through the bronchi, or bronchial tree. The left bronchus and right bronchus branch out into smaller tubes, much like branches on a tree. Tubes of the bronchial tree lead to small air sacs of the lungs, called alveoli.

A piece of cartilage, called the epiglottis, covers the trachea like a flap to prevent food in the throat from entering the airway. This flap lifts when you breathe or talk and closes when you swallow. Have you ever choked while trying to talk and eat at the same time? That happened because the epiglottis opened to allow you to talk and food went down the wrong way, into the trachea.

Functions. The functions of the respiratory system are

• To bring oxygen into the body
• To remove carbon dioxide from the body

Oxygen is a colorless, odorless gas, found naturally in the air. Each cell of the body needs oxygen to survive. Carbon dioxide is a gas that is a waste product of the body.

The respiratory system provides a pathway for oxygen to enter the body and carbon dioxide to leave. This process is accomplished by **respiration** (breathing). During respiration, blood vessels in the alveoli exchange carbon dioxide that has been brought to the lungs for oxygen. Oxygen is then carried to the heart to be circulated to the cells.

The lungs are located in the chest cavity and are protected by the rib cage. The diaphragm, a muscle that separates the chest cavity from the abdominal cavity, is immediately below the lungs. Inhalation (breathing in) occurs when your diaphragm flattens, enlarging the chest cavity. This causes the lungs to expand and fill with air, which contains oxygen. Exhalation (breathing out) occurs when the diaphragm expands, decreasing the size of the chest cavity. Air containing carbon dioxide is then forced out of the lungs.

The center that controls respirations is in the brain. The rate of respirations is affected by the amount of carbon dioxide in the blood. The faster you move, the more carbon dioxide is produced, and the faster you must breathe to eliminate it. Think about what happens to your breathing rate when you run.

Changes of Aging. The rib cage, which normally expands, becomes more rigid, and muscles weaken. These changes limit the lungs ability to fill. With increased activity, the older person has to breathe harder and faster to get enough air. There is a decrease in the elasticity of the lungs (their ability to

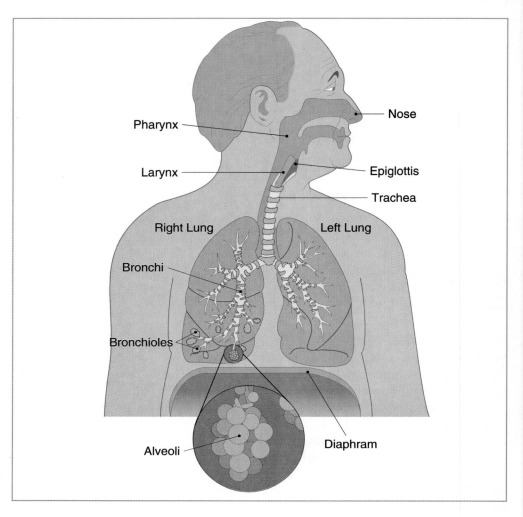

Fig. 11-9
The major structures of
the respiratory system.

stretch). The ability to resist disease is low-ered. Changes in the larynx may weaken the voice and cause it to sound different. Any change in the respiratory system that reduces the amount of oxygen brought into the body will affect all the systems.

The Circulatory System

Structure. The circulatory system includes the heart, blood, and blood vessels. Together they form the body's transportation and delivery system. The heart moves blood through the blood vessels, carrying oxygen and other substances to and from the cells. The circulatory system can be compared to any transportation system. The heart is the "pumping station," at the center of the system. The blood is the vehicle that delivers products to and from the cells by traveling through the blood vessels, which are the "roadways."

Function. The functions of the circulatory system are to

• Carry food, water, oxygen, and other sub-stances to the cells
• Carry waste products away from the cells
• Help regulate body temperature
• Protect the body against disease
• Maintain fluid balance

The Heart. The heart is an organ about the size of your fist that is composed of cardiac muscle. It is located in the chest slightly to the left of the midline, between the two lungs. The rib cage protects the heart, as it does the lungs. The function of the heart is to pump blood throughout the body. The heart is divided into four chambers that are separated by muscular walls and one-way valves. The two upper chambers are the right and the left atrium. The function of the atria is to receive blood from the body. The two lower chambers are the right and left ventricles. Their function is to pump blood out of the heart to other parts of the body.

The Cardiac Cycle. The heart moves blood through the body in a continuous one-way direction. It does this in precise, coordinated movements, called the cardiac cycle. The cycle is divided into two stages: diastole and systole. **Diastole** is the stage of the cardiac cycle when the heart is resting and filling with blood. **Systole** is the stage when the heart is contracting and pumping out the blood.

The blood returning from the rest of the body is low in oxygen and high in carbon dioxide. Most of the oxygen has been delivered to the cells and exchanged for carbon dioxide. The blood enters the right atrium of the heart through large veins called the inferior and superior vena cava. From the right atrium, the blood enters the right ven-

tricle. The right ventricle contracts and pumps unoxygenated blood into the pulmonary artery, through which it flows to the lungs. In the alveoli of the lungs, the carbon dioxide is exchanged for oxygen.

The blood returns from the lungs to the left atrium of the heart and passes into the left ventricle. The left ventricle contracts and pumps the blood into the aorta, the largest blood vessel in the body. The blood then circulates through a series of blood vessels to all parts of the body, before returning to the heart. Look at Fig. 11-10, and trace the flow of blood through the heart.

The Blood. Blood is the part of the body that actually carries oxygen, food, wastes, and other substances. The average adult has from four to six quarts of blood, which is composed of plasma and cells. Although plasma is mostly water, it also contains many other important substances.

The three main types of blood cells are

- Red blood cells
- White blood cells
- Platelets

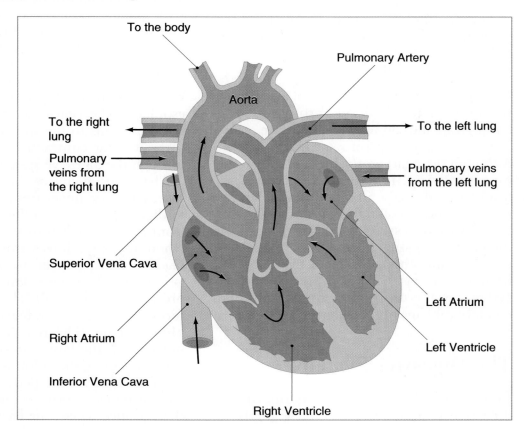

Fig. 11-10
The flow of blood through the heart.

To the body

Pulmonary Artery

Aorta

To the right lung

To the left lung

Pulmonary veins from the right lung

Pulmonary veins from the left lung

Superior Vena Cava

Left Atrium

Right Atrium

Left Ventricle

Inferior Vena Cava

Right Ventricle

Red blood cells carry oxygen to the cells. They give blood its red color. White blood cells help to fight disease and are a part of the body's immune or defense system. Platelets help the blood to clot. Blood cells only live for a short time and must be replaced by new ones.

The Blood Vessels. Blood vessels are tubes that transport blood throughout the body. They are the "roadways" of the circulatory system. The major types of blood vessels are arteries, veins, and capillaries:

- Arteries carry blood away from the heart.
- Veins carry blood back to the heart.
- Capillaries connect arteries to veins.

Arteries carry oxygen-rich blood, except for the pulmonary artery. The pulmonary artery carries blood from the heart to the lungs, where it receives oxygen. Veins carry oxygen-poor blood, except for the pulmonary veins, which return oxygenated blood from the lungs to the heart. Capillaries are very small blood vessels that allow food, oxygen, and other substances, including waste products, to enter and exit the bloodstream.

The circulatory system, the respiratory system, and the nervous system are essential to life. A malfunction of any one of the three can cause immediate death.

Changes of Aging. Changes of aging slow the movement of blood throughout the body. Heart muscle weakens with age, causing the heart to pump with less force. Although the heart works harder to keep the blood moving, it is less effective. This results in a decrease in blood flow. Changes in the blood vessels also slow the flow of blood. Blood vessels that harden and lose their ability to stretch become narrow. Fatty deposits and other substances may clog the narrowed vessels. Changes in the circulatory system are the cause of many physical and mental problems of the elderly.

The Digestive System

Structure. The primary organs of the digestive system are the mouth, pharynx (throat), esophagus, stomach, small intestine, and large intestine. These structures form a long, continuous tube that extends from the mouth to the anus (the opening to the rectum)(see Fig. 11-11). This tube, called the alimentary canal, is lined with mucous membrane. The accessory organs of the digestive system are the teeth, tongue, salivary glands, liver, gallbladder, and pancreas. The gastrointestinal (GI) system is another name for the digestive system. "Gastro" means stomach and "intestinal" refers to the intestines. The name indicates that this is the system of the stomach and intestines.

Function. The functions of the digestive system are to

- Prepare food for the body's use
- Eliminate wastes

The process of preparing food for the body's use is called digestion. Digestion begins in the mouth, with the assistance of the teeth, tongue, and salivary glands. The teeth bite and chew the food into pieces that are small enough to be swallowed. The salivary glands secrete saliva to add moisture and chemicals. Taste buds on the tongue allow a person to enjoy the food. The tongue also helps during swallowing by pushing the food into the pharynx, which contracts and moves the food into the esophagus. Peristalsis moves the food from the esophagus to the stomach. **Peristalsis** is the muscular contractions that move food through the digestive system.

The stomach churns the food into smaller pieces. Gastric juices from the stomach help to digest the food. The food mixture moves from the stomach into the small intestine, where digestive juices from the liver, gallbladder, and pancreas are added. Digestion is completed in the small intestine, where projections called villi absorb the digested food particles and release them into the bloodstream. The rest of the food mass moves into the large intestine (the colon). The purpose of the colon is to remove water from the food for the body's use. The material that remains forms a solid waste product that is called **feces**. The feces is stored in the rectum until it leaves the body through the anus (the opening of the rectum).

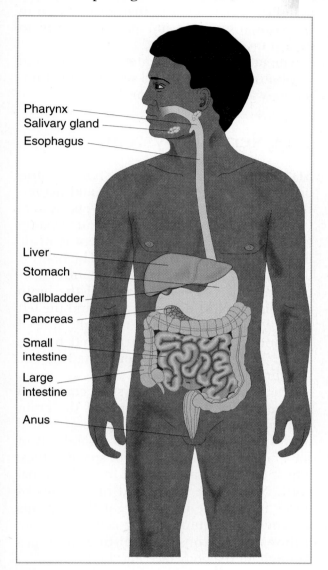

Pharynx
Salivary gland
Esophagus

Liver
Stomach
Gallbladder
Pancreas
Small intestine
Large intestine
Anus

Fig. 11-11 The digestive system.

Changes of Aging. Many changes of aging occur in the digestive system. A decrease in saliva and in the number of taste buds leads to a decrease in appetite. The elderly often have difficulty chewing and swallowing. A weakening of the gag reflex increases the risk of choking. Muscles weaken and lose their tone. A reduction in digestive juices makes food harder to digest. The absorption of vitamins and minerals is reduced. Peristalsis slows throughout the system. These changes cause the process of digestion to be less efficient in the elderly.

The Urinary System

Structure. The main structures of the urinary system are the kidneys, ureters, bladder, and urethra. The kidneys are two bean-shaped organs located in the upper abdomen, toward the back, on either side of the spine. A ureter leads from each kidney to the bladder. The bladder is a muscular sac that is located in the front of the lower abdomen. The tube that leads from the bladder to the outside of the body is called the urethra. The external (outside) opening of the urethra is called the urinary meatus (see Fig. 11-12).

Function. The functions of the urinary system are as follows:

- Remove waste products from the bloodstream
- Eliminate liquid waste products from the body
- Help maintain the body's water and chemical balance
- Produce hormones

The major function of the kidneys is to filter and remove waste products from the blood. This is accomplished through a complicated system of tubes and blood vessels. Filtration takes place in the nephrons, which are located in the outer layer of each kidney. Each kidney may have a million or more nephrons. The kidneys produce urine from filtered wastes and water. The ureters carry the urine from the kidneys to the bladder.

The bladder is a muscular, expandable sac. Urine, which is continuously produced by the kidneys, is held in the bladder until it is eliminated from the body. The average adult bladder can hold about one quart of urine. When the bladder is approximately one-third full, the brain sends a signal causing an urge to urinate. The amount the bladder can hold without discomfort, and the length of time between signals from the brain, varies from one person to another.

The urethra allows urine to pass from the bladder to the outside of the body through the urinary meatus. The elimination of water and waste products by the urinary

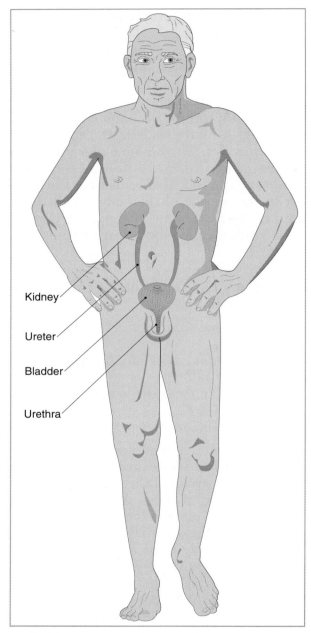

Fig. 11-12 The urinary system.

system help to maintain the fluid and chemical balance of the body.

Changes of Aging. The kidneys do not filter as efficiently in the elderly person because there is a decrease in the number of functioning nephrons. Slowed circulation also delays the filtering of the blood. This can cause waste products and toxins (poisonous substances) to build up in the body.

A decrease in the muscle tone of the bladder leads to a loss of elasticity (ability to stretch). The bladder holds less urine for shorter periods of time and may not empty completely. The muscle that keeps urine in the bladder weakens and may allow urine to escape involuntarily.

The urinary, integumentary, digestive, and respiratory systems are all involved in eliminating waste products from the body.

The Nervous System

Structure. The nervous system is composed of the brain, spinal cord, and nerves. It is divided into the central nervous system (CNS) and the peripheral nervous system (PNS). The central nervous system is made up of the brain and spinal cord. The brain is divided into sections that each control specific functions. The right side of the brain controls the left side of the body, and the left side of the brain controls the right side of the body. The brain is protected by the skull. The spinal cord is protected by the vertebral (spinal) column.

The peripheral nervous system consists of all the nerves that are outside of the brain and spinal cord. There are 12 pairs of cranial nerves, which carry messages in and out of the brain. There are 31 pairs of spinal nerves, which carry messages to and from the spinal cord. Nerves are composed of bundles of nerve fibers. The basic unit of the nervous system is the neuron (nerve cell). There are billions of neurons transmitting messages throughout the body (see Fig. 11-13).

Function. The function of the nervous system is to control and coordinate the body's activities. It is the body's communication center. The special senses of sight, hearing, smell, taste, and touch receive messages from the environment. Nerves carry those messages along the spinal cord to the brain, where they are processed. The brain then sends instructions for a response through the nerves to the appropriate body part. For instance, if you put your finger against a hot iron, nerves take that message to the brain. The brain then directs you to remove your finger from the iron. The entire process may take only a fraction of a second.

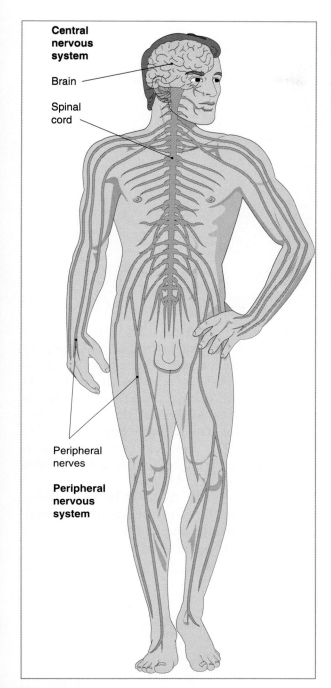

Central nervous system

Brain

Spinal cord

Peripheral nerves

Peripheral nervous system

Fig. 11-13 The nervous system.

Changes of Aging. The number of neurons decreases with aging. Unlike other body cells, nerve cells do not reproduce and are not replaced by new cells if they are destroyed. Slowed circulation also affects the nervous system. These factors of aging delay the transmission of messages through the body, resulting in slower responses and reflexes.

There is a decrease in the sensitivity of nerve endings in the skin. Numbness may interfere with the ability to handle small objects and the sense of touch is not as accurate.

Elderly persons are often more forgetful. They may forget information that is stored in short-term memory, such as names, dates, telephone numbers, or items on lists. It once was thought that there was a decrease in intelligence and awareness with aging because of a decrease in brain cells. Later studies have shown that elderly people who stay active and involved with others do not show this decline.

The Special Senses

The five special senses are sight, hearing, smell, taste, and touch. Nerve endings (receptors) in certain parts of the body transmit received information to the brain. For example, receptors in the eye allow you to see.

The Eye. The eye is the sense organ for vision. The structure of the eye includes the following:

- Eyeball: the globe-shaped part of the eye
- Orbit: the cavity in the front of the skull that contains and protects the eyeball
- Muscles: tissue that connects the eye to the orbit and allows it to move
- Eyelids: skin fold that protects the eye from injury
- Conjunctiva: mucous membrane that protects the eyeball
- Optic nerve: band of tissue that carries sight messages to the brain

The eyeball is composed of three layers. The outer layer contains the sclera (the white part of the eye) and the cornea (which helps to focus light rays). The middle layer contains the iris (the colored part of the eye). In the center of the iris is the pupil, a round, dark opening that changes size to control the amount of light that can enter. Behind the iris is the lens, which focuses light images onto the retina. The inner layer of the eyeball is the retina, which contains

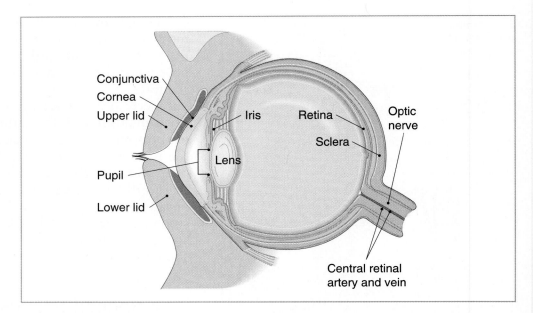

Fig. 11-14
The structure of
the eye.

sight receptors called rods and cones (see Fig. 11-14).

All these structures work together to allow you to see. Light images enter through the cornea and the pupil and pass through the lens, which projects the images onto the retina. These sight messages are received by the rods and cones of the retina and are carried to the brain by the optic nerve.

The Ear. The ear is the sense organ for hearing and balance. It is divided into three parts: the outer ear, the middle ear, and the inner ear. The auricle and auditory canal compose the outer ear. The auricle is the outer part of ear that surrounds the opening to the auditory canal. The tympanic membrane (eardrum) separates the outer ear from the middle ear. Located in the middle ear are three small bones, the malleus, the incus, and the stapes. These bones are called the ossicles. The inner ear contains semicircular canals filled with fluid and nerve receptors (see Fig. 11-15).

Sound waves are received by the auricle, which reflects them into the auditory canal. They flow through the auditory canal to the eardrum, causing it to vibrate. The vibra-

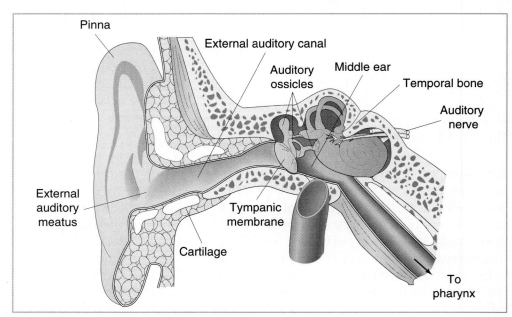

Fig. 11-15
The structure of
the ear.

tions of the eardrum set the ossicles into motion. The motion of the ossicles moves fluid in the semicircular canals of the inner ear, causing waves of fluid to stimulate tiny nerve receptors. Nerve impulses are initiated and travel to the brain by way of the auditory nerve.

The semicircular canals also contain nerve receptors for balance. Changes in the position of your head cause the fluid in the semicircular canals to move. The nerve impulses for balance are initiated by this fluid movement and are transmitted to the brain.

The Nose. While the major function of the nose is to bring oxygen into the body, it also contains the receptors for smell. Messages from the receptors in the upper part of the nose are carried by the olfactory nerve to the brain. Although the senses of smell and taste are closely related, smell is the more accurate.

The Tongue. The receptors for taste are located on the tongue. They are called taste buds. The taste buds for sweet and salty are on the tip of the tongue. Sour receptors are on the sides of the tongue, and those for bitter are located on the back of the tongue. The taste buds help you to enjoy food.

The Skin. Nerve cells located in the dermis layer of the skin act as receptors for pressure, heat, cold, pain, pleasure, and touch. The tactile (touch) receptors permit you to identify objects by touching them. They send messages to the brain, which directs a response. The sense of touch increases your awareness of the environment, allowing you to protect yourself, stay comfortable, and avoid danger.

Changes of Aging. Aging affects the special senses in many ways. The eyes take longer to adjust to changes in light, distance, and direction. Some people have trouble reading small print and must have brighter light to see. Many older people wear glasses. Atrophy of nerve fibers and receptors in the ear cause hearing loss. The receptors become less sensitive, causing sound to be distorted. The sense of balance may be affected. Smell receptors deteriorate with age, affecting the accuracy of smell. Taste becomes less distinct because there is a decrease in the number of taste buds. A decrease in the sensitivity of receptors in the skin means the sense of touch may be ·changed.

These sensory changes may interfere with the elderly persons' ability to communicate, protect themselves, and enjoy life.

The Endocrine System

The endocrine system works with the nervous system to regulate and control the activities of the body. The nervous system uses electrical impulses and chemicals for control, while the endocrine system acts only by chemicals, called hormones.

Structure. The endocrine system is composed of glands that secrete chemicals directly into the bloodstream. These chemicals are called hormones. The major endocrine glands are as follows:

- Pituitary gland
- Adrenal glands
- Thyroid gland
- Pancreas (islets of Langerhans)
- Parathyroid glands
- Gonads (testes in the male; ovaries in the female)
- Thymus

See Fig. 11-16 for the location of the major endocrine glands in the body.

Function. The function of the endocrine system is to control and regulate body functions by secreting hormones. Each gland produces different hormones, and each hormone has a specific purpose.

The Pituitary Gland. The pituitary gland is often called the "master" gland, because it regulates the other glands. It produces hormones, which regulate growth, water balance, and reproduction.

The Thyroid Gland. The thyroid gland, located in the neck, secretes hormones that affect body growth and development. This gland also regulates metabolism. **Metabo-**

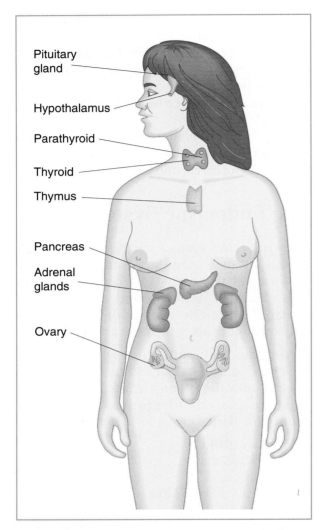

Fig. 11-16
The major endocrine glands.

glands produce hormones that help to regulate water balance and the metabolism of some foods. Small amounts of sex hormones are also secreted. The adrenals produce hormones that control the body's response to stress. One of these hormones is epinephrin (adrenalin), which allows the body to quickly produce great amounts of energy in an emergency.

The Pancreas. The pancreas produces hormones that are necessary for the metabolism of sugar. Clusters of cells in the pancreas, called "the islets of Langerhans," produce insulin and glucagon. These hormones are needed to convert sugar to energy.

The Gonads. The gonads control human reproduction. In the male, the testes produce testosterone. The ovaries of the female produce estrogen and progesterone. These hormones are involved in reproduction, and in the development of male and female characteristics.

The Exocrine Glands. All glands are not part of the endocrine system. Exocrine glands secrete substances into organs or outside the body, *not* directly into the bloodstream. The sweat glands, oil glands, and parotid glands, for example, are exocrine glands.

Changes of Aging. Changes of aging in the endocrine system affect the levels of hormones in the body. For example, there is a decrease in the production of estrogen and progesterone. Some hormones, like insulin, become less effective. The changes in hormone levels decrease the endocrine system's ability to regulate body activities.

The Reproductive System

All living things must have a method to reproduce themselves. A single cell does this by splitting or dividing itself. Human beings reproduce by sexual reproduction, a method requiring a male and a female. Each has special cells, organs, and hormones that work together to accomplish reproduction.

The Female Reproductive System. The major structures of the female reproductive

lism is the combination of all body processes. All body functions are affected by changes in metabolism.

The Parathyroid Glands. The parathyroids are located on the back of the thyroid gland. They secrete a hormone that regulates calcium in the body. Calcium levels affect nerve and muscle function.

The Thymus. The thymus produces a hormone that assists in the immune process. The immune system helps the body resist germs and disease. White blood cells that regulate the immune function also develop in this gland. They are called "T-cells."

The Adrenal Glands. The adrenal glands are located on top of the kidneys. These

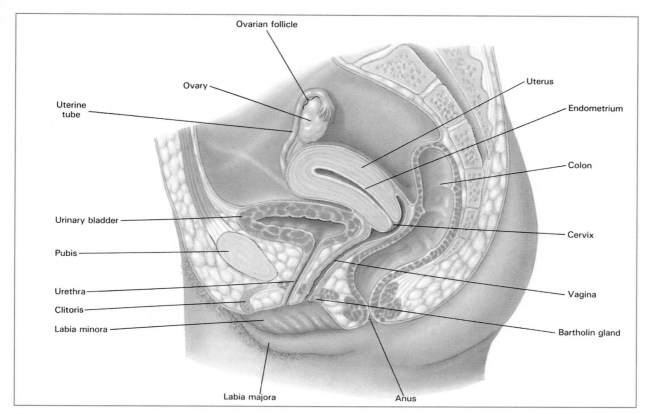

A The organs of the female reproductive system. (Frederic Martini, *Fundamentals of Anatomy and Physiology, 2e,* © 1992, pp. 918, 929. Reprinted by permission of Prentice Hall, Englewood Cliffs, New Jersey.)

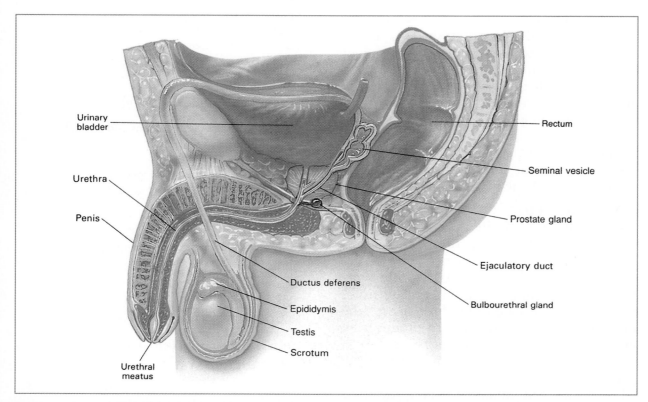

B The organs of the male reproductive system. (Frederic Martini, *Fundamentals of Anatomy and Physiology, 2e,* © 1992, pp. 918, 929. Reprinted by permission of Prentice Hall, Englewood Cliffs, New Jersey.)

Fig. 11-17 The reproductive system.

system are the ovaries, fallopian tubes, uterus, and vagina. The breasts are also considered part of this system. See Fig. 11-17A for the location of the structures of the female reproductive system.

The ovaries are located on each side of the uterus in the pelvic cavity. The major function of the ovaries is to produce ova (eggs), the female reproductive cells. They also secrete the female hormones, estrogen and progesterone. The fallopian tubes are attached on each side of the uterus and end near each ovary. Their functions are to carry the ova to the uterus and to assist in uniting the male and female sex cells. The uterus is a hollow, muscular organ in the pelvic cavity, above the bladder and in front of the rectum. The functions of the uterus are

- To protect and nourish the fetus during pregnancy
- To expel the fetus during childbirth
- To discharge the unused lining of the uterus (menstruation)

The vagina acts as a passageway for birth of the fetus and menstruation. It is also a receptacle for the male penis during sexual intercourse. During intercourse, the sperm enters through the vagina into the uterus and the fallopian tubes. If it unites with an ovum (egg), pregnancy occurs, and the fertilized ovum passes from the fallopian tube to the uterus. If pregnancy does not occur, the ovum will die and be discharged from the body with the menstrual flow.

The Male Reproductive System.
The major structures of the male reproductive system are the testes, scrotum, penis, seminal vesicles, and prostate gland. The external sex organs include the penis and the scrotum, which contains the testes. The functions of the testes are to produce sperm (the male reproductive cells) and to produce the male hormone testosterone. The scrotum contains two sacs and is located behind the penis. The penis becomes enlarged and erect when sexually stimulated. Semen, the fluid that contains the sperm, is released from the penis during sexual intercourse. The seminal vesicles and the prostate gland both secrete fluids that become part of the semen. See

Fig. 11-17B for the location of the structures of the male reproductive system.

Changes of Aging.
In women, menstruation ends with menopause, and pregnancy can no longer occur. A decrease in the pro-

---

PHYSICAL CHANGES OF AGING

INTEGUMENTARY SYSTEM
Hair thins and loses color
Dry, thin, fragile skin
Wrinkles and liver spots
Loss of fatty tissue
Decrease in feeling
Thick, hard nails

MUSCULOSKELETAL SYSTEM
Muscles weaken and lose tone
Body movements slow
Stiff joints
Brittle bones
Changes in posture, loss of height

RESPIRATORY SYSTEM
Rib cage more rigid
Muscles weaken
Decrease in elasticity of lungs
Voice weakens

CIRCULATORY SYSTEM
Heart pumps with less force
Blood vessels harden and narrow

DIGESTIVE SYSTEM
Decrease in saliva and taste buds
Decrease in digestive juices
Difficulty chewing and swallowing
Peristalsis slows
Reduced absorption of vitamins and minerals

URINARY SYSTEM
Decrease in kidney filtration
Decrease in bladder muscle tone

NERVOUS SYSTEM
Decrease in nerve cells
Message transmission slows
Slowed responses and reflexes
Decreased sensitivity of nerve endings
Short term memory loss
Decrease in vision
Hearing loss
Loss of smell receptors

ENDOCRINE SYSTEM
Decrease in hormones
Reduced regulation of body activities

REPRODUCTIVE SYSTEM
Menopause in women
Drying and thinning of vaginal walls
Enlargement of male prostate gland
Change in male hormone levels

Fig. 11-18 Physical changes of aging.

duction of estrogen leads to a loss of calcium, causing the bones to become more brittle. Decreased estrogen also contributes to a thinning and drying of the vaginal walls. Weakened muscles cause the breasts to be less firm. In men, there is a change in hormone levels and a decrease in sperm. The prostate gland enlarges and hardens, causing pressure on the urinary urethra. Although the female reproductive cycle ends with menopause, sexual needs continue for both men and women.

Conclusion

Remember these important points:

1. The basic building block of the body is the cell.

2. All the body systems are interdependent. A change in one body system will affect the others.

3. All body systems tend to slow with aging.

4. The major function of the skin is protection.

5. Muscles work with bones and joints to allow body movement.

6. The main function of the respiratory system is to bring oxygen into the body.

7. The primary functions of the circulatory system are to carry oxygen to the cells and to assist in the elimination of waste.

8. Slowed circulation occurs with aging and affects all the body systems.

9. The functions of the digestive system are to prepare food for the body's use and to eliminate waste.

10. The functions of the urinary system include removing waste products and maintaining fluid balance.

11. The nervous system is the body's communication system.

12. The five special senses are sight, hearing, smell, taste, and touch.

13. The endocrine system secretes hormones that regulate body functions.

14. The immune process helps the body to resist germs and disease.

15. Changes in the reproductive system do not eliminate sexual needs.

Discussion Questions

1. What is meant by the phrase "all the body systems are interdependent"?

2. In what ways does the integumentary system provide protection?

3. How can changes of aging in the musculoskeletal system interfere with independence?

4. How do changes in the respiratory system affect all other systems?

5. Why is the circulatory system called the body's transportation system?

6. Why is digestion less effective in the elderly?

7. Why do changes in the special senses interfere with the elderly person's ability to communicate?

8. What is the immune process?

9. What is the difference between endocrine glands and exocrine glands?

Application Exercises

1. Divide the class into nine groups. Each group or individual will discuss a body system, explaining its structures, functions, and changes of aging. Charts, pictures, or other props may be used.

CHAPTER 12

Common Health Problems of the Elderly Resident

OBJECTIVES

Upon completing this chapter, you will be able to do the following:

1. Identify two common problems of the musculo-skeletal system, the respiratory system, the circulatory system, and the nervous system.

2. Identify two common sensory problems of the elderly.

3. Identify four complications of diabetes.

4. List four nursing measures to follow when caring for the diabetic resident.

5. Identify the seven signs of cancer.

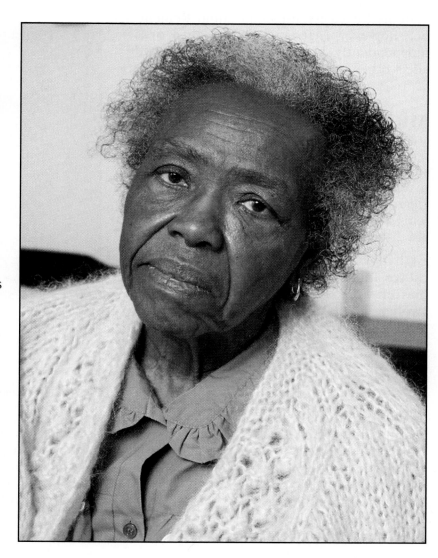

VOCABULARY

The following words or terms will help you to understand this chapter:

Inflammation	Aspiration	Hemiplegia	Comatose
Fracture	Edema	Paraplegia	Obese
Amputation	Hypertension	Quadriplegia	Hyperglycemia
Dyspnea	Dementia	Seizure	Hypoglycemia
Cyanosis	Paralysis		

Although residents in long-term care may suffer from many diseases, some health problems are more common than others. These problems will be grouped by body systems for easier understanding. Remember, however, that since no system works independently, a problem in one system will affect other systems as well.

Musculoskeletal Problems

Diseases and injuries of the musculoskeletal system create special problems because they often interfere with the ability to move. Decreased mobility results in further problems or complications. These complications are discussed later, in Chapter 17.

Arthritis. Arthritis is a chronic disease that causes inflammation of the joints. **Inflammation** means that the body part is red, swollen, hot, and painful. Perhaps you have seen someone whose hands are crippled with arthritis. Although there are several types of arthritis, the two most common are osteoarthritis and rheumatoid arthritis.

Osteoarthritis: Osteoarthritis causes breakdown of cartilage in the joints. The weight-bearing joints, such as the knee and hip, are most often affected. Joints are stiff and sore as a result of tissue damage. Because movement causes pain, people who have this condition may be less active. Osteoarthritis affects many elderly people and can lead to a loss of function and independence.

Rheumatoid Arthritis: Rheumatoid arthritis can affect people of any age, even children. It usually begins in the hands and

fingers. The inflammation may spread to other tissues. Rheumatoid arthritis is sometimes called "crippling arthritis" because of the changes it causes in body structure.

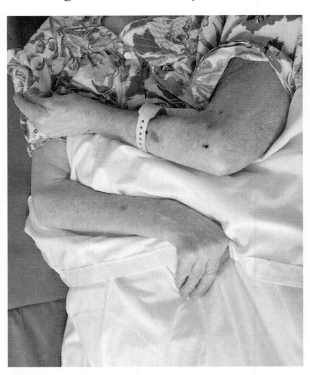

Fig. 12-1 Contractures are a complication of arthritis.

Sometimes arthritic joints are replaced in surgery by a prosthesis (an artificial body part). Hip or knee replacements are often successfully performed on an elderly person. A person who has had this type of surgery may be admitted to a long-term care facility to recover from the surgery.

Osteoporosis. Osteoporosis is a disease in which loss of calcium causes bones to become brittle. ("Osteo" means bone;

"porosis" means a condition of pores or openings.) The spine is usually affected, causing curvature and a loss of height. The major complication of osteoporosis is a **fracture** (broken bone). Hip fractures are often seen in the elderly. Brittle bones break easily when a person falls. Sometimes the brittle bone breaks first, causing a fall. Osteoporosis is more common in women because of hormonal changes.

Fractures. There are many types of fractures, but the most common are open fractures and closed fractures. In an open fracture, the skin is open, the bone is broken, and there may be severe tissue damage. This type of fracture (also called a compound fracture) requires surgical repair. In a closed fracture, the bone is broken, but the skin is intact or closed. This type of fracture does not usually require surgery.

A fractured bone must be immobilized (kept from moving) until it heals. This is often done by applying a cast. Cast care is discussed in Chapter 24.

Amputation. **Amputation** is the removal of a body part, usually by surgery. Amputation may be the result of an injury or a disease such as diabetes. The amputee may wear a prosthesis, such as an artificial leg. The person with an amputated leg may use crutches or a wheelchair.

Respiratory Problems

The term chronic obstructive pulmonary disease (COPD) is used to describe many of the problems that affect the respiratory system. This phrase is easier to understand if you first define each word. A "chronic disease" is a disease that lasts a long time. "Obstructive" means blocking or stopping something. "Pulmonary" refers to the lungs. Therefore, COPD is a disease that blocks the lungs and lasts for a long time. Emphysema is an example of COPD.

Emphysema. Emphysema is a chronic disease in which changes in the structure of the lungs cause breathing problems. Lung tissue loses its elasticity, and the alveoli remain expanded. Mucus obstructs or plugs the bronchi and bronchioles, making it difficult to get air in and out of the lungs. The lungs gradually enlarge in size. These changes lead to a decrease in the exchange of oxygen and carbon dioxide. The person with emphysema breathes harder and faster in an attempt to get more air. This is called **dyspnea**, which means difficult breathing ("dys" means difficult and "pnea" means breathing).

A decrease in the amount of oxygen affects all systems of the body. Residents with emphysema may be too weak to eat or care for themselves. The mouth may have an unpleasant odor that affects taste and smell. Nutrition is affected as appetite decreases. A person with breathing difficulties must assume a body position that allows maximum lung expansion. This is usually a sitting or upright position. Fear and anxiety are common. Unfortunately, the more upset a person becomes, the more difficult it is to breathe. Have you ever had trouble breathing? If so, were you frightened? How did you act?

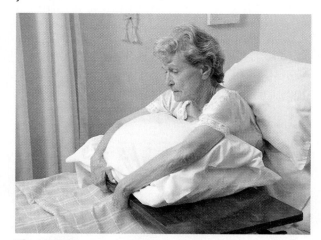

Fig. 12-2 An upright position helps the resident with COPD to breathe easier.

The resident with emphysema is constantly struggling to breathe. Coughing and wheezing are common. The skin is usually pale or there may be **cyanosis** (a blue color caused by a lack of oxygen). Emphysema can result in restlessness, confusion, respiratory failure, coma, and death.

Pneumonia. Pneumonia is an acute infection of the lungs. It often follows a cold or other upper respiratory infection. Symptoms include chills, fever, chest pain, cough, headache, and weakness. Pneumonia can progress to coma and death.

Pneumonia can be treated with antibiotics and other medications. If diagnosed and treated early, it is usually curable. Pneumonia can be serious or fatal in the elderly resident, who may already be weakened from some other condition.

Aspiration pneumonia: Aspiration pneumonia is caused by food or fluid entering the airway, instead of the stomach. **Aspiration** means choking. This can happen to someone who is not alert and oriented or to a person who is vomiting. Residents with feeding tubes are also at risk for this type of pneumonia. Residents who have difficulty swallowing may aspirate. The food or fluid causes irritation of the respiratory tract and leads to infection.

Hypostatic pneumonia: Hypostatic pneumonia results from fluid collecting in the lungs. This type of pneumonia is often a complication of limited activity. Failure to turn and move allows fluid to collect in the lungs. Think about what happens when a wet sponge is placed on a surface. Where does the water settle in the sponge?

Circulatory Problems

Diseases of the heart and blood vessels can range from mild to severe. They can be acute or chronic and may involve all age groups. Some people are born with heart disorders. Heart disease is a leading cause of death in the United States.

Coronary Artery Disease. Coronary artery disease (CAD) causes a narrowing of the coronary arteries in the heart. Changes in the lining of the arteries obstruct the blood vessels. Atherosclerosis or arteriosclerosis (hardening of the arteries) contribute to coronary artery disease. In these situations, the blood supply to the heart muscle is reduced. The heart muscle requires more oxygen than the blood vessels can supply. Blood pressure may be affected by coronary artery disease.

Angina. Angina is an episode of chest pain that occurs when narrowed blood vessels do not allow enough oxygenated blood to reach the heart muscle. The pain often occurs after exercise, eating, or an emotional experience.

Symptoms of angina begin with a sudden, acute pain in the chest. Pain sometimes travels or radiates down the left arm. It usually lasts only a few minutes. This pain can range from mild to agonizing. Treatment is aimed at relieving pain. Rest, diet, and a

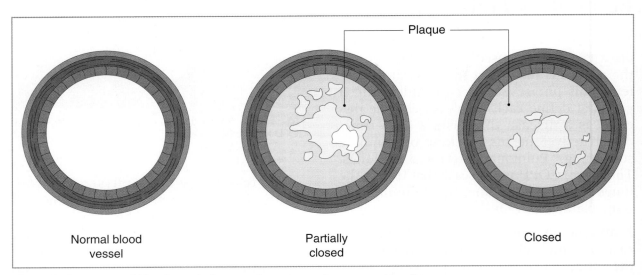

Normal blood vessel   Partially closed   Closed

Fig. 12-3 Narrowed blood vessels decrease the amount of oxygen to the cells.

healthy lifestyle help to reduce the frequency of attacks. During an angina attack, the person is anxious and fearful that a serious heart attack may be occurring. Although a person could die in an attack, most angina sufferers can live for years with proper care.

Myocardial Infarction. A myocardial infarction (MI) is a major heart attack that often results in death. "Myo" means muscle, "cardio" means heart, and "infarction" means death of tissue. Thus a myocardial infarction literally means death of heart muscle. It occurs when there is a sudden blockage of blood flow to the heart muscle. This can be caused by a blood clot or other material blocking the blood vessel. A myocardial infarction sometimes follows an angina attack.

Symptoms of a myocardial infarction generally begin with a sensation of pressure or a sudden, severe, crushing pain in the chest and dyspnea (difficult breathing). The skin is pale or cyanotic (bluish colored). Although the person may be sweating, the skin feels cold to touch. There may be nausea and vomiting. Fear and anxiety may be high.

A myocardial infarction is a life-threatening situation that requires immediate medical attention. The person will usually be taken to a hospital for intensive treatment. Death can occur suddenly. How quickly treatment begins, and the amount of heart damage, determine the outcome.

Congestive Heart Failure. Congestive heart failure (CHF) occurs when the heart fails to pump efficiently. Blood and other body fluids tend to pool or congest in the body. One of the first symptoms observed in CHF is edema. **Edema** is the swelling of a body part with fluid. It is most noticeable in body parts that are farthest from the heart, such as the hands and feet. There is usually weight gain. Since the heart and lungs are congested (filled with fluid), breathing is labored, and the pulse may be irregular. Urine output is usually decreased, because the body is holding fluid. Pain, nausea, and vomiting may be present.

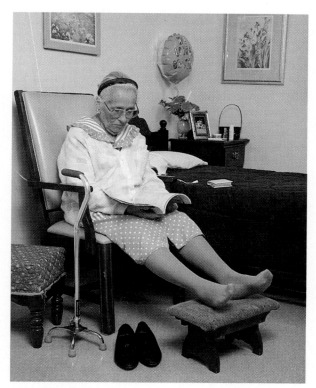

Fig. 12-4 Edema can result from poor circulation.

CHF can become a chronic illness, with acute episodes. An acute attack can result in death.

Hypertension. **Hypertension** is high blood pressure ("hyper" means high; "tension" means pressure). A blood pressure of 140/90 or above is considered high. Although the exact cause of hypertension is not known, factors that contribute to it include heredity, diet, weight, and lifestyle. Hypertension is common in heart disease and diabetes and can lead to other complications, such as a stroke.

Nervous System Problems

Problems of the nervous system may involve the brain, spinal cord, or nerves. These structures control and regulate the activities of the body. Diseases of the nervous system may interfere with thinking, talking, and moving. People with mental or nervous disorders may or may not have other physical problems as well. Mental illness is difficult for families and friends to understand, because their loved one may look healthy and yet be unable to function normally.

Dementia. **Dementia** is an impairment of mental function. Mental illnesses such as schizophrenia cause dementia. It can also be caused by a severe stroke or a series of small strokes. The death of brain cells, due to interruption of blood flow, leads to a loss of mental function.

Residents with dementia are confused and disoriented. The ability to cope is decreased. They are often irritable and angry as they try to adapt to a changing world. The inability to understand what is happening causes them to focus on themselves. As their world narrows, they may appear demanding and thoughtless. It is frightening to lose control of both self and environment. While mental illness is usually treated in mental health facilities, many people with dementia are residents in long-term care facilities.

Alzheimer's Disease. Alzheimer's disease is a progressive nervous disorder that eventually destroys all mental function. Progressive means the disease keeps getting worse. Alzheimer's not only affects old people, but younger age groups as well. It accounts for approximately 50 percent of dementia in the United States. The disease causes problems in thinking, communication, and behavior. As the disease progresses, physical symptoms appear that eventually lead to death.

The first noticeable symptom of Alzheimer's is usually a loss of memory. It is unlike the normal memory loss that may come with aging. As people get older, they often have difficulty remembering names and telephone numbers. The person with Alzheimer's may not remember where home is, or who family members are. Eventually self-identity may be lost. Most residents with Alzheimer's disease are confused and disoriented. They may be anxious or paranoid (overly suspicious). Their attention span is short, because their ability to concentrate is decreased. Impaired judgment prevents the person from knowing right from wrong or safe from unsafe.

Many behavior problems are seen in people suffering from Alzheimer's. They become chronic wanderers, constantly on the move, stopping for a few moments here and there, without purpose. In the long-term care facility, they may enter other residents' rooms or staff areas. When an outer door opens, they may be outside in a flash, with no regard for traffic or other dangers.

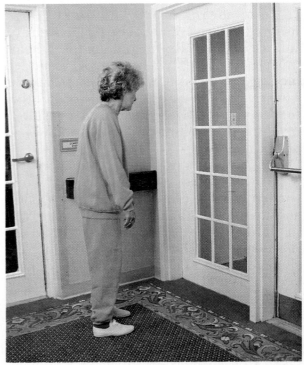

Fig. 12-5 Protecting the resident with Alzheimer's disease is challenging.

Communication skills decrease, and in later stages the person may not talk or appear to listen. Some use the same words or phrases over and over or mumble meaningless words. Socialization becomes difficult or impossible.

The physical symptoms of Alzheimer's include decreased appetite, weight loss, weakness, and loss of mobility. It is difficult to maintain adequate nutrition for a person who loses interest in food and forgets to eat. Hunger pangs go unnoticed. The resident with Alzheimer's may be fed through a tube into the stomach. Many of the normal reflexes are lost as mental and physical deterioration progress. Eventually, the

Alzheimer's resident becomes bedridden. The lack of adequate nutrition and loss of mobility may lead to pneumonia, which is often the cause of death.

Many people who have Alzheimer's are in long-term care facilities. The care they require is so time consuming that caring for them at home is extremely difficult. Many of them were cared for at home until the caregiver became physically and emotionally exhausted.

There is no "typical" Alzheimer's resident. Some are angry and agitated, while others are sweet and gentle. Some endlessly pace the floor, while others sit in one spot for hours. Personality and behavior can change quickly. Much depends on the stage of progression of the disease. Care of the resident suffering from Alzheimer's disease is addressed in a later chapter.

Cerebrovascular Accident. Cerebrovascular accident (CVA) is the correct term for what is commonly called a stroke. "Cerebro" means brain; "vascular" means blood vessels. A cerebrovascular accident is an accident in the blood vessels in the brain. Either something blocks a blood vessel, or the vessel ruptures (breaks open). Frequently, the cause is a blood clot. The affected area of the brain is left without a blood supply and, therefore, without oxygen. The oxygen-deprived brain cells die.

A stroke may occur because the blood pressure is too high. In this situation, the person often complains of a headache and dizziness. This might continue for hours or days before the pressure damages the blood vessel. However, a stroke may also happen suddenly, with no warning. Symptoms may vary from a mild dizzy spell to coma and death.

A stroke is always serious. Strokes are not only a leading cause of death in the United States, they cause a large number of illnesses and disabilities. The type of disability depends on the area of the brain involved and the amount of damage to the area. A CVA in one side of the brain will affect the opposite side of the body. There are areas of the brain that control speech, thinking, and

movement. A CVA in the speech center will affect the ability to speak. A CVA in the area that controls movement will affect the ability to move. **Paralysis**, the inability to move a body part, is common.

The resident who has had a stroke can have many problems, affecting any of the body systems. Difficulties in swallowing, digestion, and elimination are common.

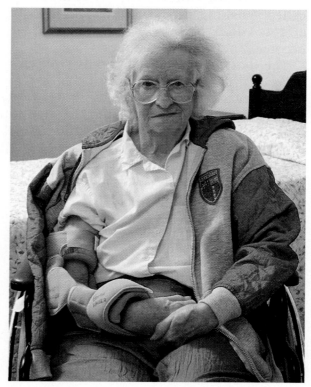

Fig. 12-6 A CVA may result in weakness or paralysis of one side of the body.

Multiple Sclerosis. Multiple sclerosis (MS) is a progressive disease that primarily affects the brain and spinal cord. Myelin, the substance that insulates nerve fibers, deteriorates and is replaced by scar tissue. The scar tissue interferes with the transmission of nerve impulses. This results in numbness, tremors, staggering gait, weakness, paralysis, and loss of balance and coordination. The resident with MS may be in a wheelchair. There may be vision and speech problems. Although intelligence is usually not affected, there may be emotional instability. Because of these problems, residents with MS may be unable to care for themselves.

MS usually begins at an early age, between 20 and 40. Although the person's condition progressively gets worse, there may be periods of time when the disease symptoms level off or seem to disappear. This makes appropriate treatment difficult.

Parkinson's Disease. Parkinson's disease is a chronic disease that causes loss of control of motor function. It is commonly called "shaking palsy." Parkinson's usually affects older people, and its symptoms become more severe as the years pass.

The most noticeable symptoms are trembling, stiffness, and a shuffling walk. The person with Parkinson's usually shows very little facial expression, causing the face to look like a mask. There is difficulty swallowing and handling oral secretions. The person may have trouble performing activities of daily living (ADLs) independently. Communication problems are common. The disease can progress very slowly, so you might see a resident in long-term care in any stage of Parkinson's.

Nervous System Injuries. Most injuries of the nervous system involve either the brain or the spinal cord. These injuries may be caused by falls, vehicular accidents, sports accidents, or bullet wounds. Many of the younger residents of a long-term care facility are there because of an injury to the nervous system.

An injury to the nervous system may result in one of the following forms of paralysis:

- **Hemiplegia** (paralysis of one side of the body)
- **Paraplegia** (paralysis of the lower half of the body)
- **Quadriplegia** (paralysis of both arms and legs)

Don't be overwhelmed by the "plegias." "Plegia" means paralysis. That gives you the first clue. "Quad" means four. You have four extremities (arms and legs). That makes understanding quadriplegia easy. "Hemi" and "para" both mean half, so how do you tell them apart? A "paraplegic" puts on a "pair of pants" over the legs, so a paraplegic has both legs paralyzed. A hemiplegic is paralyzed on one side.

Brain injuries may result in severe bleeding, blood clots, and swelling. These complications can cause further damage. Symptoms of a brain injury will depend on the location and severity of the damage. Any part of the body may be affected. Weakness, dizziness, headache, loss of coordination, spasms, or seizures may occur. A **seizure** (convulsion) is a sudden spasm of muscle contractions and relaxations. Partial or complete paralysis may occur. Vision and hearing problems are common. Mental changes may include irritability, restlessness, confusion, or amnesia (loss of memory). The person with a brain injury may be comatose. **Comatose** means unconscious or unable to respond.

Spinal cord injuries most often affect young males between the ages of 10 and 25. Symptoms depend on whether the spinal cord is damaged or severed (cut in two). If the cord is damaged, there may be weakness, spasms, or paralysis. There may not be complete paralysis in this situation. However, if the cord is severed, the result will be total paralysis of body structures below the injury. Paralysis can result in the inability to control urine or bowel movements. Most paraplegics and quadriplegics in long-term care have suffered a spinal cord injury.

Sensory Problems

The most common problems of the sensory system involve loss of vision or hearing. The majority of elderly people are affected to some degree by one or both of these disorders. This can result in communication difficulties and a loss of independence.

Ears. Hearing problems can range from slightly hard-of-hearing to total deafness. One or both ears may be affected. The loss might involve low-, medium-, or high-pitched sounds, or a combination. There are two basic types of hearing loss. One kind can be helped by a hearing aid, which makes sounds louder. The other type of hearing loss is not usually helped by a hearing aid.

Hearing loss can be caused by disease, noise, or injury. It is also affected by the changes of aging. Communicating with, and caring for, the hearing-impaired resident is discussed in other chapters.

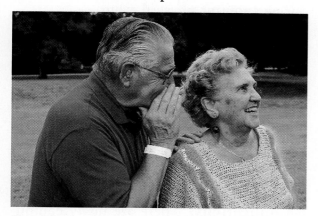

Fig. 12-7 A hearing aid makes communication easier for the resident who is hearing impaired.

Eyes. People of all ages, including children, may have vision problems. They may be nearsighted (can see things that are near but distant vision is poor) or farsighted (can see things that are far away but have difficulty with close vision). Many people who have good vision in their younger years become farsighted as they get older. They have difficulty seeing small print and tend to hold reading material at a distance in an attempt to see better. Although some of these conditions may respond to surgery, people who have these problems usually wear eyeglasses or contact lenses.

There are two other eye conditions that are frequently seen in elderly people.

Cataracts: A cataract is a clouding of the lens of the eye. As the lens loses its transparency, there is a gradual loss of vision that can lead to blindness. A person may have a cataract in one or both eyes.

Cataracts can be caused by disease, injury, or aging. The main symptom is a gradual decrease in vision. The condition is usually not painful. As the cataract progresses, the pupil of the eye appears white and cloudy.

Treatment of cataracts includes corrective eyeglasses, contact lenses, or surgery. Surgery involves removing the diseased lens and implanting a new one. Because it is a

relatively quick, safe procedure, cataract surgery can be done on even a frail, elderly resident.

Glaucoma: Glaucoma is a disease in which pressure within the eye gradually destroys the optic nerve. There are several kinds of glaucoma, and it can be acute or chronic. Although the cause is unknown, high blood pressure and diabetes are related factors. It tends to occur in members of the same family, and the chance of developing glaucoma increases with age.

Symptoms of glaucoma include headaches and a decrease in the field of vision. Some complain of seeing "halos." However, in early glaucoma there may be no symptoms at all. Treatment includes eye drops and other medications. Surgery is sometimes helpful.

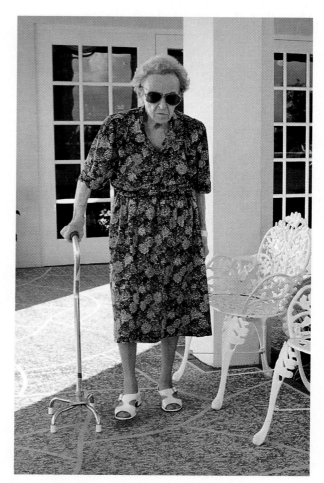

Fig. 12-8 The person who is blind can still be independent.

Diabetes Mellitus

Diabetes mellitus is a chronic disease that results when insulin is not produced or not used properly by the body. Insulin is a hormone, produced in the pancreas, that changes sugar to energy for the body's use. When the body can't use sugar, it will use fat. The breakdown of fat produces acetone (ketones). The ketones and unused sugar can build to toxic levels in the blood. The disease is commonly called "sugar diabetes" or just "diabetes."

Types of Diabetes. There are several types of diabetes, but the most common are Type I and Type II.

Type I Diabetes: Type I diabetes causes the diabetic to be insulin dependent. Because the body produces little or no insulin, it must be given by injection. Type I used to be called juvenile diabetes because it primarily affected young people. Only a small percentage of diabetics are Type I.

Type II Diabetes: Type II diabetes does not cause insulin dependence. This diabetic may produce a normal amount of insulin, but for some reason, the body can't use it. Type II diabetes is often controlled with diet and exercise. Oral medication or insulin may also be needed. This type of diabetes affects an older age group—people in their fifties and sixties. Ninety percent of all known diabetics are Type II.

Cause of Diabetes. The exact cause of diabetes is not known. However, there are certain factors that contribute to the development of the disease. Diabetes is hereditary, which means that it can be passed from generation to generation. The primary risk factor is obesity. **Obese** means very fat. The majority of Type II diabetics are overweight. Women are more at risk than men, and the risk increases with age.

Symptoms of Diabetes. The symptoms of diabetes include frequent urination, thirst, and hunger. The diabetic tires easily and may have weight loss, even though food intake has increased. There may be vision problems or sores that won't heal. Some dia-betics are depressed. Women may complain of vaginal itching. Tests will show a high level of sugar in the blood. Type I diabetics are usually diagnosed in an emergency setting at an early age. Type II is often detected during a routine physical exam.

Treatment of Diabetes. Although there is presently no cure for diabetes, many complications can be prevented. Treatment for diabetes includes diet, exercise, oral medication, and insulin. Treatment begins with an individually planned diet and exercise program. Oral medications are sometimes effective. Some diabetics must have insulin injections. The goal in managing diabetes is to keep the blood sugar level within a normal range.

Complications. There are many complications of diabetes. Some are short term, occur quickly, and may be relieved by prompt treatment. Hyperglycemia and hypoglycemia are examples of short-term complications.

When the blood sugar is high, or above normal, it is called **hyperglycemia**. ("Hyper" means high, "glyc" means sugar, and "emia" means blood). It can result from eating too much, eating the wrong foods, or not exercising enough. High blood sugar may also lead to diabetic coma. Hyperglycemia is treated with medications to decrease the amount of sugar in the blood.

Low blood sugar is called **hypoglycemia**. It can be caused by skipping a meal (not eating enough), too much exercise, too much medication, or an illness. People with low blood sugar may go into insulin shock. The treatment for hypoglycemia is simple sugar, such as candy, sweetened orange juice, or administration of glucose.

Either of these reactions to blood sugar level can result in coma or death. It is important that you know the symptoms of hyperglycemia and hypoglycemia. The chart in Fig. 12-9 will help you to understand the difference in the two reactions.

Long-term complications occur gradually and may go unnoticed. Most problems occur as a result of years of uncontrolled diabetes. They can lead to blindness, amputation, and death.

	HYPERGLYCEMIA (Diabetic Coma)	**HYPOGLYCEMIA** (Insulin Shock)
Behavior	Sluggish	Irritable, excited, dizziness, coma
Skin	Hot, dry, flushed	Cold, clammy, pale
Breathing	Deep, fruity odor	Shallow
Pulse	Slow to normal	Rapid, thready
Speech	Slurred	Normal
Urine	Glucose and acetone present	No glucose or acetone
Possible Causes	Overeating, infection, vomiting, not enough insulin	Not eating enough, excessive exercise or activity, too much insulin

Fig. 12-9 Signs and symptoms of hyperglycemia and hypoglycemia.

One of the most serious long-term complications involves the circulatory system. Changes in the blood vessels slow the flow of blood throughout the body. Because of this, the diabetic is more prone to heart attacks, high blood pressure, and strokes. Kidney problems often occur. Slowed circulation means that sores don't heal and infection frequently occurs. Impaired circulation to the feet and legs results in infection that may turn to gangrene (a serious infection that causes tissue death). Gangrene can lead to amputation.

Nerve damage results in a loss of sensation in the nerve endings. A feeling of numbness may occur, placing the diabetic at risk for burns and other injuries. Diabetics have vision problems that can lead to blindness. Personality changes, confusion, and disorientation may occur. Diabetics who keep their disease under control can avoid many of these complications.

Nursing Care. The nursing assistant plays an important role in the care of the diabetic resident. The resident will be on a diabetic diet to maintain correct blood sugar levels. Encourage the resident to eat all the food that is served. The daily diet is divided between three meals and snacks. If the resident does not eat all the food, hypoglycemia may result. Let the nurse know which foods were not eaten, so the proper supplements can be offered. Remember that snacks are included in the total count. The diabetic diet is discussed in detail in Chapter 21.

Serve the resident's food on time. The diabetic must eat at regular intervals to keep the blood sugar at normal levels. If the resident doesn't like a certain food, check with the nurse to determine a substitute. The resident should avoid foods that are not included in the dietary plan. However, some diabetics may insist on eating foods that are not allowed on their diet. Do not argue or take food away from the resident. Remember that the resident has the right to refuse dietary or any other treatment. Let the nurse know if there is a problem.

Encourage the resident to be active. Exercise is part of the treatment for diabetes. It provides physical and emotional benefits to the resident. Activity also builds appetite and aids digestion. Report any change in the resident's normal activity.

Observing and reporting are important responsibilities of the nursing assistant. Report any signs or symptoms of hyperglycemia or hypoglycemia. Note any change in the resident's mood, behavior, or personality. Watch for skin problems and signs of infection.

You may be asked to perform a urine test for sugar and acetone. The procedure is discussed in Chapter 24.

Foot Care. Slowed circulation and nerve damage place the feet and legs of the diabetic resident at risk for injury, infection, and gangrene. The feet require special attention to prevent complications.

GUIDELINES FOR PROVIDING FOOT CARE FOR THE RESIDENT WITH DIABETES

- Examine the feet at least once daily and observe for discoloration or injury.
- Report any injury immediately, no matter how slight it may be.
- Wash the feet daily and dry thoroughly, especially between the toes.
- Toenails must be carefully trimmed. In many states, nursing assistants are not allowed to cut toenails. Follow facility policy.
- Encourage regular exercise.
- Keep bed linens loose over the resident's feet to prevent pressure.
- Check to see that shoes and socks fit well. Socks should not be elastic.
- Inspect shoes and socks for tears or objects that might injure the foot.

Cancer

Cancer (CA) is a disease that can affect any system of the body. It begins with a body cell that changes to a cancer cell. Cancer cells grow and divide rapidly. They use food and oxygen that are needed by normal cells. Cancer cells group to form tumors. A tumor is a mass of tissue that grows in the body and performs no useful function. Tumors can be benign or malignant. A benign tumor is not cancerous, grows slowly, and does not spread. A malignant tumor grows rapidly and spreads to other body tissues. Cancer cells form malignant tumors and can metastasize (spread to other parts of the body). As they grow and spread they interfere with normal body functions. For example, a malignant tumor in the lung will interfere with breathing.

Cancer affects all age groups, from newborn babies to the very old. However, over 50 percent of cancer patients are elderly. Although cancer can be treated and sometimes cured, it remains one of the leading causes of death in the United States. Although the cause of cancer is unknown, research indicates that a number of factors are involved. These factors include viruses, immune response, diet, and heredity.

Exposure to certain substances (carcinogens) is known to cause cancer. Some carcinogens include tobacco smoke, asbestos, pesticides and other chemicals, sunlight,

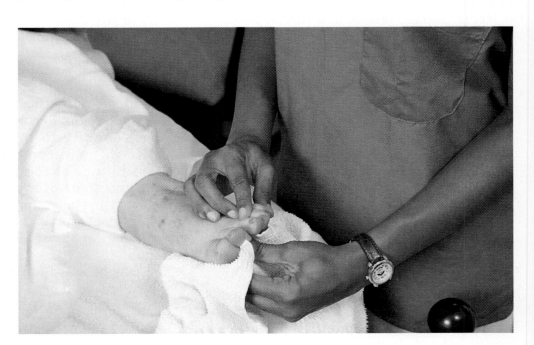

Fig. 12-10
Proper foot care can help prevent some of the complications of diabetes.

X- rays, and other types of radiation. We are exposed to many carcinogens in our normal, everyday life. They are found in the environment—in our food, water, and air. Some carcinogens are present because human activities have polluted the environment. Cigarette smoke has been shown to cause lung cancer, not only in the smokers, but in the people around them. When people stop smoking, there is a decrease in the occurrence of lung cancer. Prevention of pollution reduces the number of carcinogens in the environment.

A resident with cancer may have many problems. Weakness, loss of appetite, and skin breakdown can occur. A decrease in mobility and independence are common. Some cancers cause pain. Confusion and disorientation may result.

A diagnosis of cancer causes many anxieties and fears. Anxiety concerning treatment, fear of death, and fear of the unknown can affect the resident, the family, and the health care workers. They may be influenced by some of the false beliefs about cancer. For example, some may be afraid that cancer is contagious. Many people believe that a diagnosis of cancer is a death sentence. The person with cancer may ask many questions. Will there be pain? Will I be disfigured and look abnormal? Will the treatments make me sicker than I already am? Will I lose my hair? Will my family still love me? Am I going to die? There is concern about the possible loss of independence and control. Death is always a possibility.

Cancer can be treated by surgery, radiation, chemotherapy, or a combination of those methods. The goal of treatment is to prevent the spread of cancer cells by destroying them. Both radiation and chemotherapy can also harm normal tissue. The side effects of these types of treatment include nausea, diarrhea, and hair loss.

Today, many types of cancer can be cured. Early diagnosis and treatment can mean the difference between life and death. According to the American Cancer Society, early warning signs of cancer are:

- A change in bowel or bladder habits
- A sore that does not heal
- Unusual bleeding or discharge
- A lump or thickening in the breast or elsewhere in the body
- Indigestion or difficulty swallowing
- An obvious change in size or shape of a wart or mole
- A nagging cough or hoarseness

It is your responsibility to observe early warning signs of cancer in the resident. You may be the first to notice them. You can help prevent cancer by careful observation and reporting.

Conclusion

Remember these important points:

1. A problem in one system will affect other systems.

2. Diseases and injuries of the musculoskeletal system often interfere with mobility.

3. The most common problem of the respiratory system is chronic obstructive pulmonary disease.

4. Heart disease is a leading cause of death in the United States.

5. Alzheimer's is a disease that eventually destroys all mental function.

6. Multiple sclerosis causes loss of balance and coordination.

7. The most common problems of the sensory system involve loss of vision or hearing.

8. Diabetes is a chronic disease that affects the body's ability to use insulin to change sugar to energy.

9. Many of the complications in diabetes are the result of impaired circulation.

10. The feet of the diabetic resident require special attention to prevent complications.

11. Cancer can affect any system of the body.

12. The prevention of pollution reduces the number of carcinogens in the environment.

13. Early diagnosis of cancer is very important.

14. Everyone should be aware of the seven early warning signs of cancer.

Discussion Questions

1. Do you know anyone who has breathing problems? How do they act? What emotions do they show?

2. What are some of the complications that you might observe in a person who has had a stroke?

3. How do you think a paralyzed young man would feel if he were admitted to a long-term care facility?

4. The diabetic resident asks you to buy her a candy bar. She says that she gets "jittery" sometimes, and the candy makes her feel better. What would you do?

5. What are some of the emotions you would feel if a loved one was diagnosed with cancer?

Application Exercise

1. The students will work as a group to write questions and answers that will be used for a game of "Jeopardy," concerning common health problems of the elderly. They will then divide into teams and compete. A team response unit may be used.

Psychosocial Needs of the Resident

OBJECTIVES

Upon completing this chapter, you will be able to do the following:

1. List the five basic needs of all human beings.

2. Explain the concept of caring for the "whole" person.

3. Describe the effect of culture, spirituality, and religion upon the resident's basic needs.

4. Describe the effects of major psychosocial changes upon the elderly.

5. Identify four examples of restorative care that help to meet the resident's psychosocial needs.

6. Identify four facts about sexuality of the elderly.

7. List three guidelines for care of the resident with Alzheimer's disease.

8. Identify four possible causes of each of the following: confusion, depression, and aggressiveness.

9. Describe the care required by confused, depressed, and aggressive residents.

10. Describe reality orientation and validation therapy.

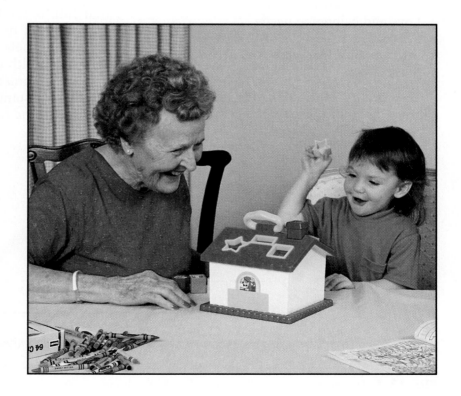

VOCABULARY

The following words or terms will help you to understand this chapter:

Physical needs
Psychosocial needs
Self-actualization
Adapt

Stimuli
Disruptive behavior
Disorientation
Dementia

Sundowner's syndrome
Reality orientation (RO)
Validation therapy
Rapport

Basic Needs

Physical needs and psychosocial needs are two types of basic needs shared by all human beings. **Physical needs** are the needs of the body. You may remember the meaning of the word physical by recalling that a "physical" exam is an examination of the body, just as physical needs are needs of the body. **Psychosocial needs** are emotional, social, and spiritual needs. "Psycho" means thoughts and emotions; "social" means contact and involvement with others. Many psychosocial needs are met through interaction with others. Basic human needs include

- Physical needs
- Safety and security needs
- Love and belonging needs
- Self-esteem needs
- Self-actualization needs (the need to prove oneself)

The quality of life depends upon the fulfillment of all of these basic needs.

Abraham Maslow, a scientist, listed the five basic needs in the order of their importance. As you can see in Fig. 13-1, he illustrated these needs by using a pyramid. The most basic needs are the foundation that supports all other needs. If the physical needs of the foundation are not met, the pyramid will crumble and the upper portion (the higher levels) will fall.

The Whole Person. In nursing, it is important to care for the "whole" person, which includes caring for both the physical and the psychosocial needs of the resident. You will spend much time learning procedures for the care of the resident's body, because physical care is very important. However, it is also important to provide care that fulfills the resident's emotional, social, and spiritual needs. To have quality of life, the psychosocial needs must be met. Perfect physical health does not mean much if it is not accompanied by emotional health. As a nursing assistant you will find it challenging to meet all the residents' needs.

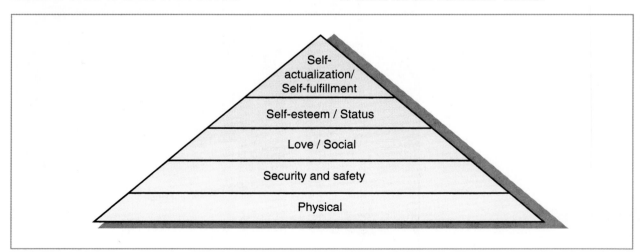

Fig. 13-1 Physical needs are the foundation for all other human needs.

Physical Needs. The most basic needs are the physical needs, which include oxygen, food, water, rest, and hygiene. These needs must be met to prevent death. If the physical needs are not met, other, higher needs become unimportant. An individual can be concerned with higher needs, only when physical needs have been met, and life is not in danger. For example, a resident who is having difficulty breathing may not want to leave the room to socialize. When breathing improves, the need for social contact will become important again. The resident may then decide to attend social activities. Social contact fulfills the need for love and belonging, which is one of the higher needs.

The Need for Safety and Security. The second level of basic needs is the need for safety and security. Being safe and secure means that an individual is free from harm. Having money, a job, and a safe place to stay meet a person's need for security. Being able to trust others and to trust one's environment increases a person's feelings of safety and security.

The Need for Love and Belonging. The need for love and belonging is the need for affection and to feel "connected" with others. This need may be met by belonging to a group such as a family, a church, or an organization. Meaningful relationships with other people fulfill the need for love and belonging.

The Need for Self-Esteem. This is the need to feel good about oneself. Feeling important and useful helps to meet the need for self-esteem. Self-esteem is fulfilled by the roles we hold throughout life. When we are needed by others we feel that we are important. Being able to care for oneself also improves self-esteem.

The Need for Self-Actualization. This is the highest need and can be met only when all other needs are fulfilled. When something is "actual" it is "real" and has been proven by facts. With this definition in mind, you might think of **self-actualization** as "proving yourself." Accepting challenges and meeting goals that you have set are examples of self-actualization. Spiritual fulfillment is also self-actualization. Learning, creating, and striving to achieve all help to meet the need for self-actualization. Completion of a class is an example of self-actualization.

The following example might help you understand the importance of meeting the lower basic needs first. Completing a class (self-actualization) would be difficult or impossible if some of your lower needs were unmet. Illness (unmet physical needs) may affect your ability to study and learn. If your safety is threatened (loss of safety) or you don't have enough money (loss of security), you may have difficulty concentrating. A divorce (loss of love and belonging) might cause a student to drop out of class. If you don't believe you can learn (loss of self-esteem), then you might not have enough confidence to enter a class. Your success in class might be less important than other problems.

Sometimes you may be able to meet higher needs without first meeting all the lower needs. However, the higher needs would lose importance, because one's energy and attention would be turned to meeting the more basic needs first.

The resident's unmet needs are included in the care plan. Many of the approaches that will be used to meet these needs will be the responsibility of the nursing assistant. Be familiar with the resident's care plan, and review it often, to fulfill your role in assuring that all basic needs are met.

Culture, Spirituality, and Religion

Each person's needs, and methods for meeting those needs, are influenced by culture, spirituality, and religion. Culture is passed to future generations through customs, values, and beliefs. Examples of cultural groups (also referred to as ethnic groups) include nationalities, races, religions, families, and social groups. A group of people who have the same cultural background usually share the same values and beliefs. They may also share customs, clothing, and food preferences.

There are many cultures. You may get a better understanding of the difference in cultures by thinking of someone from another country. Consider the differences that exist. What kind of clothing do they wear? Are their favorite foods the same as yours? Do family roles and interactions differ from yours? Remember that a person's nationality is not the only cultural influence.

Religion and spirituality are part of one's cultural background. Religion, however, is not the only type of spiritual expression. Expressing spirituality gives a sense of fulfillment, joy, and emotional energy. You may be familiar with the phrase, "My spirits are high." Each person will express spirituality in a unique and individual way. This may be accomplished by creative efforts, by service to others, or by religious practices.

For many people, religious practices express spirituality. A group of people with similar beliefs and spiritual needs may join to form an organized religion. Religion may also be practiced through personal beliefs, without participation in a group. Culture and religion influence a person's beliefs and practices in regard to health. Beliefs about the cause and cure of disease may be influenced by religion and culture. Many find comfort in religion in times of illness. One's spirit is as individual as one's personality.

Psychosocial Changes Affecting the Elderly

In the course of a lifetime, each of us fills many roles that help us meet our psychosocial needs and form our personalities. One person may be a mother or father, a daughter or son, a civic leader, and a career person. As we proceed through life, our circumstances and roles change, and we must adapt. To **adapt** means to change or adjust. Although roles change, an individual's personality usually remains fairly stable throughout life.

Major adjustments are necessary as a person ages. The elderly must adapt to many stressful role changes. The younger person is usually not faced with so many changes at one time. Significant psychosocial changes such as retirement, loss of income, loss of a spouse, loss of health, and loss of home may have a severe effect upon the emotional health of the elderly person. In these situations psychosocial needs may become difficult to meet. For example, being unable to drive or to afford a car makes it difficult to socialize and be independent.

In America we have been taught to value youth and usefulness. Growing old, without an important role to play, leaves some elderly individuals with low self-esteem and a poor sense of self-worth.

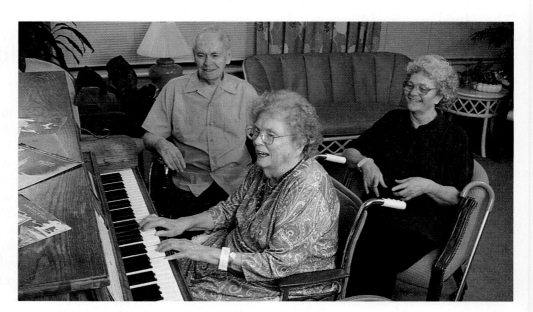

Fig. 13-2

Music is an expression of spirituality, joy and emotional energy.

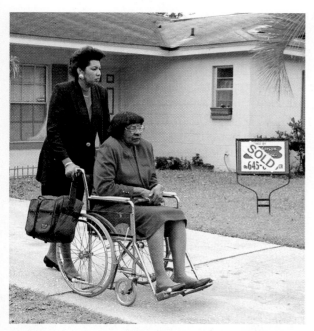

Fig. 13-3 As a person ages, major adjustments are necessary.

Psychosocial Needs of the Resident in the Long-Term Care Facility

Some elderly people who become chronically ill and dependent must be admitted to a long-term care facility. Leaving one's own environment to enter a facility causes problems. It is difficult to feel loved when you are separated from your loved ones. Being dependent upon others affects self-esteem. Sharing living quarters with many others makes it difficult to maintain one's privacy and individuality. Can you recall a time when you lived among a large number of people? Did you find that it was difficult to find privacy, or to have time alone?

It is your responsibility as a nursing assistant to help the resident be independent and maintain, or regain, a sense of self-esteem. The resident's safety and security depend upon you. You are a daily source of love, and you are the one who will help to accomplish goals. Report any signs of unmet needs that you observe, so they can be addressed in the resident's care plan. You are the resident's life line to health, happiness, and well-being.

Restorative Measures to Meet the Resident's Psychosocial Needs

Helping the resident to regain independence is a basic step toward helping to meet many other psychosocial needs. Self-esteem, privacy, and freedom to socialize are all influenced by the ability to do things for oneself. Encouraging the resident's independence is an invitation to use your creativity.

Allowing and encouraging residents to make decisions, assist with their own care, and be as active as possible are restorative measures that can challenge your imagination. Noticing and drawing the resident's attention to the smallest act of independence is a finely tuned talent that you can develop. Successfully assisting the resident to achieve independence and improve self-esteem will meet your own need for self-actualization. Your self-esteem will increase by helping another succeed.

Safety and Security. Being in control of your own safety is reassuring, whereas having to depend on others for safety and security is frightening. Can you imagine how frightening it would be to know that you were helpless to protect yourself from harm? Many of the residents are totally dependent upon the staff for survival. Their need for safety and a sense of security can be met by following safety rules. These include the safe use of equipment and side rails, using proper body mechanics, preventing the spread of infection, and identifying residents correctly. Safety measures are discussed in an earlier chapter.

It is important to provide a sense of security by developing trusting relationships with residents. If you carry through on your promises to them, they will feel more secure. They will know that they can count on you when it is necessary. Showing them your concern for their welfare, encouraging them to discuss their concerns with you and listening carefully, will reassure them of their safety.

Love and Belonging. Nursing assistants help to meet the residents' need for love by caring about them and being sensitive to their needs. Taking time to talk with residents, giving encouragement and praise, and listening attentively helps them to feel loved and appreciated. While you are using verbal communication skills, remember the importance of nonverbal skills. A smile, a touch on the shoulder, and a hug all communicate love. Love is usually returned to you through the residents' responses to your care.

Some residents have very few visitors, which increases their need to interact with other residents, staff members, and volunteers. Communicating with others and participating in social activities helps to restore the sense of belonging. For many residents, staff members and other residents become "family." Remember to introduce residents to people they don't know.

While you are encouraging the resident to socialize, remember the importance of hearing aids and clean glasses. Without these, some residents would be "alone" in a crowd. Their efforts to reach out to others might be useless. Remember, also, that you must assist many residents to attend activities that help to fulfill the resident's need for love and belonging. Assisting with ambulation or providing a wheelchair or walker may be necessary to help the resident socialize. Have you realized how important your assistance is? The resident who feels the most unloved and isolated may not be able to be with others unless you help with small details.

Self-Esteem. The resident's self-esteem is improved by many of the same things that help you feel better about yourself. Helping the resident to be well groomed, to keep things in order, and to feel loved and useful are self-esteem builders. Encouraging the resident to be independent also helps self-image. An increase in independence promotes a sense of well-being. Treating the resident as an individual and giving praise for accomplishments, leads to a feeling of value. Knowing that someone has an interest in you and wants to know more about you, may raise your self-esteem. Do you like to be listened to when you have something to share?

Our interactions with others pass through a "self-esteem filter." If others' reactions are positive toward us—then we tend to feel good about ourselves. If those reactions from others are negative or unkind—then our self-image may be affected in a negative way. Be aware of your attitudes and interactions with residents, and make sure you send positive esteem messages to them.

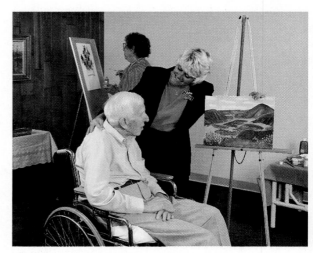

Fig. 13-4 Giving praise helps the resident feel valued.

Self-Actualization. Provided that more basic needs have been met, the resident may be ready to pursue some higher goals that will increase their joy in life. Your creativity will be useful in helping the resident find ways to meet the need for self-actualization. Helping the resident toward goals will be rewarding for both of you. A resident might work toward meeting a health care goal such as walking, grooming, or eating without assistance. Specific goals will be written in the care plan of each resident.

Social activities provide many opportunities for self-actualization. Creative projects such as painting, writing poetry, or participating in a music group provide a way for residents to feel that they have accomplished something. Participating in committee work, or helping to plan a project, may be satisfying to some. Remembering and sharing life stories and events helps restore a sense of pride in their accomplishments earlier in life.

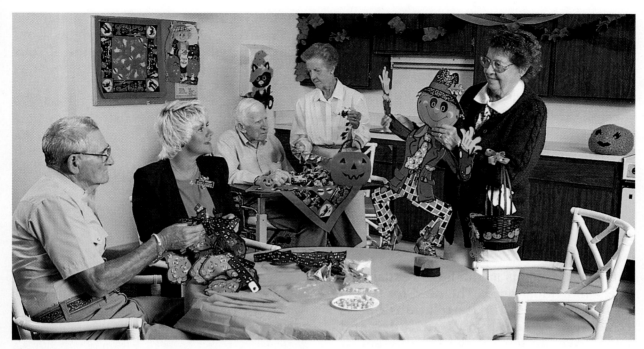

Fig. 13-5 Working together on a project helps to meet higher needs.

Religious expression is an important part of meeting the need for self-actualization. The nursing assistant must respect and accept each resident's religious and spiritual beliefs. Do not attempt to influence the resident with your own spiritual beliefs. Assist the resident to meet spiritual needs according to personal desire. Requests for visits by religious representatives or clergy should be reported to the nurse without delay. Provide privacy for the visit.

Assist the resident who wants to attend religious services and activities. Listen respectfully if the resident wishes to discuss spiritual concerns. Learning about the religious beliefs and practices of others will help you understand and gain respect for them. Be respectful of clothing and objects that may have religious importance to the resident.

Feeling that we have accomplished something, and that we have produced some "goodness" in our lives, is important. Remember that all of us are encouraged by compliments, praise, and attention from others. Your interest in the resident's accomplishments helps to restore a sense of value and worth.

Remember, also, that a positive self-image contributes to a person's motivation. Can you recall a time when you felt so good about yourself that you wanted to take on a new challenge, or do something exciting? You had a need for self-actualization. As you help the residents to succeed, be aware of your own feelings of pride, joy, and success. This is an opportunity for one of the most satisfying rewards of nursing.

Sexuality and the Elderly

Sexuality is as much a part of the whole person as spirituality. Each of us is born a sexual being. Beyond birth our sexuality is influenced psychosocially. Usually girls are encouraged to acquire feminine actions and participate in feminine activities, while boys are encouraged to practice masculine actions and activities. Interest in dolls and sports, housework and mechanics, makeup, hairstyles, and dress help to influence sexuality. Can you recall some of the influences on your sexual identity during childhood?

Sexual fulfillment is not only physical, it includes a need for closeness, love, and affection. Most sexual relationships include a warm and caring attitude between the partners.

Sexual Myths and Facts. Sexuality in the elderly is the subject of many myths (false beliefs). Some of these myths are

- Sex and intimacy are not important or acceptable for the elderly.
- Elderly women have no interest in sex.
- The elderly are not able to have sexual intercourse.
- Elderly men and women are not attractive to each other.
- Appearance is not important to the elderly.

These statements are all false. Sexuality is a very individual need. The need for sexual fulfillment and intimate relationships is influenced by a person's attitudes and beliefs. We are born with sexuality and it remains with us until death. The sexual needs of a person continue throughout life. Patterns of sexual fulfillment generally remain the same. The elderly person experiences many losses during old age. The need for the warmth, caring, and security of a close relationship with another may become greater.

Some changes in the elderly person's sexual activity may occur. The physical changes of aging in the reproductive system cause some problems. These changes are discussed in Chapter 11. The length of time required for arousal, erection, and orgasm may be increased as a result of the physical changes of aging. The frequency of sexual intercourse may decrease. Chronic illness, fatigue, and fear of being unable to perform sexually may interfere with sexual fulfillment. Immobility or pain may affect the elderly person's usual pattern of sexual activity. Loss of a sexual partner is a common problem for elderly individuals.

Sexuality in the Long-Term Care Facility. When an elderly person becomes a resident of a long-term care facility, additional burdens are placed upon the need for sexual fulfillment. Even though married partners may share a room, they often sleep in separate hospital beds. Privacy becomes a problem because there is always a possibility that someone may come to the room. Concern about what others may think if they stay to themselves or close the door may worry the couple.

For individuals who no longer have a spouse, finding a suitable partner may be a problem. Expression of love and affection may present obstacles for single elderly residents who develop intimate relationships with each other.

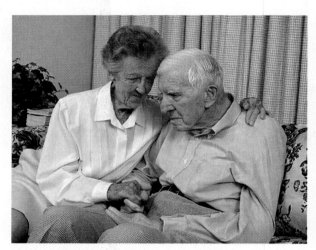

Fig. 13-6 Love and affection are satisfying.

Sexual fulfillment can be achieved in ways other than sexual intercourse. Expression of affection such as kissing, hugging, and hand-holding are also sexually satisfying. For some residents, sexual self-stimulation through masturbation may relieve tension and provide sexual satisfaction. Masturbation is a normal form of sexual fulfillment.

In the past, beliefs about sex created an attitude of nonacceptance of sexuality. Today, we know that sexuality is an important part of the whole person and must be fulfilled according to an individual's needs. Meeting the needs of the whole person assures total health and well-being.

Allowing Residents to Meet Their Sexual Needs. One of the greatest problems in dealing with sexuality in the long-term care facility is the discomfort of staff members. We may become embarrassed when confronted with the sexuality of another person. Many of us have been taught to value the privacy of sexual matters and to look with disapproval upon public display of sexuality. When the sexuality of others is brought to our attention, it is not unusual for us to feel uncomfortable. A normal tendency may be to giggle or laugh in an attempt to "lighten" our discomfort or to minimize it. Some of us might become angry and wish to immediately stop the situation that leads to our embarrassment.

As a nursing assistant you must be able to overcome these personal reactions. It is the staff's responsibility to support residents' rights by allowing the fulfillment of the resident's sexual needs. Being knowledgeable about sexuality in the elderly will help. Comfort with your own sexuality, and concern for the resident's quality of life, will also help you to handle these situations correctly. Can you imagine yourself as a resident of a long-term care facility? Would you find it difficult to fulfill your sexual needs? As you consider this, you may develop empathy for the residents.

Encouraging and assisting the resident in grooming is important. Your compliments are helpful. Personal appearance and a positive self-image are the cornerstones that support a person's sexual identity. Makeup, shaving, fragrance, and clothing make a statement about a person's sexuality. Femininity and masculinity are enhanced by these.

Protect the resident's privacy by preventing exposure of the body during care. Close the door if it seems appropriate to do so, and knock before entering a resident's room. Allow time for the resident to respond before entering. Advise other staff members if you know that the resident wants time alone.

Accept displays of affection between residents as a natural part of human relationships. Also, accept the residents' individual preferences of sexual expression. Your own standards cannot be imposed upon others. Do not be judgmental or gossip. Accept the resident's individuality. Married couples are allowed to share a room in the long-term care facility. Encourage single residents to get acquainted, and think of elderly couples in the same way that you would think of younger couples.

Handling Sexual Aggression. Some residents may attempt to meet sexual needs by making advances toward staff members. If a resident touches you inappropriately, flirts, or makes sexual comments to you, you may feel angry and embarrassed. While that is a normal way to feel, it is important that you handle your feelings correctly.

Illness, medications, confusion, poor self-image, and cultural differences may cause the resident to act this way. The resident may be responding to the caring, nurturing individual that you are. The resident may have difficulty drawing a line between care giving and affection. Because of an overwhelming need to be loved and to feel human closeness, the resident's reaction may be inappropriate. Because of poor vision or confusion, the touch may not be where it was meant to be. The resident may have mistaken you for a spouse, a loved one, or a sexual partner. Some sexual behavior may be the result of mental changes.

Some residents may approach confused or unconsenting residents for the same reasons. These residents must be protected by staff members. Sometimes residents may knowingly make inappropriate sexual advances. In all cases you must deal with sexual advances in a professional manner. The best method may vary from one situation to another.

GUIDELINES FOR HANDLING SEXUAL AGGRESSIVENESS

- Be knowledgeable about sexuality in the elderly.
- Be aware of and accept your own sexuality and reactions.
- Maintain a professional attitude.
- Be aware that your own behavior may affect the resident's sexual interest.
- Firmly and calmly tell the resident to stop the objectionable advance.
- Explain that this action is not acceptable and that it makes you uncomfortable.
- Never scold, embarrass, shame, or belittle the resident.

- Remain calm and matter-of-fact.
- Provide privacy for a resident who is sexually aroused. If a resident is sexually aroused in front of others, removal to a private area is necessary.
- Check the care plan for approaches to be used.

Anytime that you feel concern regarding sexuality of the residents, you should bring that concern to the attention of your charge nurse.

The Resident with Alzheimer's Disease

The resident with Alzheimer's disease (AD) has a progressive nervous disorder that eventually destroys all mental function. It causes problems in thinking, communication, and behavior and causes physical deterioration resulting in death. Alzheimer's disease is discussed in detail in Chapter 12.

Confusion, mood swings, depression, wandering, and poor judgment require special care that must be provided for the resident with AD. Many facilities maintain an area or unit specifically for residents with Alzheimer's disease. This area allows the specialized environment and care that is needed.

GUIDELINES FOR CARE OF RESIDENTS WITH ALZHEIMER'S DISEASE

- Provide a calm, quiet environment: Speak in short, simple sentences, and move calmly and slowly. Do not force the resident to make decisions or perform tasks that cause frustration. As the disease progresses the resident may have difficulty understanding stimuli in the environment. **Stimuli** are factors that cause a reaction. Too much stimulation causes anxiety.
- Prevent fatigue by scheduling frequent rest periods and naps. Encourage activities that require little time and do not drain the resident's energy.
- Reassure and explain frequently. Keep a scheduled routine for the resident's daily care and activities. This will prevent anxiety and decrease the occurrence of disruptive behavior. **Disruptive behavior** is behavior that interferes with normal routine.
- Observe for possible causes of behavior changes. Physical discomfort, anxiety, stimuli in the environment, or medications can cause the resident with AD to become disruptive. Report any problems to the nurse so care can be planned that will provide the resident with optimum comfort and modify (change) behavior.
- Provide emotional support for the family: They are suffering as they see the day by day death of a loved one. The resident with Alzheimer's may not even recognize them, or respond. There are support groups for families of AD patients. Refer family members to your charge nurse or the social worker for information.
- Promote safety. As a result of confusion and wandering, the resident with Alzheimer's disease is at risk of accidents and injuries. Wandering is part of the disease process and should be allowed, within a safe environment. Very close observation is necessary for residents with Alzheimer's disease.

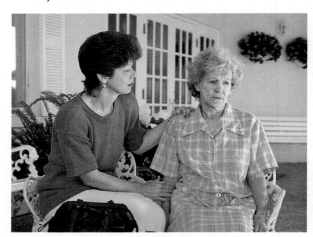

Fig. 13-7 The resident with Alzheimer's disease may not recognize family members.

The resident with Alzheimer's may eventually become totally dependent upon the staff for every part of life, as the final stage of this disease develops and death approaches. The physical care required may include hygiene and grooming, skin care, exercise and positioning, bowel and bladder management, and nutrition. This care is discussed in later chapters.

The Confused Resident

The confused resident may be disoriented. **Disorientation** means confusion about the location (place), the time, and the identities of people (including self). This is referred to as disorientation to person, place, and time. The disoriented person is not thoroughly aware of reality.

Confusion affects individuals in different ways. A person may be confused in all three areas of orientation (person, place, and time) or may be confused in one or two areas. For example, it is possible to know that you are in Florida in the winter season and yet be confused about the city that you are in or the month or date.

Have you ever awakened from a sound sleep and found yourself temporarily disoriented about where you were, or how to get to the bathroom? That was disorientation to place, and was a temporary, normal reaction to your circumstances. How did you feel during your confusion? Were you nervous or frightened?

Causes of Confusion. Physical changes in the nervous system may cause confusion. Many elderly residents of long-term care facilities suffer from Alzheimer's disease or other forms of **dementia** (an impairment of mental function). These disorders are discussed in Chapter 12.

Environmental factors may contribute to confusion for an elderly resident. Increased stress, unmet needs, changes in environment, losses, illness, and medications may cause confusion for the elderly person, whose ability to adapt to change has been impaired or slowed. Loss of vision or hearing may cause confusion. The person may not understand surroundings or what is being said. A darkened room, on a bright sunny day, may cause the resident to think that it is night or that it is cloudy. Objects and people might be mistaken for others. Words that are said may be misunderstood and therefore may lead to confusion.

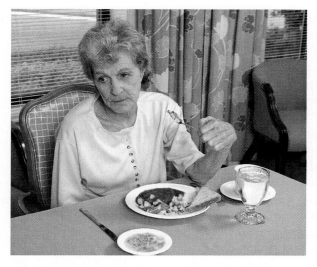

Fig. 13-8 The confused resident may not remember to feed herself.

Problems Caused by Confusion. Safety and self-care become greater problems as confusion increases. Because of an inability to recognize hunger or thirst, the resident may become dependent upon the staff for nutrition and fluids. The memory of how to get a drink or how to feed oneself may be lost. Hygiene and toileting may become the responsibility of the staff if the resident is unable to recognize those needs. Rest may not be achieved without the assistance of staff members. The confused resident may not know where to rest, and endless wandering, pacing, or other activity may prevent rest. Anxiety (worry) resulting from confusion may also prevent rest by causing the resident to cling to others. Being alone may be a frightening experience.

Behavior problems and confusion may increase as evening occurs. This is referred to as **Sundowner's syndrome**. It may be caused by fatigue and frustration that results from a day full of challenges and stimulation. The resident may not be able to communicate needs. Repeated questions may never receive a satisfactory answer. The safety of a wanderer who cannot make wise decisions requires the attention of staff.

Communicating with the Confused Resident. Communicating with the confused resident should begin with calling the resident by name to gain attention. Using short, simple, step-by-step statements and repeating them as needed promotes understanding. Ask questions that require simple answers and will not stress the resident. It is important to communicate in a quiet setting so the resident can concentrate more easily.

Stay calm, take your time, and be careful not to be demanding. Remember to give frequent encouragement and praise. Touching the resident lightly (if touch is acceptable) while you maintain eye contact may help the resident to concentrate on you. It is very difficult to fail to notice someone who is touching you. Think of how small children get mother's attention when she is busy. They call out, dance around to catch mother's eye, and pull at her clothing!

Providing Restorative Care for the Confused Resident.
The confused resident requires much empathy, patience, and reassurance. Constant wandering, poor judgment, decreased alertness, and a careless curiosity make this resident more likely to have accidents and to suffer injury. The resident must be protected from things that could be harmful. The wanderer must be distracted frequently. This can be a difficult

task. If you provide activity, a short attention span may cause the resident to forget it soon. If the resident is able to cooperate, the activity may lead to a feeling of usefulness. This might include hanging clothes, straightening drawers, or making the bed. Sometimes the resident may stay with someone who is willing to talk.

The confused wanderer may try to leave the building or interfere with other residents and their belongings. Alarms on outer facility doors often are present to warn the staff of the resident's attempt to leave. Telling the resident that leaving is not allowed may only increase the problem. You might distract the resident by offering a snack. Sometimes placing stop signs, like those used for traffic, may be useful. They are very familiar objects. The confused wanderer, who constantly forgets where the room is, may be helped by having the door marked in some very obvious way. A large, brightly colored sign may be used. The staff must frequently remind the resident to look for the sign.

Spending time in one-on-one interaction with the confused resident helps you get acquainted with each other. This makes the

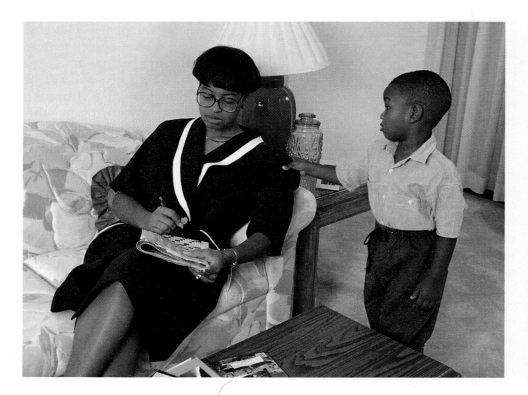

Fig. 13-9
Touch is important to communication.

resident more comfortable and builds trust. A trusting relationship helps to control wandering and other unacceptable behavior. It is important to be able to adapt to frequent, sudden behavior changes. Be aware of behavior patterns, and notice events that may result in behavior changes. Report these observations to the nurse.

Restlessness and wandering may be a reaction to discomfort or and unmet needs. Being able to determine the source of discomfort is very helpful. The resident who is thirsty but can't communicate this need, or can't get his own water, may become restless and wander. Excessive stimulation, hunger, and the need to change position also cause restlessness. Other causes of restlessness include pain, temperature, the need to use the toilet, and the need for human contact and affection.

The resident who becomes more confused will become less able to accomplish self-care. The nursing assistant must be able to recognize physical causes for behavior. It is also important to provide assistance and care as needed.

While assisting the resident, you must maintain a restorative approach. The basis of this approach is encouragement and praise. The resident must be encouraged to do as much as possible, but must not be challenged to the point of frustration. If there is no challenge, because everything is done for the resident, there will be no reason to think and function. Mental function may be lost sooner than if the resident was required to think and to do things. How much challenge is healthy for the confused resident will depend upon the stage of confusion. This information can be found in the care plan.

Mental functions will deteriorate if they are not used, just as unused physical functions decline. For example, what happens to math or language skills learned in school if you stop using them for a period of time? Are you able to solve math problems or to diagram sentences as easily as you did while you were practicing them? Probably you would be a little slow, and you might need to relearn those skills.

Provide the disoriented resident with a predictable (expected) world. Imagine how you would feel if you had no idea what to expect from one day to the next. It is comforting to be able to live with some predictability. How would you feel if you didn't know that you would have a job the next day? How important is it to be able to count on friends and relatives? If you had new people to interact with every day, and no contact with familiar ones, how would it affect you? Is being able to choose the foods you eat, the clothes you wear, and your recreational activities important to you? Being able to make choices increases predictability and a sense of control.

To provide as much predictability as possible, it is important for the resident to have contact with the same staff members daily. Maintaining a routine that is the same from day to day helps the resident feel secure and oriented. Inform the resident frequently of what to expect, of who you are, and the location.

If the resident is able to make decisions, choices should be provided. These may need to be small choices such as deciding between two pieces of clothing. If unable to decide, the resident may be helped by a simple suggestion such as "I like the green shirt. Would you like to wear it today?" or "Are you ready for bed? I'd like to help you now." Making choices creates a sense of control over one's life.

Care for the confused resident must be provided in a restorative manner, which emphasizes independence and self-care. The resident's care plan will address specific needs and actions to be taken. Sometimes you may be responsible for every detail of care and activities of daily living (ADLs). You must be consistent, observant, patient, and creative. To meet the demands of caring for the confused resident, you must be well rested and healthy. You must also be able to cope well with stress and maintain a positive attitude.

Nursing assistants who possess the special qualities needed to care for these residents love their work. They possess enough energy and enthusiasm to give of themselves tirelessly. They are the special people who care enough to give, without expecting a response from the resident. They find a reward in the awareness that they have given their best.

Approaches to use in caring for the confused resident can be found in Fig. 13-10.

CARE FOR THE CONFUSED RESIDENT

1. Distract the wanderer
2. Provide activities
3. Build a trusting relationship
4. Observe for causes of behavioral changes
5. Avoid frustration
6. Provide a regular routine
7. Use patience and understanding
8. Provide a calm, quiet atmosphere
9. Use reality orientation and validation therapy
10. Come to work rested

Fig. 13-10 General rules of care for the confused resident.

Reality Orientation and Validation Therapy

Restorative Programs for the Disoriented Resident. Programs that are designed for use with the disoriented resident include reality orientation, validation therapy, remotivation therapy, sensory stimulation, pet therapy, music therapy, and other recreational activities. The activity director has the responsibility for planning these programs. The responsibilities of the activity department are discussed in Chapter 4. The programs to be used with each resident will be included in the care plan.

Reality Orientation. Reality orientation (RO) is a technique that helps the resident to maintain awareness of person, place, and time. It assists the confused resident to stay in touch with the reality of the environment rather than the confusion of the mind. Reality orientation helps self-understanding. It also encourages the resident to perform simple ADLs. Reality orientation is used in all contact with the resident. The resident may attend RO classes.

The resident is always addressed by name, and the speakers identify themselves to the resident. The date, time, and place are repeatedly stated to the resident throughout the day. Careful explanations are given. Clocks, calendars, and bulletin boards are posted, and the resident's attention is drawn to them frequently. Familiar personal items and pictures, reading material, radio, and TV draw attention to current events. Conversations between the disoriented resident and staff members should include current topics. The following are examples of the type of interaction that might be used in reality orientation.

"Good morning Mr. Brown. I am Joe, your nursing assistant. I am going to help you get up this morning. Did you sleep well?" (Allow time for response.) "It is eight A.M., almost time for breakfast." (Open the drapes to let sunlight in.) "This is February fourteenth, and it is cold outside. The weatherman says we may have snow." (Hold the clothing in front of the resident.) "Would you like to wear this red shirt or the blue one?" (Pause for response. If there is no response, continue.) "How about the red one? This is Valentine's Day, and the red one will look perfect. There is a valentine party later."

RO should be used in all conversations with the resident, 24 hours a day and 7 days a week. A regular routine and care given by the same staff members are also important parts of RO. A familiar, calm, quiet, and unrushed atmosphere should be maintained. This decreases confusion and distraction.

If the resident makes confused or incorrect comments, the staff reaction should be based on the resident's needs. This will be indicated in the care plan. A calm, kindly approach should be used if correction is necessary. Some residents may become angry about being corrected. This could cause frustration and increase confusion. If the resident reacts with anger, do not continue. Further statements should be ignored. Never argue with the resident.

Reality orientation does not work with all disoriented residents. Some residents may become so frustrated and angry when corrected that they stop interacting with others.

They may feel rejected because a staff member disagrees with them. They may become insecure and more confused when "their reality" is threatened. These reactions to RO are harmful and unhealthy. There are other restorative programs for working with disoriented residents.

Validation Therapy. **Validation therapy** is a technique that creates a climate of acceptance by encouraging the confused resident to explore personal thoughts. The confused resident may withdraw, especially if others seem to reject personal beliefs. An effort must be made to draw the resident out of isolation. Validation therapy helps to do this. To validate is to approve or support. Instead of indicating that the resident is not correct, the nursing assistant should ask questions about what the resident is saying, thinking, and feeling. By doing so, the nursing assistant is drawing the resident into conversation. Validation therapy is an attempt to restore the resident's comfort in interacting with others. It helps to validate the emotions being experienced.

It is never correct to encourage or add to the resident's false beliefs or statements. When using validation therapy you are not agreeing with false beliefs. You are simply encouraging the resident to explore and discuss them. This helps the resident to feel accepted. Feeling accepted and participating in conversation is a normal healthy part of life. Exploration of false thinking may lead to more normal thinking and reduce stress. For example, if the resident says, "I have to go home and make dinner for the children." An appropriate response might be, "You must have been a very good mother." or "What was your family's favorite meal?" Validation therapy helps the resident to maintain self-esteem and dignity.

The Aggressive/Combative Resident

Residents may be physically or verbally aggressive. A combative resident is one who struggles and fights. Some residents interfere with their care because they are so combative. It is difficult to work with them.

Causes of Combative Behavior. Combativeness usually occurs as a result of anger or fear. Residents who are confused may be combative because they believe that someone will harm them. They may mistake a person for someone else with whom they are angry. Residents with hearing loss or vision loss may not understand what is said or what is happening. This may lead to anger. Residents who are not confused or impaired may also be angry. Can you think of anything that you might be angry about if you were an elderly resident?

Losing control over one's life, having to live by a daily schedule that someone else has set, having to depend on someone else, or being rushed could cause the resident to become angry. Physical discomfort, changes in the nervous system, illness, and medications may also cause aggressiveness.

Awareness of the cause of combative behavior will help you develop empathy and understanding. Understanding the reason for behavior is the basis for dealing with it. It is very important to be aware of behavior that indicates possible combativeness. If you think about the signs of anger, you will have awareness of the clues to aggressive behavior. Muscle tension may be seen in a clenched jaw, glaring eyes, clenched fists, or rigid posture. Activity such as pacing, rocking, or kicking often indicate tension and possible combativeness. Speech may be loud and rapid or changeable.

Recognizing the signs of anger will help you to protect yourself and the resident (see Fig. 13-11). You will know that you are dealing with a person who could become combative. Often the combative behavior occurs very suddenly. The tension and anger are usually visible before action occurs. When you are working with an aggressive resident, always trust your intuition or "gut" feelings. Those feelings are usually correct.

Providing Restorative Care for the Aggressive Resident. Be sure that the resident understands what you are going to do

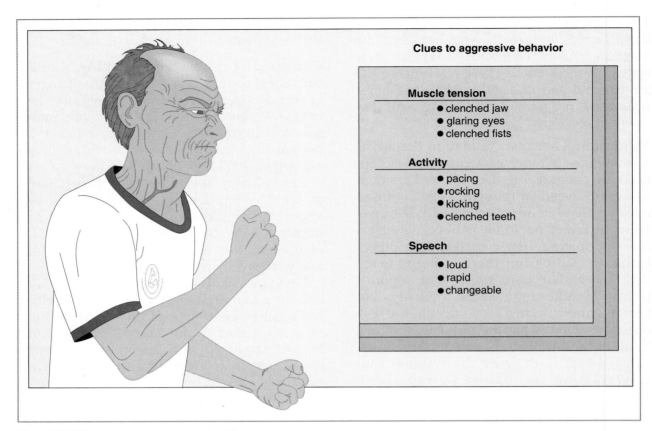

Clues to aggressive behavior

Muscle tension
- clenched jaw
- glaring eyes
- clenched fists

Activity
- pacing
- rocking
- kicking
- clenched teeth

Speech
- loud
- rapid
- changeable

Fig. 13-11 Learn to recognize signs of anger.

before you do it. Many residents have a short attention span and must be reminded frequently. If not reminded, they may forget what is being done and react with anger. Use the communication skills that are suggested in Chapter 8. What reaction would you have in the following situation? Imagine that you couldn't hear well or see well. As you sat in a wheelchair, unaware of the presence of another, someone suddenly began to move you down the hall. What would you do?

Allowing the angry resident a chance to choose and make some decisions helps provide a sense of control and may help relieve anger. Provide the resident with a predictable schedule. When you are talking, don't stand over, or talk down to, the resident. Speaking with a soothing voice will often calm the resident. Keep your movements calm and slow. Be respectful and watch your reactions.

It is normal to feel some fear when dealing with an aggressive person. Don't take the resident's angry words or actions personally. Remind yourself of possible reasons for the angry behavior. Use body language that is nonaggressive. Hand gestures may be useful to aid in communicating with an angry resident. If you are unable to calm the resident, call on someone who has rapport (a mutually trusting relationship). This may be a family member or other staff member. Offering food sometimes has a soothing effect. It may distract the resident from anger. Be sure that what is offered cannot be used as a weapon.

Restraints must be used only as a last resort. Restraint removes all control from the angry individual, who is already experiencing a loss of control. The combative behavior will worsen.

If you encounter a combative resident, you must protect yourself. Don't allow the resident to feel cornered. Don't turn your back, and stay an arm's length away, when possible. Try to build a trusting relationship. Taking time and effort to build rapport with your resident affects the comfort with which you care for him. If touch is acceptable to the resident, patting or holding a hand may be calming. Don't stop a resident who is pacing, because pacing is an outlet for emotional energy.

Be sure to report all signs of anger and aggressiveness to the nurse. Get help in working with the combative resident. You may find it helpful to talk about your feelings with the charge nurse or a counselor. All staff members should be familiar with the care plan for the combative resident, because it is important to use a consistent approach.

The Depressed Resident

Many elderly residents are depressed. Facing the losses they have suffered often overwhelms their emotional strength. Being unable to be independent, and to run their own lives, in addition to physical illness or impairments, may burden them to the point of giving up. They may lose the motivation to participate in any part of life.

Symptoms of Depression. Symptoms of depression include deep sadness, low self-esteem, feelings of worthlessness, lack of interest in activities, social withdrawal, negative reactions, and difficulty in decision making. Physical symptoms resulting from decreased energy include poor hygiene and grooming, slow movement, sleep problems, poor appetite, and weight loss. Constipation and fatigue also occur with depression. Severe depression can lead to confusion, chronic illness, and death. Observing and reporting signs of depression are important in preventing its negative effects on the quality of the resident's life. Be sure to report objective information, such as, "The resident is crying." It would not be correct to report, "The resident is depressed." Reporting comments about suicide helps to protect the resident's well-being.

Providing Restorative Care for the Depressed Resident. Encourage the depressed resident to talk about feelings. Talking about the problems may help. Once the resident begins to talk, listen attentively. If the resident cries, you may feel helpless. You may find yourself wanting to stop the resident's crying, but crying is helpful, and the resident should be allowed to do so.

No matter how uncomfortable you may be when the resident expresses sadness and

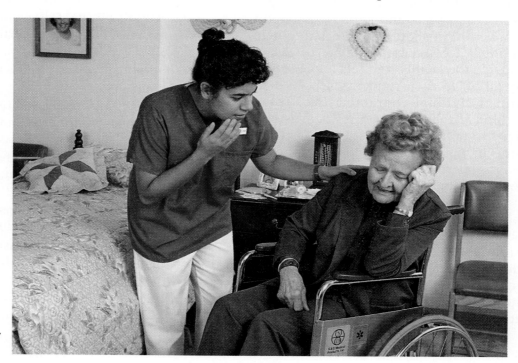

Fig. 13-12 If the resident cries, you may feel helpless.

frustration, you can help most by being there and taking time to listen. Hushing the resident or making comments like, "It will be all right" or "I'd like to see a smile now" only prevents the resident from working through the problems. Can you remember a time when you were depressed and needed to talk about your problems? Did you find that it was helpful if someone listened and allowed you to talk? Can you remember when someone hushed you and told you that everything would be all right instead of listening? Which situation helped you to feel better?

The activity department plays a major role in providing activities to stimulate and remotivate the depressed resident. The nursing staff must help to make planned activities a part of daily life for the resident. Encouraging the resident to prepare for and attend activities is a responsibility of the nursing assistant. You can help by showing interest. Ask the resident questions about the activities.

The supportive relationship that is provided by a sensitive and caring nursing assistant can be a great help in overcoming depression. Because the depressed resident feels unloved and alone, having someone who can be depended upon for social contact, acceptance, and support is important. Conversation should be directed to help the resident feel accepted, relate to the world outside the facility, and feel appreciated. Pay attention to each resident's special qualities and individual characteristics. It is also helpful if the depressed resident is encouraged to talk to other residents. Getting outside in the fresh air and sunshine, when possible, relieves depression. As always, encouragement and praise are important.

The depressed resident needs another person to help, just as each of us needs someone to help us out of our own depression. Remember, the earlier you notice depression and try to help the depressed resident, the easier it will be to overcome. Just as with all restorative care, begin early, stress ability, and encourage activity.

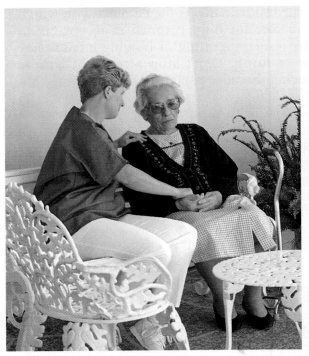

Fig. 13-13 Spending time outside with a caring person can help the depressed resident.

Conclusion

Remember these important points:

1. The basic needs of all human beings are physical, safety and security, love and belonging, self-esteem, and self-actualization.

2. The most basic needs are the physical needs.

3. Fulfillment of basic needs affects the quality of one's life.

4. Culture, spirituality, and religion influence an individual's basic needs and the way in which those needs are fulfilled.

5. The many psychosocial changes and losses experienced by the elderly cause emotional stress.

6. Independence helps the resident gain self-esteem, privacy, and the freedom to socialize.

7. The nursing assistant must send messages that help to improve the resident's self-esteem.

8. The nursing assistant's interest in the resident's accomplishments helps to meet the resident's need for self-actualization.

9. Sexual fulfillment helps meet the need for closeness, love, affection, and belonging.

10. Unwanted sexual advances must be handled in a professional manner.

11. Residents with Alzheimer's disease, or other types of confusion, require a quiet calm environment, frequent rest, and predictability.

12. Causes of confusion may include dementia, changes of environment, unmet needs, illness, stress, and medication.

13. Reality orientation and validation therapy are restorative programs that may be included in the confused resident's plan of care.

14. Understanding the reasons for aggressiveness will help the nursing assistant to work with aggressive residents.

15. Inviting the resident to talk and being a good listener are important restorative measures to use for the depressed resident.

16. Encouraging the dependent resident to participate in planned activities is important.

Discussion Questions

1. Can you recall a time when unmet lower needs interfered with higher needs?

2. How do you feel about expressions of sexuality among the elderly in the long-term care facility?

3. What are important steps to be taken in communicating with the confused resident?

4. When you are angry, what increases your anger? What calms you?

5. What makes you feel better when you are depressed? How could you help the depressed resident?

Application Exercises

1. The class will plan a cultural day in which the students will explore their cultural diversities. The students may wear clothing that represents their individual cultures. Each student will share elements of their cultural background that they feel are unique. These elements might include social activities, food preferences, family traditions, and family roles.

2. Students will interview grandparents or other elderly relatives to determine the effects of psychosocial changes on their lives. Questions might include

    a. What changes have taken place?

    b. Which changes were most stressful?

    c. How they responded to those changes?

    d. What are their plans for the future?

The Resident's Unit

OBJECTIVES

Upon completing this chapter, you will be able to do the following:

1. Describe what is meant by a restorative environment.

2. List six pieces of furniture and equipment that might be found in the resident's unit.

3. Identify five guidelines for cleaning equipment.

4. Identify three methods to prevent waste and contain costs.

5. Explain the responsibility of the nursing assistant in maintaining the resident's unit.

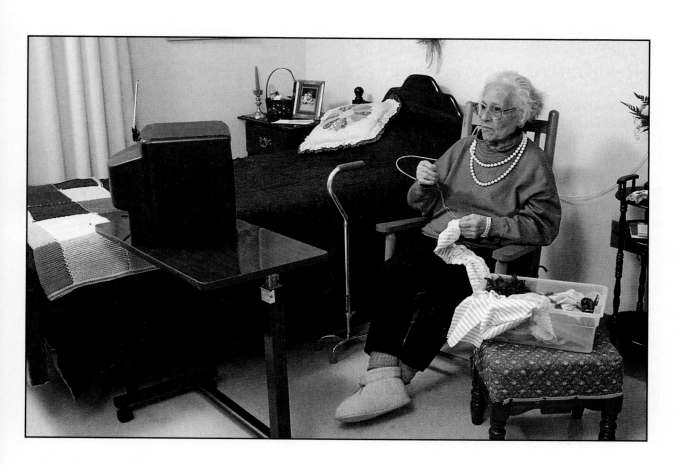

VOCABULARY

The following words or terms will help you to understand this chapter:

Restorative environment	Emesis basin	Emesis
Urinal	Disinfection	Sterile

The resident's unit refers to the room or area that contains the resident's furniture and belongings. It is a private space—a retreat. The resident lives in the unit. When you enter the resident's unit, you are entering a home.

Think about how you would be expected to behave when you visit the home of someone who lives in your neighborhood. First, you would knock on the door and wait for permission to enter. While you were there, you would treat their furniture and belongings with care. You would behave courteously, respect their privacy, and be a well-mannered guest in their home. The same courtesies should be demonstrated when you enter the resident's unit. You are a guest in that home as well.

A Restorative Environment

A **restorative environment** is one that promotes independence. It is arranged in a way that allows for self-care as much as possible. Furniture and equipment are placed for convenience and safety. Adequate lighting is provided, with switches or controls that are within the resident's reach. A call signal is available that allows the resident to call staff members with a minimum of effort.

Safety is very important. The call signal must always be within reach, even if the resident is confused or comatose. The bed is positioned close to the floor, so that getting in and out of it will be easier. The wheels on the bed are locked at all times. Emergency signals and safety bars are provided in the bathroom. A person who does not have to depend on others for safety feels more secure. A feeling of security promotes independence.

Privacy is protected in a restorative environment. Drapes or blinds at the windows provide privacy as desired. If the resident does not have a private room, screens or curtains separate the individual units. Each unit is complete, with its own furniture and equipment. Although the bathroom may be shared, doors can be closed to provide privacy. Maintaining privacy increases the resident's feeling of self-worth.

A restorative environment is one that provides a peaceful atmosphere. It is kept as free from loud noise as possible. It is climate controlled to provide a comfortable temperature at any time of the year. However, residents should be able to adjust the temperature in their own rooms.

Cleanliness and neatness are important to a restorative environment. Housekeepers clean the unit daily and as needed. Maintenance employees keep the furniture and equipment repaired. All staff members follow aseptic practices to prevent the spread of infection. These precautions help to keep the resident healthy and free from disease, making it is easier to maintain independence.

A restorative environment is familiar and homelike to the resident. Walls may be wallpapered or painted in soft colors. Wall-hangings, drapes, and bedspreads are coordinated for beauty. The resident is encouraged to bring family pictures and mementos from home. A favorite afghan or cushion might be placed on the bed. When space permits, the resident may want to use a rocking chair, chest of drawers, or other personal furniture. The resident should be able to look around the unit and recognize familiar objects. It is comforting to awaken at night and see a picture of a loved one on the bedside table.

The Effects of a Restorative Environment. A restorative environment creates feelings that flow in a continuous cycle through self-esteem, motivation, indepen-

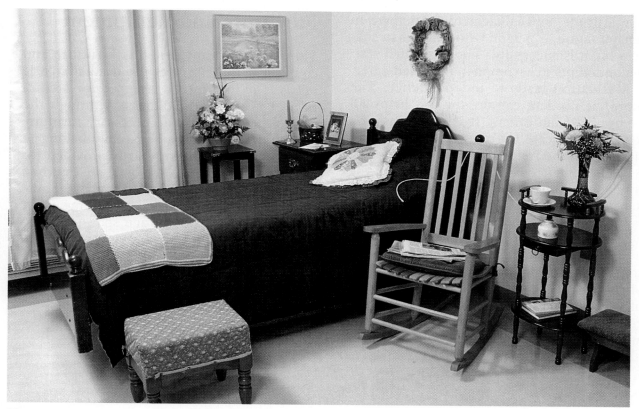

Fig. 14-1 The resident's unit should be familiar and homelike.

dence, and self-worth (see Fig. 14-2). These positive feelings occur over and over again, with each one supporting the other. It is difficult to know where one ends and the other begins. Each are equally important and the cycle could begin with any one of them.

A restorative environment increases the resident's self-esteem. Dignity and privacy are protected. Living in a clean, attractive room, with many personal belongings, helps to maintain the resident's identity. A caring supportive staff strengthens the resident's self-confidence. The resident is encouraged to provide self-care as much as possible.

The resident with high self-esteem is more likely to be motivated. Motivation is an inner feeling that causes a person to take action. The motivated resident has a posi-

Fig. 14-2
A restorative environment creates a continuous cycle of positive feelings.

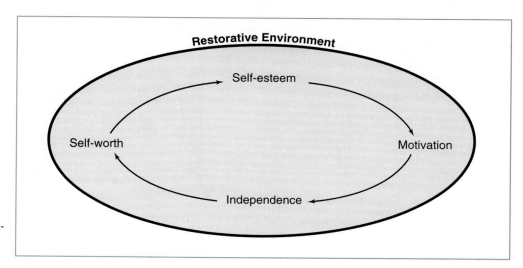

tive attitude, and is eager to participate in rehabilitation. A person who believes in success often is successful. The motivated resident attempts to accomplish more self-care.

Motivation leads to independence. The more the resident can do, the less help will be needed from others. It is very satisfying to be able to care for oneself. Making decisions helps the resident to maintain control. As independence is gained in one area, the resident becomes motivated to be independent in others. One success leads to another.

Independence increases feelings of self-worth. It is difficult to feel valuable and worthwhile when one is dependent on someone else. The person with a high level of self-worth feels important and deserving of success. Increased self-worth raises self-esteem. A restorative environment nurtures and maintains these positive feelings.

Furniture and Equipment

The resident's unit contains furniture and equipment to help meet the resident's basic needs. The furniture is designed for promotion of health and wellness. Although the facility furnishes all the necessary furniture and equipment, some items may belong to the resident. Furniture that is provided for the resident includes a bed, an overbed table, a bedside stand, and a chair. Some rooms might also have a chest of drawers or a desk. Closets and storage space are provided for each unit.

The Overbed Table. The overbed table is sometimes used for the resident's meals. It is also used for treatments and personal care. This table is a clean area. Contaminated (soiled) linens or equipment (such as bed-

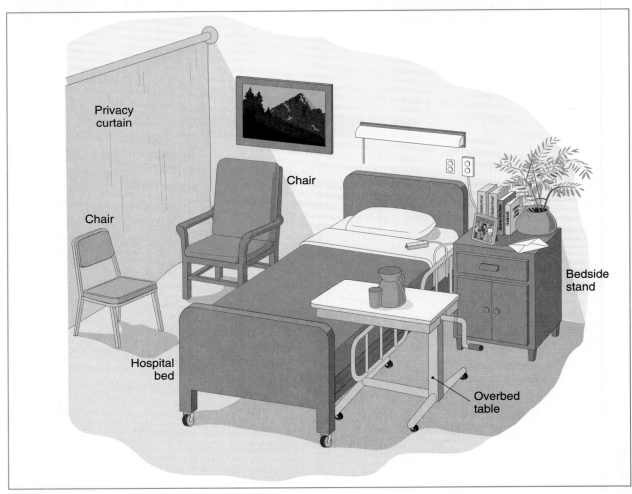

Fig. 14-3 Furniture is provided in each unit to meet the resident's basic needs.

pans) should not be placed on it. Do not put anything on the overbed table that you would not feel comfortable placing on your own dining table.

The Bedside Stand. The bedside stand provides storage for personal care equipment such as wash basins and bedpans. It also provides a convenient place for small personal items, such as a toothbrush, toothpaste, hairbrush, hearing aid, and eyeglasses. The water pitcher and cup are often found on top of the bedside table. Personal mementoes may also be placed there.

The Call Signal. The facility provides a call signal for each unit. This allows the resident to call for assistance as needed. The call signal may be a light or a bell, which is connected to an intercom at the nurses station. When the resident pushes a button, a light will go on outside the door and at the nurses' station. Sometimes an alarm will also ring. The nurse may be able to talk to the resident through the intercom. It is important to always keep the call signal within the resident's reach and promptly answer all call lights.

In some facilities, each room has a bathroom. If the room is not a private room, the bath will be shared by the residents who occupy that room. In other facilities, the bathroom may be located between two rooms and is shared by the occupants of those rooms.

Standard equipment that is usually provided in a resident's unit includes a wash basin, emesis basin, bedpan, and urinal. These items are used for personal care. An **emesis basin** is a small kidney-shaped pan into which the resident spits or vomits (**emesis** is vomitus). The curved edge of the basin is designed to fit the curve of the resident's chin. The emesis basin may also be used for mouth care. A **urinal** is a container that the male resident uses when urinating. It is used for the resident who cannot go into the bathroom.

A water pitcher and glass may also be furnished. Most residents bring their own toothbrush, toothpaste, comb, brush, and other personal care items. Although some residents may have their own bar of soap, most facilities provide liquid soap in dispensers. The facility will also provide lotion for residents who do not bring their own.

Sometimes a resident will require special equipment to be used for administering oxygen, tube feedings, or IV fluids. This type of equipment is returned to the appro-

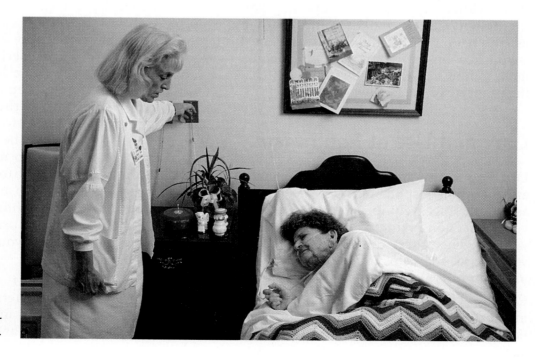

Fig. 14-4
The call signal allows the resident to call for assistance as needed.

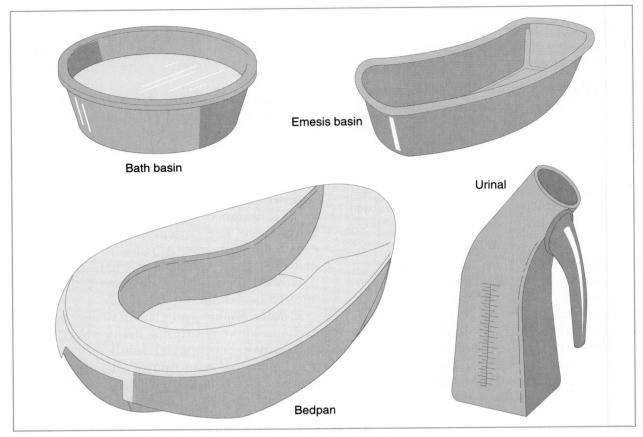

Bath basin

Emesis basin

Urinal

Bedpan

Fig. 14-5 Examples of standard equipment that will be in the resident's unit.

priate storage area when not in use. Wheelchairs are available for residents who need them. However, some residents may have their own. Canes, walkers, and crutches usually belong to the individual resident. It is your responsibility to know which equipment belongs to the resident and which is the property of the facility.

Care and Use of Equipment

Learning to use and care for equipment is an important responsibility of the nursing assistant. Using equipment correctly prevents infection or injury to the resident or yourself. The proper care of equipment prevents waste and helps to hold down the cost of health care.

Correct Use of Equipment. The correct method for using many pieces of equipment is taught in nursing assistant training classes. The use of other equipment is explained during orientation to the long-term care facility. You can refer to the procedure book for the proper care and use of equipment. The procedure book includes every procedure that is performed in the facility. This book will be located at the nurse's station. Step-by-step directions tell you exactly how to use the equipment. Manufacturers' instructions are often included. Always follow the correct steps when using equipment. Do not take shortcuts. Shortcuts often lead to accidents. If you do not know how to use a piece of equipment, ask your charge nurse to explain. Do not attempt to perform a procedure with equipment that you do not know how to use.

Disposable Equipment. Much of the equipment used in a long-term care facility is disposable. Disposable means that the equipment will be thrown away after it has

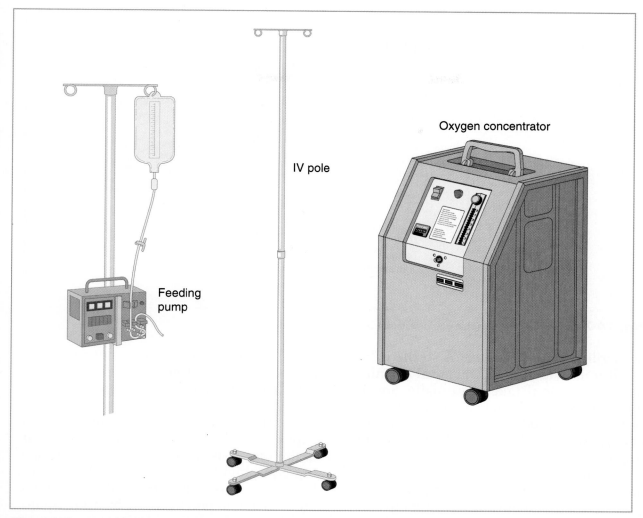

Fig. 14-6 Examples of special equipment that might be needed.

been used. Some of this equipment is used once and discarded. Latex gloves are an example of this type of equipment. Other equipment, such as wash basins, bedpans, and urinals, may be used by the resident for a period of time before being discarded.

Disposable equipment is used to prevent the spread of microorganisms. Residents should not share personal equipment. Sharing increases the risk of infection. Always discard disposable equipment in the proper container in the dirty utility room.

Nondisposable Equipment. Larger and more expensive equipment is usually not disposable. It must be cleaned before reuse. Cleaning reduces the number of microorganisms on the equipment. Always rinse equipment with cold water before cleaning.

This is done to remove feces (bowel movement) or other material. Do not use hot water in this step. Hot water causes the material to become thick, hard, and difficult to remove. Guidelines for cleaning equipment follow:

GUIDELINES FOR CLEANING EQUIPMENT

- Wear gloves and follow universal precautions.
- Rinse equipment in cold water.
- Wash with soap and hot water.
- Use a brush if necessary.
- Rinse and dry.
- Disinfect or sterilize.

Disinfection is the use of chemicals to destroy pathogens. It does not kill all microorganisms. Some equipment must also

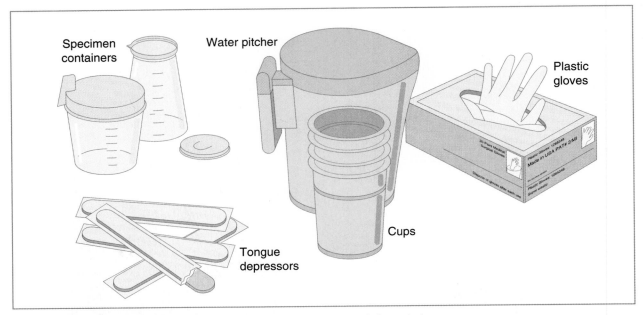

Fig. 14-7 Examples of disposable equipment that is used once and discarded.

be sterilized. An object that is **sterile** is free of all microorganisms. Chemical disinfectants are toxic if taken internally. Special precautions must be taken while using and storing these products. Always be sure that disinfectants are kept out of the residents reach.

Do not use equipment that is defective or damaged. Defective equipment can cause accidents. For example, a broken footrest on a wheelchair could result in a serious injury to the resident. Check equipment very carefully before you attempt to use it. Report defective equipment immediately.

Preventing Waste. Medical equipment is expensive. This is one of the reasons that health care costs so much. Buying and replacing equipment contributes to the cost of health care. It is your responsibility, as a nursing assistant, to prevent waste by using equipment correctly and carefully. Using proper

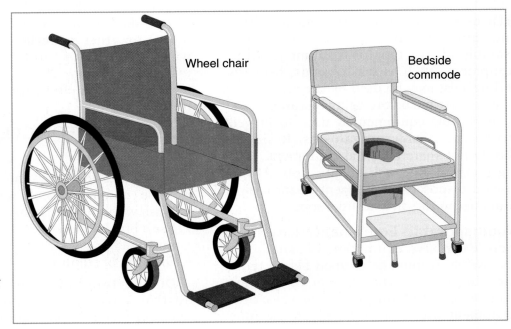

Fig. 14-8
Some equipment is not disposable and must be cleaned before using.

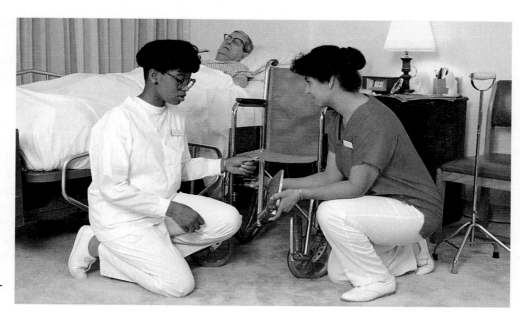

Fig. 14-9
Report defective equipment immediately.

cleaning techniques also helps equipment last longer. Compare the use of equipment to the use of your car. If you do not maintain your car properly, it will not run efficiently, and you may have to replace it. The same thing is true of health care equipment.

Do not be wasteful with equipment. Use only what you need. Some packages come with more than one item. Close the package carefully to protect the unused items. Return items you have used to their proper places. Many times new equipment must be obtained because the original was misplaced. For example, a resident may have three or four partly used bottles of lotion, because the nursing assistant was unable to find the original bottle. Waste costs money. The resident's money, the facility's money, and the taxpayer's money are all affected.

Cost containment in health care is an important issue in health care today. You can do your part in keeping costs down by the correct care and use of equipment. All of us bear the burden of the cost of health care.

Responsibilities in Maintaining the Resident's Unit

Nursing assistants in long-term care have many responsibilities regarding the resident's unit. They help to keep it clean and neat. After providing care to the resident, equipment is cleaned and put away. The rules of safety and asepsis must be followed. One of your most important responsibilities is to maintain a restorative environment. You can take the suggestions from the resident's plan of care and make them work. In doing so, you will experience the joy and satisfaction of improving the resident's quality of life.

Conclusion

Remember these important points:

1. The resident's unit is a home.

2. Treat the resident's belongings with respect and care.

3. A restorative environment increases the resident's self-esteem.

4. Increased self-esteem motivates the resident to participate in rehabilitation.

5. A restorative environment creates positive feelings.

6. It is important to keep the call signal within the resident's reach and to answer lights promptly.

7. Using equipment correctly prevents injury to the resident and yourself.

8. If you do not know how to use a piece of equipment, ask the nurse to explain.

9. Always discard disposable equipment in the dirty utility room.

10. Report equipment that is defective or damaged immediately.

11. Using equipment correctly and carefully saves money and prevents waste.

12. Maintain a restorative environment for the residents.

Discussion Questions

1. How do you feel when someone treats your belongings carelessly?

2. What can you do to help the resident maintain a restorative environment?

3. What effect might a restorative environment have on a depressed resident?

4. How can you, as a nursing assistant, help keep down the cost of health care?

Application Exercise

1. The instructor will divide students into pairs and assign each pair to a resident unit. The students will visit with the resident or residents in that unit and observe evidence of a restorative environment. Each pair of students will make a report to the class that includes the features that contributed to a restorative environment.

Bedmaking

OBJECTIVES

Upon completing this chapter, you will be able to do the following:

1. Maintain physical safety and emotional comfort for the resident when making a bed.

2. Use correct body mechanics when making a bed.

3. Apply the rules of asepsis when making beds.

4. Identify four restorative measures to use while making beds.

5. Explain the use of communication and observation during bedmaking.

6. Make a closed bed, an open bed, and an occupied bed.

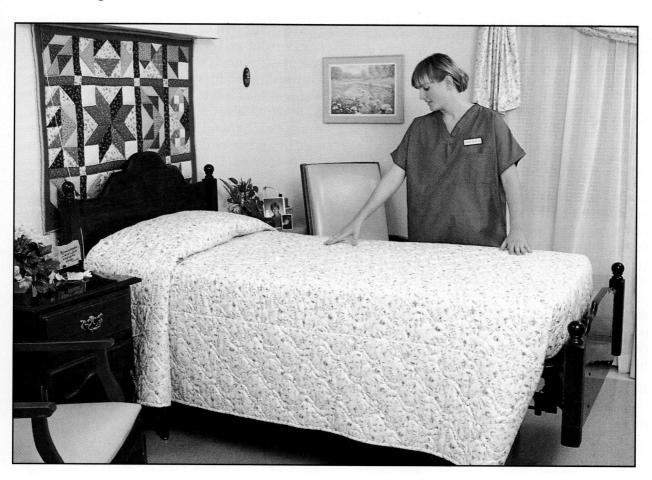

The following words or terms will help you to understand this chapter:

Body alignment
Pressure sore (decubitus ulcer)
Occupied bed

Gatch handle
Draw sheet

Closed bed
Open bed

The Purpose of Bedmaking

Bedmaking is important because it provides comfort, ensures resident safety, and offers a pleasing, professional appearance. Comfort is a priority because some residents spend a lot of time in their beds. A bed will be more comfortable if the linen is clean and free from wrinkles. Follow safety rules to protect the resident and yourself. The appearance of the bed is very important. Remember, the facility is the resident's home, and we all like to see our homes neat and clean. A neat, clean bed can increase the resident's self-esteem. Just think of how good it feels to get into a nice, clean bed!

Safety

The following safety factors should be considered when making a bed:

Body Mechanics. Always use correct body mechanics while making a bed. Raise the bed to a height that is comfortable for you. Stand with your feet apart and your back straight. Bend at your knees, not at your waist. Avoid twisting motions by turning your whole body at once when you change directions. It is quicker and less tiring to make one side of the bed before beginning the other side. Review the guidelines for using correct body mechanics in Chapter 6.

Body Alignment. **Body alignment** means maintaining a normal or correct anatomical position. This helps the resident look and feel more comfortable. Use pillows, pads, and other special equipment to support the body and prevent bony areas, like the knees, from rubbing together.

Skin Protection and Prevention of Pressure Sores. A **pressure sore (decubitus ulcer)** is a breakdown of tissue that occurs when blood flow is interrupted. It is sometimes called a bedsore. Correct bedmaking helps to prevent pressure sores. Anything that might cause pressure on the resident's skin must be avoided. The linen must be kept free of wrinkles, small objects, or crumbs. A wet or dirty bed must be changed immediately, as it can also cause skin problems. Pressure sores are discussed in detail in a later chapter.

Most facilities use mattresses with a waterproof covering. However, some may use plastic sheets to protect the mattress and bottom linen. Plastic must never touch the resident because it can cause damage to delicate skin. If protective pads are used, they must be changed as soon as they become wet or dirty. Avoid excessive padding, as it causes pressure.

Furniture and Equipment. Before you leave the room, return the bed to its lowest position and lock the wheels. The gatch handles should be positioned out of the way, so that no one will be injured. A **gatch handle** is a crank that is used to change the position of the bed (see Fig. 15-3). Be sure the call signal is within the resident's reach. If the resident is out of the room, fasten it to the bedding or place it where it is readily available.

Asepsis and Infection Control

Following universal precautions and the rules of asepsis help to prevent the spread of infection.

Hand Washing. You may need to wash your hands several times during the bed-making procedure. Remember, hand washing is the best way to prevent the spread of infection. Always wash your hands before you begin, before handling clean linen, after handling soiled linen, and before leaving the room. Hands must be washed before applying, and after removing, gloves.

Removing Dirty Linen. Even though used linen may look clean, it is contaminated and must be handled properly. You must wear gloves when handling linen that is contaminated with any body fluid. In many facilities, gloves are worn when handling all dirty linen. Linen should not be shaken and must be held away from your uniform. When removing linen from the bed, the linen should be folded away from you, with the side that touched the resident on the inside.

Never place dirty linen on the overbed table or on the floor. When possible, place dirty linen directly into a dirty linen hamper. If bags are provided, the linen must be emptied from the bag into the hamper. If the bag is disposable, it is then discarded. Follow facility policy regarding placement of dirty linen. Remember to wash your hands after handling dirty linen.

The Dirty Linen Hamper. The dirty linen hamper contains contaminated items, so it should be kept away from food, medicine carts, and clean linen carts. It must be emptied regularly and be kept covered. The dirty linen hamper should be returned to the dirty utility room after the beds are made. Wash your hands after touching the dirty linen hamper.

Handling Clean Linen. Clean linen should be placed on a clean surface, such as the overbed table. Do not place the linen on another resident's bed because germs may be transferred from one bed to another. Keep the linen from touching the floor. Keep it away from your uniform, and avoid shaking it. Remember to wash your hands before handling clean linen.

Clean Linen Cart. Most facilities have a cart in the hall that holds clean linen. This prevents extra trips to the linen closet. Because the cart sits in the hall, it could become a source of infection unless everyone uses it with care. Keep it covered, and do not allow linen on the lower shelf to touch the floor. Position the clean linen cart away from dirty linen hampers, housekeeping carts, and trash containers.

Extra Linen. Take only the linen you will need into the resident's room. Unused linen that is in the room should be placed in the dirty linen hamper. It cannot be taken from one room to another. Do not borrow linen

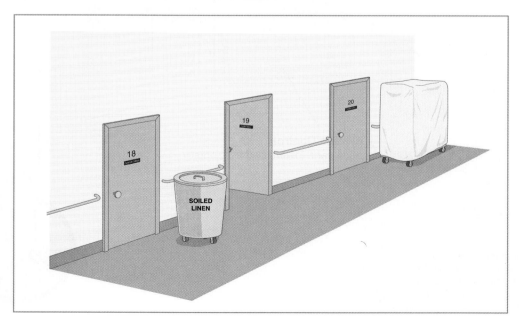

Fig. 15-1
The clean linen cart and the dirty linen hamper are spaced an appropriate distance apart.

from another room. If you need more linen, get it from the clean linen cart.

Types of Beds

There are many types of beds in long-term care facilities. Some are electric and some are manual (operated by hand). Electric beds are easier to operate, but they are more expensive. The electric controls may be located so the resident can operate the bed, or they may be at the foot of the bed, out of the resident's reach (see Fig. 15-2).

Manual beds are equipped with gatch handles to change the position of the bed. Usually, there are three controls. One raises and lowers the entire bed. The second handle operates the head of the bed, and a third one operates the foot of the bed (see Fig. 15-3). A facility may have more than one kind of bed. There might also be beds that have both electric controls and gatch han-

dles. Handles or cranks must be folded under the bed or positioned out of the way to prevent injuries.

Most beds are on wheels to allow moving them as needed. The wheels should have locks, which must be used to prevent injury. A bed on wheels will move very easily and quickly.

Side Rails. There are also many kinds of side rails. Although they may not look alike or work in the same way, they all have the same purpose—to protect the resident. It is not correct to raise the side rails on all residents' beds, because side rails are a form of restraint. Familiarize yourself with facility policies, and identify residents requiring the use of side rails.

Mattresses. Mattresses tend to slide toward the foot of the bed. This can make the resident uncomfortable when the head of the bed is raised. Before you make the bed, you must slide the mattress to the top

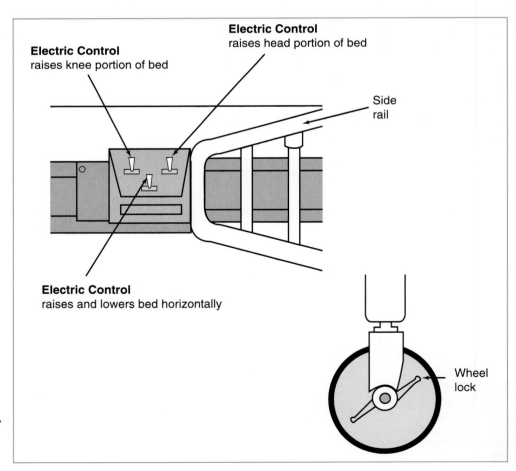

Electric Control raises knee portion of bed

Electric Control raises head portion of bed

Side rail

Electric Control raises and lowers bed horizontally

Wheel lock

Fig. 15-2
An electric bed may have the controls located where the resident can operate them, or they may be at the foot of the bed. The wheels will have locks.

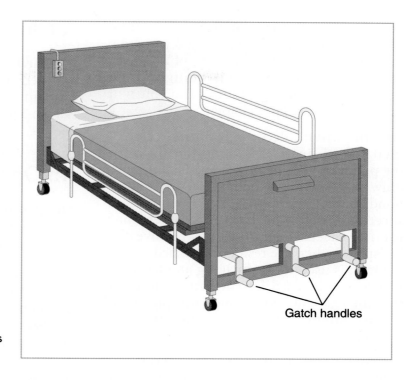

Fig. 15-3
The manually operated bed has gatch handles
to change the position of the bed.

of the bed. If the mattress does not have handles, move the mattress by grasping it underneath. You may need to do this several times a day for a bedbound resident. If necessary, ask a coworker to help. A mattress pad may be used between the mattress and the bottom sheet to make the resident more comfortable.

Linen

Organization of linen is important when you make a bed. Collect the linen in the order in which it will be used. The mattress pad, if you are using one, will be on the bottom of the stack and the pillowcase will be on the top. Collect the linen in this order:

- Mattress pad
- Bottom sheet
- Draw sheet
- Top sheet
- Blanket
- Bedspread
- Pillowcase

Carry the linen to the resident's unit, holding it away from your uniform. Place the linen on a clean surface, turning the

entire stack over so that the linen is in the order in which it will be used. The mattress pad will now be on top.

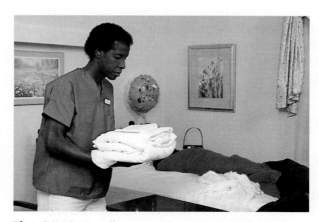

Fig. 15-4 A well-organized nursing assistant gets his work done quickly and efficiently.

Draw Sheets. A **draw sheet** is a small sheet that is placed across the middle of the bottom sheet (see Fig. 15-8). It is also known as a pull sheet or turning sheet. When the draw sheet is tucked in, it helps keep the bottom sheet in place and free of wrinkles. When it is not tucked in, it can be used to move and position the resident. Your facility may have special sheets for this purpose. If not, a regular flat sheet can be folded to the size needed. Usually a draw sheet is about one-half the size of a regular sheet. The procedures for using a draw sheet to move and position a resident will be explained in a later chapter.

Use of Linen. Because facilities differ in their use of linen, it is important to learn the policy of your facility. Some facilities use draw sheets, while others use disposable or nondisposable pads. Although fitted bottom sheets are used in many places, others may use flat sheets. Many facilities remove the bedspread when the resident is in bed.

Linen is used for bedmaking and bathing. It may also be used for comfort, or to position the resident. Do not mop up spills with linen. Sheets are not to be used as restraints.

Linen Changes. In many long-term care facilities a complete change of linen is not made daily. Most of the residents are up and about during the day and only use their beds at night. Some facilities change part of the linen every day. Beds are changed more often for residents who spend most of their time in bed. All beds are changed immediately if they become wet or dirty. It is your responsibility to learn the policy in your facility.

Stripping a Bed

Before clean linen is placed on a bed, the dirty linen must be removed. This procedure is called stripping a bed. Many times, the bed is stripped as soon as the resident is up. If the bed is dirty or wet, you will want to strip the bed and dispose of the linen right away. Wipe the bed with disinfectant before applying clean linen. Let the nurse know if the mattress is damaged.

Check carefully for personal items that may be in the bed. Residents sometimes put jewelry, glasses, or dentures under their pillows. These items may be lost or ruined if they go through the laundry.

A Closed Bed

A **closed bed** is fully made with a blanket and bedspread in place. It is made for the resident who is up for the day. A closed bed is also made when the bed will not be in use.

An Open Bed

An **open bed** is made with the linen turned down. Open beds are made for residents who will be returning to the bed, after being up for a short while. The bed is made while the resident is out of it. The linen is turned down, and the bed is ready for the resident. An open bed may also be prepared for a new admission. Usually, a bedspread is not used on an open bed.

An Occupied Bed

Making a bed with the resident in it is called making an **occupied bed**. This is done when a resident is not able to get out of bed. Critically ill or comatose (unconscious) residents are residents for whom you may need to make an occupied bed.

You should always encourage the resident to help in turning and moving. Movement and exercise are important to the resident's health and well-being. Using this restorative approach will encourage the resident to participate as much as possible. Effective communication skills are important for this procedure. You must explain what you are going to do, even to the unconscious resident. Always assume that an unconscious resident can hear. Even a resident who is very ill may be able to cooperate if you explain first. Remember that touch is a form of communication. Handle the resident gently and carefully. Observe and report any changes in the resident's condition.

A bedspread may not be needed for this procedure. It is usually folded and put away when the resident is in bed.

Stripping a Bed

Before any procedure you must always follow the five basic steps: wash your hands, collect the equipment, identify the resident, explain the procedure, and protect privacy.

Follow universal precautions and wear gloves when appropriate.

1. Raise the bed to a comfortable working height.
2. Loosen the linen all around the bed.
3. Remove the pillow from the pillowcase.
4. If the bedspread and blanket are dirty, roll them up with the rest of the linen. If they are to be reused, fold them separately, using the following steps.
   a. Grasp the bedspread at the top center edge and the corner nearest you. Fold it by bringing the top edge of the spread to the bottom edge of the spread.
   b. Grasp the center of the folded edge with one hand and the corner nearest you with the other hand. Fold the bedspread again by bringing the folded edge to the bottom edge of the spread.
   c. Fold the spread by grasping the edges nearest you and bringing these edges to the edges of the spread on the other side of the bed.
   d. Fold the spread over the back of the bedside chair.
   e. Repeat the steps for the blanket.
5. Roll or fold the rest of the linen away from you with the side that touched the resident inside the roll (see Fig. 15-5).
6. Place the soiled linen in the dirty linen hamper immediately.
7. If a bag or pillowcase is used for the linen, it must be emptied into the hamper; discard the bag if it is disposable.
8. Wipe the mattress with disinfectant, if it is wet, and observe for damage.
9. Wash your hands.

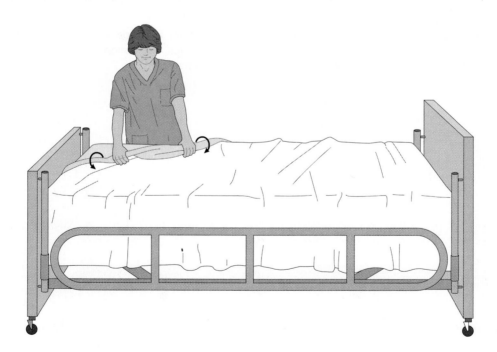

Fig. 15-5 Roll the soiled linen away from you, with the side that touched the resident inside the roll.

PROCEDURE

Making a Closed Bed

Before any procedure you must always follow the five basic steps: wash your hands, collect the equipment, identify the resident, explain the procedure, and protect privacy.

Follow universal precautions and wear gloves when appropriate.

1. Place the clean linen in the order in which it will be used, on a clean surface in the resident's room.
2. Raise the bed to a comfortable working height.
3. If you have not stripped the bed, you must do so at this time (refer to the procedure for stripping a bed).
4. Slide the mattress to the top of the bed.

Working from one side of the bed, use the following steps:

5. Put the mattress pad on the bed.
6. Place the bottom sheet in the center of the bed.
7. Check to see how the sheet is folded. Unfold the sheet and place the narrow hem at the bottom, even with the foot of the mattress. The wide hem will be at the top (see Fig. 15-6).

8. Smooth the side nearest you.
9. Tuck the sheet under the top of the mattress at the head of the bed on the side nearest you.
10. Make a mitered corner (see Fig. 15-7).
    a. Grasp the edge of the sheet 10-12 inches from the top of the bed and fold it onto the mattress (see Fig. 15-7A).
    b. Tuck the part of the sheet that is hanging down under the mattress (see Fig. 15-7B).
    c. Bring the folded part down over the edge of the mattress (see Fig. 15-7C).
    d. Tuck the entire side of the sheet under the mattress (see Fig. 15-7D).
11. If a draw sheet is to be used, place it on top of the sheet, about 12 inches from the top edge of the mattress (see Fig. 15-8).
12. Tuck the draw sheet under the mattress on the side nearest you.
13. Put the top sheet on the center of the bed.
14. Unfold the sheet with as little movement as possible.
15. Center the top sheet with the wide hem even with the top of the mattress and the stitched or seamed side up.
16. Smooth the side of the bed nearest you. Do not tuck the bottom of the top sheet under the mattress yet.

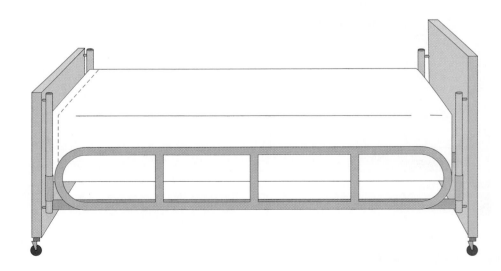

Fig. 15-6 The bottom sheet is placed on the bed with the narrow hem at the bottom.

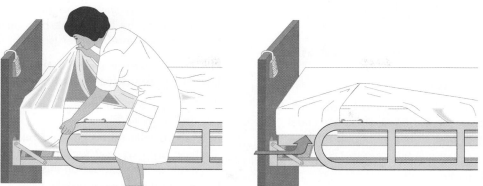
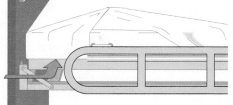

A Grasp the edge of the sheet 10-12 inches from the top of the bed and fold it onto the mattress.

B Tuck the part of the sheet that is hanging down under the mattress.

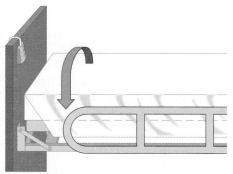
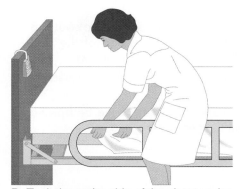

C Bring the folded part down over the mattress.

D Tuck the entire side of the sheet under the mattress.

Fig. 15-7 The nursing assistant is making a mitered corner.

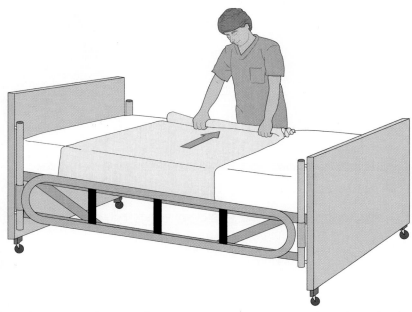

Fig. 15-8 The draw sheet is placed on top of the bottom sheet. It should be pulled tight and tucked under the mattress.

Making a Closed Bed (cont.)

17. Place the blanket over the top sheet as follows:

    a. Unfold and center it.

    b. The top of the blanket should be about 6–8 inches below the top edge of the top sheet.

    c. Smooth the blanket on the side nearest you.

    d. Fold the top sheet down over the top of the blanket to make a cuff.

18. Place the bedspread over the blanket as follows:

    a. Unfold and center it.

    b. Place the bedspread so that about 18 inches extends over the head of the bed (this will be used to cover the pillow).

    c. Smooth the bedspread on the side nearest you.

    d. Turn about 24–25 inches of the bedspread back from the head of the bed.

19. Tuck in the top sheet, the blanket, and the bedspread at the foot of the bed on this side, and make a mitered corner (see Fig. 15-7).

    Go to the other side of the bed to finish the procedure as follows:

20. Tuck in the bottom sheet at the head of the bed (see Fig. 15-9).

    a. Make a mitered corner and pull the bottom sheet tight as you tuck it under the entire length of the mattress on this side.

    b. Smooth it to remove wrinkles.

21. Pull the draw sheet tight and tuck it under the mattress.

22. Straighten the top linen, working from the top to the foot of the bed.

23. Tuck the top linen under the foot of the mattress. After smoothing and tightening it, make a mitered corner.

24. Finish turning the top of the bedspread down about 24–25 inches. Turn the top of the sheet over the top of the blanket.

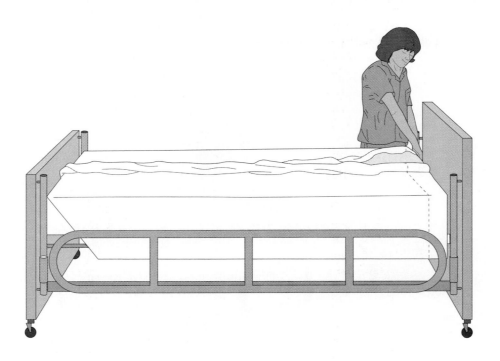

Fig. 15-9 Go to the other side of the bed and tuck in the bottom sheet at the head of the bed.

25. Place the pillow on the bed, and put it into the pillowcase, using the following steps (see Fig. 15-10):

 a. With one hand, grasp the pillowcase at the center of the seamed end (see Fig. 15-10A).

 b. Turn the pillowcase back over that hand with your free hand (see Fig. 15-10B).

 c. Grasp the pillow at the center of one end with the hand that is inside the pillowcase (see Fig. 15-10C).

 d. Pull the pillowcase down over the pillow with your free hand (see Fig. 15-10D). Line up the seams of the pillowcase with the edge of the pillow.

 e. Straighten the pillowcase, making sure that the corners of the pillow are in the corners of the pillowcase (see Fig. 15-10E).

 f. Fold the extra material of the pillowcase under the pillow.

26. Place the pillow on the bed so that the open edge of the pillowcase is facing away from the door.

27. Cover the pillow with the bedspread.

28. Place the call signal in reach of the resident. Attach it to the bed if the resident is out of the room.

29. Lower the bed to its lowest level and tidy the room.

30. Wash your hands.

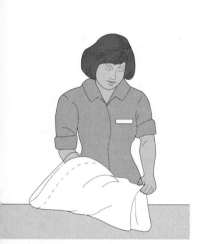

A With one hand, hold the pillowcase at the center of the seamed end.

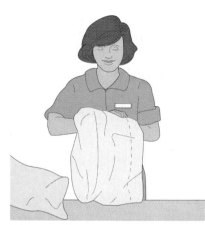

B Turn the pillowcase back over that hand with your free hand.

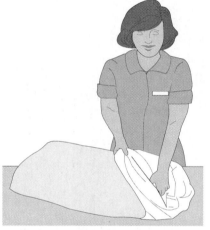

C Grasp the pillow at the center of one end with the hand that is inside the pillowcase.

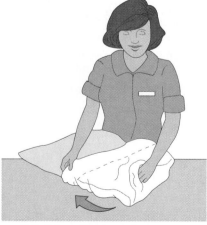

D Pull the pillowcase down over the pillow with your free hand.

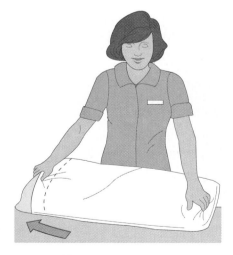

E Straighten the pillowcase.

Fig. 15-10 The nursing assistant is putting the pillow into the pillowcase.

PROCEDURE

Making an Open Bed

Before any procedure you must always follow the five basic steps: wash your hands, collect the equipment, identify the resident, explain the procedure, and protect privacy.

Follow universal precautions and wear gloves when appropriate.

1. Place the clean linen in the order in which it will be used, on a clean surface in the resident's room.

2. Raise the bed to a comfortable working height.

3. If you have not stripped the bed, you must do so at this time (refer to the procedure for stripping a bed).

4. Slide the mattress to the top of the bed.

Working from one side of the bed, use the following steps:

5. Put the mattress pad on the bed.

6. Place the bottom sheet in the center of the bed.

7. Check to see how the sheet is folded. Unfold the sheet and place the narrow hem at the bottom, even with the foot of the mattress. The wide hem will be at the top (see Fig. 15-6).

8. Smooth the side nearest you.

9. Tuck the sheet under the top of the mattress at the head of the bed on the side nearest you.

10. Make a mitered corner (see Fig. 15-7).

    a. Grasp the edge of the sheet 10–12 inches from the top of the bed and fold it onto the mattress (see Fig. 15-7A).

    b. Tuck the part of the sheet that is hanging down under the mattress (see Fig. 15-7B).

    c. Bring the folded part down over the edge of the mattress (see Fig. 15-7C).

    d. Tuck the entire side of the sheet under the mattress (see Fig. 15-7D).

11. If a draw sheet is to be used, place it on top of the sheet, about 12 inches from the top edge of the mattress (see Fig. 15-8).

12. Tuck the draw sheet under the mattress on the side nearest you.

13. Put the top sheet on the center of the bed.

14. Unfold the sheet with as little movement as possible.

15. Center the top sheet with the wide hem even with the top of the mattress and the stitched or seamed side up.

16. Smooth the side of the bed nearest you. Do not tuck the bottom of the top sheet under the mattress yet.

17. Place the blanket over the top sheet as follows:

    a. Unfold and center it.

    b. The top of the blanket should be about 6–8 inches below the top edge of the top sheet.

    c. Smooth the blanket on the side nearest you.

    d. Fold the top sheet down over the top of the blanket to make a cuff.

18. Tuck in the top sheet and the blanket at the foot of the bed on this side, and make a mitered corner (see Fig. 15-7).

Go to the other side of the bed to finish the procedure as follows:

19. Tuck in the bottom sheet at the head of the bed (see Fig. 15-9).

    a. Make a mitered corner and pull the bottom sheet tight as you tuck it under the entire length of the mattress on this side.

    b. Smooth the sheet to remove wrinkles.

20. Pull the draw sheet tight and tuck it under the mattress.

21. Straighten the top linen, working from the top to the foot of the bed.

22. Tuck the top linen under the foot of the mattress. After smoothing and tightening it , make a mitered corner.

23. Turn the top of the sheet over the top of the blanket.

24. Place the pillow on the bed, and put it into the pillowcase, using the following steps (see Fig. 15-10):

    a. With one hand, grasp the pillowcase at the center of the seamed end (see Fig. 15-10A).

    b. Turn the pillowcase back over that hand with your free hand (see Fig. 15-10B).

    c. Grasp the pillow at the center of one end with the hand that is inside the pillowcase (see Fig. 15-10C).

    d. Pull the pillowcase down over the pillow with your free hand (see Fig. 15-10D). Line up the seams of the pillowcase with the edge of the pillow.

    e. Straighten the pillowcase, making sure that the corners of the pillow are in the corners of the pillowcase (see Fig. 15-10E).

    f. Fold the extra material of the pillowcase under the pillow.

25. Place the pillow on the bed so that the open edge of the pillowcase is facing away from the door.

26. Grasp the top of the sheet and blanket, and fold it to the foot of the bed (see Fig. 15-11).

27. Attach the call signal to the bed. If the resident is in the chair, be sure that it is within reach.

28. Lower the bed to its lowest level.

29. Tidy the room.

30. Wash your hands.

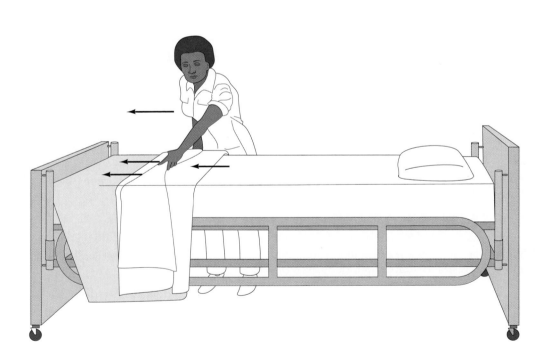

Fig. 15-11 Grasp the top of the sheet and blanket and fold them to the foot of the bed.

PROCEDURE

Making an Occupied Bed

Before any procedure you must always follow the five basic steps: wash your hands, collect the equipment, identify the resident, explain the procedure, and provide privacy.

Follow universal precautions and wear gloves when appropriate.

1. Place the clean linen in the order in which it will be used, on a clean surface in the resident's room.

2. Pull the curtain around the bed and close the door.

3. Raise the bed to a comfortable working height and lock the wheels.

4. Lower the head of the bed, being sure to maintain a height that is safe and comfortable for the resident.

5. Lower the side rails on the side of the bed nearest you. Be sure the rail is up on the opposite side of the bed.

6. Loosen the top linen at the foot of the bed.

7. Remove the blanket.

   a. If it is dirty, remove it by rolling or folding it away from you, with the side that touched the resident, inside the roll.

   b. If it is to be reused, fold it over the back of the chair.

8. Cover the resident with a bath blanket, using the following steps:

   a. Unfold the bath blanket over the top sheet.

   b. Ask the resident to grasp the top of the bath blanket, or tuck the top edge under the resident's shoulders to keep it in place (see Fig. 15-12).

   c. Grasp the sheet under the bath blanket, and slide it out at the foot of the bed, rolling it with the side that touched the resident on the inside. Place it with the dirty linen.

   d. If you do not have a bath blanket, leave the top sheet in place over the resident, or use a clean top sheet. The resident must be kept covered for warmth and privacy.

9. Move the mattress to the top of the bed.

10. Assist the resident to turn to the far side of the bed.

    a. Help the resident to maintain correct body alignment.

    b. Adjust the pillow as needed.

    c. Be sure the resident is not too close to the side rail.

11. Loosen the bottom linen on this side of the bed and fold it to the resident's body. Tuck it under the resident's body (see Fig. 15-13).

Working from the side of the bed nearest you, use the following steps:

12. Put the mattress pad on the bed.

13. Place the bottom sheet in the center of the bed, next to the resident.

14. Check to see how the sheet is folded. Unfold the sheet and place the narrow hem at the bottom, even with the foot of the mattress (see Fig. 15-6).

15. Smooth the side nearest you, and tuck the sheet under the top of the mattress at the head of the bed.

16. Make a mitered corner (see Fig. 15-7).

17. If a draw sheet is to be used, place it on top of the sheet, about 12 inches from the top edge of the mattress (see Fig. 15-8).

18. Tuck the draw sheet under the mattress.

19. Fold the clean linen toward the resident, next to the dirty linen (see Fig. 15-14).

20. Raise the side rail on this side.

21. Ask the resident to turn or move toward you to the clean side of the bed. Assist as necessary.

    a. Explain that the resident will roll across the folded linen.

b. Be sure the resident is not too close to the rail.

c. Adjust the pillow.

Go to the opposite side of the bed.

22. Lower the rail on this side.

23. Loosen the used bottom linen, roll it away from you with the side that touched the resident on the inside, and place it with the other dirty linen.

24. Unfold the clean linen that is in the center of the bed.

25. Straighten the bottom sheet, and tuck it in at the head of the bed.

    a. Make a mitered corner.

    b. Tuck the sheet under the mattress while pulling it tight.

26. Straighten the draw sheet, and tuck it under the mattress while pulling it tight (see Fig. 15-15).

27. Assist the resident to a comfortable position.

28. Put the top sheet on the center of the bed.

29. Unfold the sheet with as little movement as possible.

30. Center the top sheet so that the wide hem is even with the top of the mattress and the stitched or seamed side up.

31. Smooth this side of the bed. Do not tuck the bottom of the top sheet under the mattress yet.

32. Place the blanket over the top sheet as follows:

    a. Unfold and center it.

    b. The top of the blanket should be about 6–8 inches below the top edge of the top sheet with the top sheet folded down over it.

    c. Smooth the blanket on this side.

33. Ask the resident to hold the clean top sheet and blanket as you remove the dirty sheet or bath blanket, by pulling it from under the clean linen at the foot of the bed. Roll the dirty linen with the side that touched the resident to the inside.

    a. If the resident cannot hold the sheet, you may tuck it beneath the shoulders.

    b. Place it with the dirty linen that has already been removed.

34. Tuck the top linen under the bottom of the mattress on this side of the bed, and make a mitered corner.

35. Put the side rail up on this side of the bed.

    Go to the other side of the bed and lower the side rail.

36. Complete the bed by straightening the top linen and tucking it in at the bottom of the mattress (see Fig. 15-16) and making a mitered corner.

37. Raise the side rail.

38. Check the tightness of the linen over the resident's feet. Loosen it by pulling up on the top linen (see Fig. 15-17).

39. Place the pillow on the bed, and put it into the pillowcase (see Fig. 15-10).

40. Place the pillow on the bed so that the open edge of the pillowcase is facing away from the door.

41. Position the resident comfortably and in correct body alignment.

42. Attach the call signal so it can be reached by the resident.

43. Lower the bed to its lowest level.

44. Tidy the room.

45. Pull the curtain from around the bed and open the door.

46. Dispose of the linen in the dirty linen hamper, if you have not already done so.

47. Wash your hands.

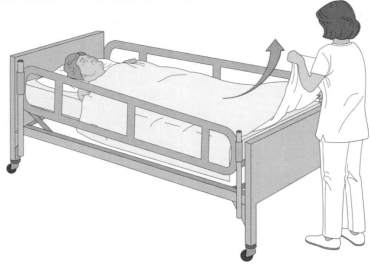

Fig. 15-12 Tuck the top edge of the bath blanket under the resident's shoulders to hold it in place while you slide the top sheet out from under the blanket.

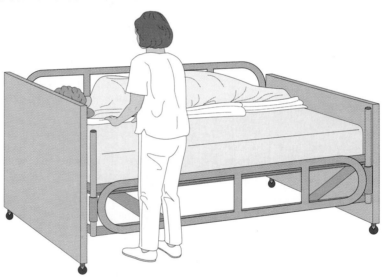

Fig. 15-13 The dirty bottom linen is folded to the resident's body and tucked under to hold it in place.

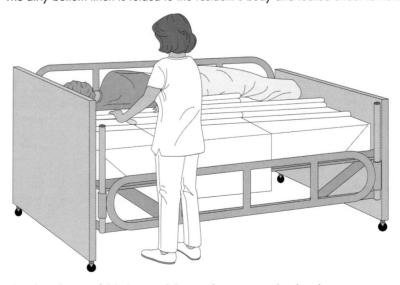

Fig. 15-14 The clean linen is folded toward the resident, next to the dirty linen.

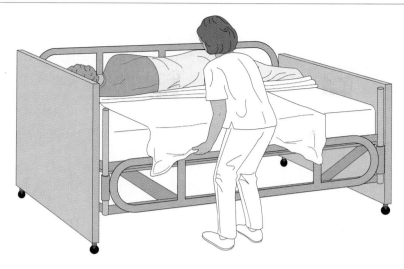

Fig. 15-15 The draw sheet is straightened, pulled tight, and tucked under the mattress.

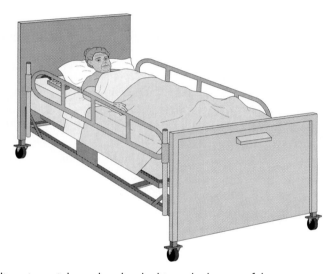

Fig. 15-16 The top linen is straightened and tucked in at the bottom of the mattress.

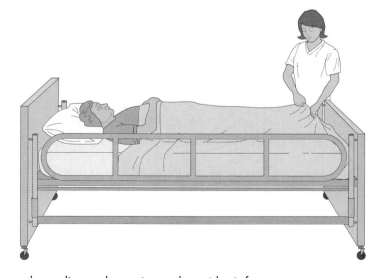

Fig. 15-17 Pull up on the top linen to loosen it over the resident's feet.

A Restorative Approach to Bedmaking

There are many opportunities to use restorative measures while making the resident's bed. Some residents may be bedbound and will have to stay in the bed while it is being made. If this is the case, explain clearly, as you assist the resident to move and turn. Residents who are able to get out of bed should be encouraged to do so. Assist them as needed and encourage independence.

A clean neat bed and a tidy room help to create a restorative environment for the resident. Leaving the bed at a safe, low level, with the call signal in easy reach, promotes safety and independence. A restorative environment is comfortable, safe and homelike.

Communication and Observation. Bedmaking provides an excellent time for communicating with the resident. You will have the perfect opportunity to help maintain the resident's sense of individuality and self-esteem. Talk about current events and ask questions. Show your interest and give encouragement. You may hear verbal complaints and problems that cannot otherwise be observed. Remember how important it is to be a good listener. Your visual observations of movements and posture are possible at this time. Be alert for nonverbal signs of distress. Gestures and facial expressions may communicate more than words.

Conclusion

Remember these important points:

1. Collect and organize the linen.
2. Always provide privacy for the resident.
3. Raise the bed to a comfortable working height, and use correct body mechanics.
4. Complete one side of the bed at a time, as much as possible.
5. Change linen immediately if it is soiled.
6. Never place dirty linen on a clean surface or on the floor.

7. Carry clean linen away from your uniform.
8. Don't shake clean or dirty linen.
9. Frequent handwashing is the best way to prevent the spread of germs.
10. Follow universal precautions and wear gloves when appropriate.
11. Keep the bed wrinkle free and smooth.
12. Communicate with the resident during bedmaking.
13. Talk to all residents, including those who are unconscious.
14. Handle the resident gently, and position in correct body alignment.
15. Leave the call signal within the resident's reach.
16. Raise the side rails when appropriate.

Discussion Questions

1. *What effect can a clean, neat bed have on the resident?*
2. *What are some safety measures that you should take to protect the resident from injury? How can you protect yourself?*
3. *How can you prevent the spread of germs while you are making a bed?*
4. *Why are communication skills necessary during bedmaking?*
5. *How can bedmaking be restorative?*

Application Exercises

The class will divide into three groups, with each group selecting a leader.

Group 1: Make a list of safety measures to be followed while making a bed.

Group 2: Make a list of aseptic practices to be used when making a bed.

Group 3: Make a list of restorative measures that can be used while making a bed.

Each leader will present the group's list to the class. The lists can be written on the blackboard. Each leader should ask the class for additional suggestions.

Admission, Transfer, and Discharge

OBJECTIVES

Upon completing this chapter, you will be able to do the following:

1. Describe the emotional impact of admission to the long-term care facility.

2. List four responsibilities of the nursing assistant in the admission process.

3. List four responsibilities of the nursing assistant in transferring a resident.

4. List four responsibilities of the nursing assistant in the discharge process.

5. Identify four restorative approaches to use when admitting, transferring, or discharging a resident.

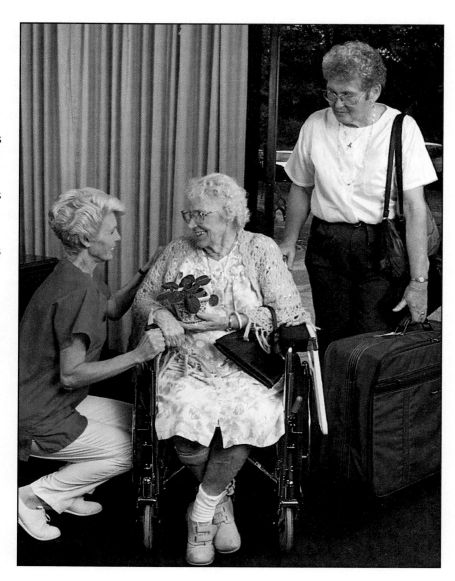

The Emotional Impact of Admission

Admission to a long-term care facility can cause anxiety for the new residents and their families. Many have suffered losses such as health, spouse, home, possessions, and independence. Residents who have lost independence require assistance with activities of daily living (ADLs). They may be ill and need the care of medically trained personnel. Some will stay in the facility until they die. Others may get better and return home.

Events prior to admission may have been stressful. Admission often means giving up a home, familiar routines, and the closeness of family, friends, and pets. Not only must losses be faced, a new environment may cause uncertainty and fear. Can you imagine yourself moving, without your family and friends, to an unfamiliar place? Would you have any fears? If you were ill or unable to do things for yourself, would you worry about how you would survive and who would help you? If you couldn't choose your own roommate, your privacy and security might be threatened.

Admission to a long-term care facility involves many concerns for the resident and family. Most families would prefer to care for relatives at home, and some have promised to do so. However, it is sometimes necessary to admit a loved one, regardless of the desire to provide care at home. The confused wanderer may be unsafe at home. The care and assistance that is necessary may be impossible to provide in the home setting.

Working family members may find themselves unable to attend to needs that must be met 24 hours a day. Lack of sleep can become a problem. Lifting, moving, and personal care may be to difficult for family members. Nursing care may be required, and reliable help may not be available for hire at home. The family, faced with all these problems, must make a difficult deci-

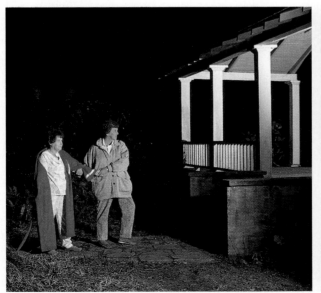
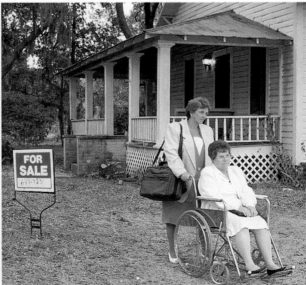

Fig. 16-1 Prior to admission, the new resident and her family may have experienced many stressful events.

sion. Many times, admission to a long-term care facility is the only choice that will provide the care that is necessary. Family members may feel guilty because they believe they have failed.

Nursing assistants play a very important role in easing the emotional stress for the resident and family. Your attitude can relieve many fears and provide a more comfortable beginning for the new resident. First impressions are lasting, so it is important to make a positive first impression on both the resident and the family.

Admitting the Resident

The admission process begins in the business office, where information about the facility is provided. Plans and arrangements for admission are made, and paperwork is completed. Often this part of the process begins before the day of admission. When that day arrives, the nursing unit will be notified.

Be prepared before the resident's arrival if you will be expected to assist with admission. Be sure to check with the nurse for necessary information such as the resident's abilities and disabilities and if food or fluids are allowed. Prepare the room to be comfortable and welcoming. Place the necessary equipment and linen in the unit. This may include a bedpan, urinal, water pitcher, glass, bath basin, towel, washcloth, and gown.

If the resident will arrive by stretcher, prepare the bed by turning down the covers and raising the bed to stretcher height. Otherwise, the bed should be left in the lowest position. Covers will be arranged as necessary for the resident. Be sure that lighting and window openings produce a comfortable degree of brightness for the new resident.

Warmly greeting the new resident by name will help create a feeling of welcome and comfort. Introduce yourself by name and title. Accompany the resident to the room. Greet the family in a friendly manner and encourage them to accompany the resident. Remember that they may also be

uncomfortable or nervous about the admission. If the resident requests privacy, suggest a comfortable place where the family might wait, and remember to invite them back when privacy is no longer necessary.

Introduce the resident and roommate to each other. Identify furniture, bathroom, and room areas to be used. Demonstrate the call signal and place it within reach. Provide ice water if allowed. Assist with unpacking. If medications have been brought, report this to the nurse. Always handle resident's belongings with respect and care. These may be all that remain of life-long belongings.

The Belongings List. The nurse will provide you with a form to list the resident's valuables and personal belongings. Describe each item and list quantities. Money should be counted and recorded. Extra money may be locked in the safe. Facility policy may determine how much money can be kept in the room. Check with the nurse regarding this procedure. Jewelry must be described by color of metal and stones. Never say "gold" or "diamonds." It is correct to say "yellow" or "gold-colored metal" and "white stones." What appears to be precious metal or stones may not be.

Another staff member should assist you with the belongings list. Your facility may require that the list be signed by two employees. The resident or responsible party may also be required to sign it. Belongings are marked according to facility policy. Family members should be instructed to advise the staff if they bring in additional items. Items that are taken from the facility must be deleted from the list.

Observation must be made of the entire body surface. Provide privacy and explain what you are going to do. Most facilities provide a form for recording observations including skin condition, tubes, bandages, amputations, injuries, and scars (see Fig. 16-2). Remember to wash your hands upon completion of the observation.

Vital signs (blood pressure, temperature, pulse, and respirations), height, and weight are usually measured and recorded upon admission. These procedures are provided

ADMISSION INFORMATION CHART

Directions: Complete all entries. Indicate all body marks, scars, and sores.

DATE OF ADMISSION _____ TIME OF ADMISSION _____

CONDITION ON ADMISSION:

TEMP: _____ PULSE: _____ RESP: _____ B.P. _____ WEIGHT: _____ HT: _____

__ AMBULATORY   __ CONFINED TO CHAIR   __ REQUIRES FEEDING   __ CONTINENT

                        __ CONFINED TO BED   __ FEEDS SELF   __ INCONTINENT

Additional remarks _____

_____

MENTAL ATTITUDE:

__ ORIENTED   __ FORGETFUL   __ DEPRESSED   __ COOPERATIVE

__ DISORIENTED   __ CHEERFUL   __ NORMAL ATTITUDE   __ UNCOOPERATIVE

Additional remarks _____

_____

CONDITION OF HAIR AND SCALP:

CONDITION OF FINGERNAILS AND TOENAILS:

CONDITION OF TEETH:

RESIDENT HAS: __ DENTURES   __ GLASSES   __ HEARING AID   __ OTHER _____

                                                                      (specify)

ALLERGIES:

GENERAL CONDITION OF RESIDENT'S BODY:

Show all body marks: scars, bruises, cuts, decubiti, ulcers, and discolorations (birth marks should not be shown).

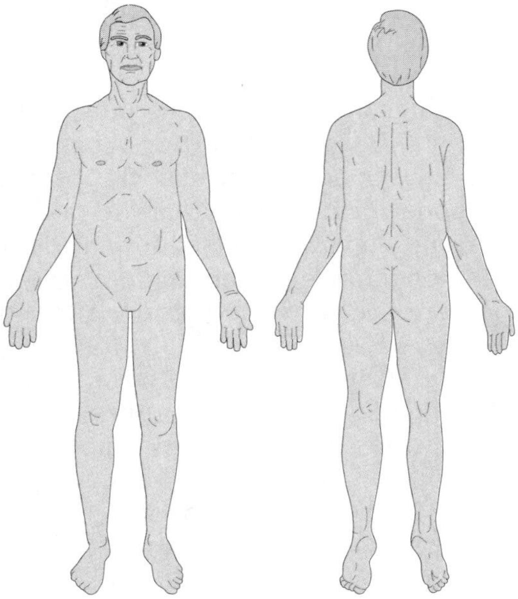

Signed _____

Fig. 16-2 A sample admission form.

in later chapters. You may find them in the index of this book. Report observations to the nurse. If the new resident complains of pain or dyspnea (difficult breathing) report these observations to the nurse immediately.

The admission is not complete until you have reported and recorded all necessary information. Listen for important information that the resident or family members say to you. Be sure to include requests and preferences that are expressed by the resident or family. This information will become a part of the resident's care plan.

Familiarizing the Resident with the Facility

Orient the resident to the facility. Mealtimes, dining locations, visiting hours, and smoking rules should be explained. Show the resident how to find the nurses desk, rest rooms, water fountains, TV rooms, recreation areas, and the chapel. Provide a general idea of daily schedules and ask about preferences. Introduce the resident to other residents and staff members.

Before leaving, assure the resident that you will be nearby and available. Explain the use of the call signal, and leave it within reach. Be sure to check back frequently, and inform the resident when you are leaving for the day. This will help to reassure and build a sense of security. Building a trusting relationship with the resident begins on admission. Your attitude, courtesy, and helpfulness are the foundation of the next phase of the resident's life. Help to make it comfortable and safe.

Transferring the Resident

The nursing assistant plays a very important role in transferring a resident. The transfer may be from room to room or from one nursing unit to another. Transfers can be very upsetting to the resident. Even a healthy resident, who is willing to move, may find that moving is both physically and emotionally distressful. An elderly resident who would prefer not to move, and who is dependent upon others, experiences an additional burden. The harsh reality is that circumstances may require a move. In addition, the resident may feel great concern about who the new care givers and roommate will be. The resident may not feel wel-

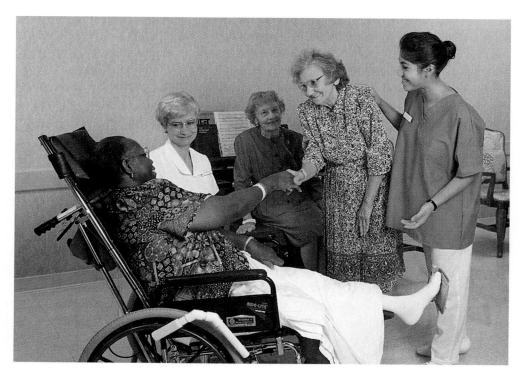

Fig. 16-3
Introduce the new resident to other residents and staff members.

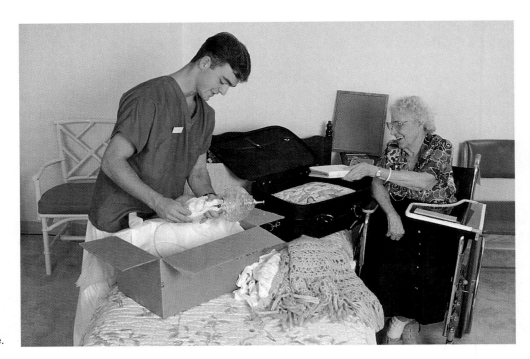

Fig. 16-4
Handle the resident's personal belongings with respect and care.

come, and may fear that needs will not be met. Emotional support will be needed from staff members in both areas of the facility.

If it becomes necessary to transfer the resident, the nurse will notify the resident and family. The nursing assistant must assist the resident to gather personal belongings. These should be handled with care and respect. Be supportive of the resident while demonstrating a positive attitude toward the new location. Remember to be a good listener, as the resident may wish to express feelings about the move.

When the nurse tells you to do so, you must move the belongings and assist the resident to the new location. The nurse will assist you if you are not sure what the exact transfer process in your facility requires. Introduce the new roommate, other residents, and staff members. Assure the resident's comfort, and place the call signal within reach. Do not leave the area without notifying the nurse on duty.

Staff members at the new location will complete the transfer process according to facility policy. A helpful, courteous, and supportive attitude is necessary upon transferring the resident. If the resident is transferred to another area within your facility, a visit from you later may be appreciated.

Discharging the Resident

Discharge is usually a happy time for the resident who has recovered enough to return home. Sometimes, however, a resident must be discharged to the hospital or another long-term care facility. Discharge is a stressful event, even in the most positive circumstances. The resident may have fears about being able to function adequately at home. Leaving old relationships can cause sadness and loneliness.

The resident may fear being discharged to the hospital. Once again, it is necessary for the nursing assistant to provide emotional support and reassurance while preparing the resident for discharge.

Discharge cannot take place until the doctor has written an order and financial arrangements have been made. The nurse will inform you of the time of discharge, after notification by the doctor and the business office. If a resident attempts to leave, and you have not been informed of the discharge, notify the nurse immediately.

Discharge planning includes the plans and arrangements for care of the resident after discharge. This plan begins on the resident's admission to the facility. The plan of restorative care usually includes the goal

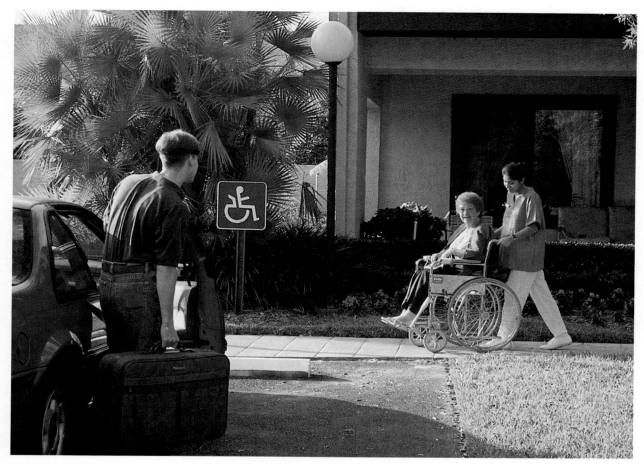

Fig. 16-5 The resident is taken to the car by the nursing assistant.

and preparation for discharge. This plan includes care provided within the facility during recovery and care after discharge. Resident and family education is a part of discharge planning.

You are responsible for care and preparation of the resident's belongings. A list of belongings that are being taken home may be required by your facility. Check with the charge nurse if you are not sure. Pack the belongings with care and respect. Allow the resident to assist.

The resident is usually released to a family member or guardian and is taken to the car in a wheelchair. You must assist the resident into the car. Never leave the resident unattended. If the resident is discharged to another facility or hospital, an ambulance may be needed. In this situation, ambulance personnel will move the resident from the bed to the transport vehicle.

Using a Restorative Approach for Admission, Transfer, and Discharge

A restorative approach to care begins upon admission to a long-term care facility. Because it is not normal to give up independence, home, and individual life-style, the resident will need to be reassured and encouraged. Restorative care must be continued throughout residence. The primary restorative goal is to return the resident to a normal life at home.

Your courteous, friendly, and helpful attitude is restorative and will help the resident to feel more secure. Although admission, transfer, and discharge may not be the resident's choice, you must always encourage participation in planning and preparing for the move. Involve the resident in settling

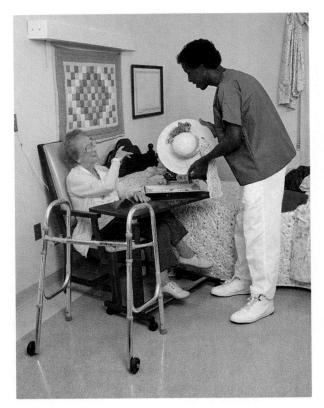

Fig. 16-6 Involve the resident in arranging her room.

into a new environment. This can be accomplished by seeking input and assistance with packing, organizing, and arranging the environment. It is normal to want control of one's environment. Imagine how you would feel if someone reorganized your home without your permission. Involvement gives the resident the opportunity for independence, control of the environment, and expression of individuality.

Conclusion

Remember these important points:

1. Admission to a long-term care facility is stressful for both the resident and family.

2. Prepare the room before the resident's arrival.

3. Greet the resident by name and introduce yourself.

4. List valuables and label clothing according to facility policy.

5. Orient the new resident to the facility and introduce residents and staff members.

6. A friendly, helpful, and reassuring attitude can reduce the stress of transferring.

7. Listen while the resident expresses feelings about moving.

8. Discharge planning begins upon admission.

9. Emotional support is necessary during admission, transfer, and discharge.

10. A restorative approach to care begins upon admission and continues through discharge.

Discussion Questions

1. *What are some fears or concerns that you might have if you were to be admitted to a long-term care facility?*

2. *How can the nursing assistant affect the impression of the long-term care facility that is made upon the new resident and family?*

3. *How would you feel if suddenly you realized you had to move?*

4. *Why might the resident feel stressed about being discharged?*

Application Exercise

1. The class will divide into groups. Members of each group will do one of the following:

   a. Obtain articles or documentaries that affect public opinion about long-term care facilities.

   b. Interview some elderly residents regarding their feelings about admission to a long-term care facility.

   c. Interview a resident who has been transferred. Ask her to share her feelings about the move.

Each group will present a report to the class for discussion.

Moving and Exercising Residents

OBJECTIVES

Upon completing this chapter, you will be able to do the following:

1. Explain the importance of activity.

2. Identify four complications of limited activity.

3. List and explain three restorative techniques for moving and exercising residents.

4. Identify four rules of body mechanics for moving and positioning residents.

5. Explain the importance of body alignment.

6. Demonstrate four basic body positions.

7. List three advantages of using a gait/transfer belt.

8. Identify four rules of safety when using a mechanical lift.

9. List six safety measures to be used when transferring a resident to and from a stretcher.

10. Describe the proper technique for using a wheelchair.

11. Explain the proper way to assist the resident to ambulate with a cane or walker.

12. Identify four safety guidelines for performing range-of-motion exercises.

13. Demonstrate the procedures described in this chapter.

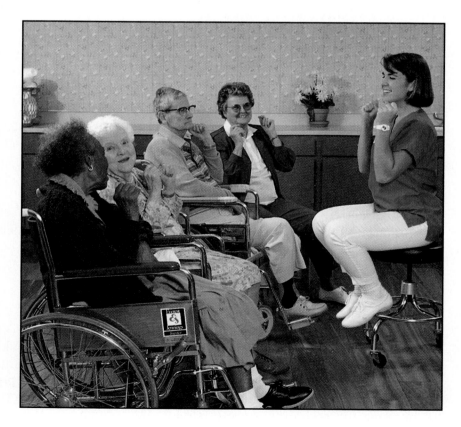

VOCABULARY

The following words or terms will help you to understand this chapter:

Pressure sore/decubitus ulcer
Contracture
Atrophy
Constipation
Fecal impaction

Extremities
Edema
Body mechanics
Body alignment
Supine position
Prone position

Lateral position
Fowler's position
Dangling
Geri-chair
Ambulate
Range-of-motion exercises

SECTION I: THE RESTORATIVE APPROACH TO ACTIVITY

The Importance of Exercise and Activity

Physical activity is necessary to maintain the well-being of all body systems. It increases muscle strength and tone. Muscles that are in tone provide better support and are less likely to be injured. Activity helps the body maintain flexibility and coordination.

Physical activity increases respiratory rate and depth. This helps to keep the airway clear of mucus and prevents pooling of fluid in the lungs. The heart responds to activity by pumping faster and harder. An increased heart rate delivers more oxygen to the brain and other tissues. Improved circulation helps to maintain healthy skin. It contributes to the immune system and helps the body resist infection. Toxins and waste products are eliminated more effectively.

Physical activity helps the digestive system function more effectively and causes an increase in the rate of peristalsis (the muscular contractions that move food through the digestive system). This allows food to be digested more quickly. Activity also improves appetite and fluid intake.

Residents who are active feel better both physically and emotionally. They have a more positive attitude. Activity also increases independence and raises self-esteem. Restorative efforts are more successful because the residents are motivated to set and reach goals. Physical activity helps them to be more alert and oriented. Studies have shown that activity slows the aging process. As you can see, activity benefits the "whole person."

Complications of Limited Exercise and Activity

When a person is not active, problems occur that may affect all the body systems. Some complications of limited activity include

Pressure sores

Contractures

Muscle atrophy

Constipation

Fecal impaction

Edema

Blood clots

Urinary tract infection

Kidney stones

Pneumonia

Confusion

Depression

A **pressure sore/decubitus ulcer** is a breakdown in skin tissue that occurs when blood flow is interrupted. If a resident lies or sits in one position too long or is positioned incorrectly, pressure will cause skin damage.

A **contracture** is a permanent shortening of a muscle due to lack of use or lack of exercise. A contracture results when a part of the body is not moved and exercised enough. Have you ever noticed a person with a paralyzed arm, holding it against the chest? If it is kept in this position for a period of time, a contracture may develop. A resident with arthritis may also keep a hand or an arm in one position, in an effort to avoid pain.

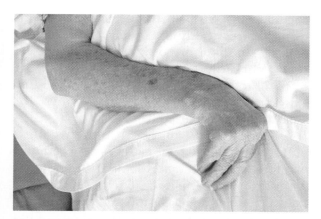

Fig. 17-1 Keeping the arm in one position for a long period of time can cause a contracture.

One form of contracture is called foot drop. Foot drop occurs when the foot is not supported in natural alignment. A contracture may be the result of paralysis or a spastic condition. However, most contractures can be prevented by exercise and proper positioning. All these measures are means of providing restorative care.

Muscle atrophy is another complication of limited activity. **Atrophy** means wasting or a decrease in size. Muscular atrophy is wasting or a decrease in the size of a muscle.

Decreased activity may slow peristalsis. When this happens, the large intestine absorbs too much water from the stool, causing it to become dry and hard. **Constipation** is the passage of hard, dry stool. A large amount of hard, dry stool is called a **fecal impaction**. An impaction fills the rectum and must be removed before the person can have a normal bowel movement.

Inactivity causes circulation to slow down and become sluggish. When blood flow slows to the **extremities** (the arms and legs), fluid collects in the tissues. This accumulation of fluid causes swelling and is called **edema**. Poor circulation is the major factor contributing to blood clots. It also plays a role in the development of pneumonia, urinary tract infections, and kidney stones.

The pneumonia that results from limited activity is called hypostatic pneumonia. If a person remains in one position for a long period of time, gravity causes the blood and other fluids to pool in one part of the lung. Infection easily occurs.

Limited activity can affect the resident's mental and emotional status. The lack of stimulation, combined with slowed circulation, may cause the resident to become confused and disoriented. Inactive people can easily become depressed. They may feel helpless and without hope. An active life is a healthy life. Inactivity damages the body and dulls the spirit.

Restorative Techniques

Restorative nursing care can prevent most of the complications of limited activity. Assisting the resident to move and exercise will allow you many opportunities to use restorative techniques. Always encourage the resident to do as much as possible. This promotes mobility and increases body strength. It also helps to build independence and self-esteem.

In this chapter, you will learn about specific restorative programs, such as range-of-motion exercises and ambulation. However, all nursing care should be carried out in a restorative manner.

Before you attempt to assist the resident in moving or exercising, assess the situation carefully. Ask yourself the following questions. What are the resident's abilities and disabilities? How much can the resident do? How is the resident's sense of balance? Is the resident strong enough to stand? What special equipment will be needed? Is the resident oriented enough to follow directions? Is the resident motivated to be active?

Once you have completed your assessment, you can begin the procedure. Keep directions simple and be consistent. Allow enough time for independent self-care, but don't let the resident become frustrated. Watch for signs of fatigue. Use praise and encouragement frequently. Emphasize the positive and concentrate on success.

Remember the principles of restorative care that were described in Chapter 4 of this text:

Treat the whole person.

Start rehabilitation early.

Stress ability—not disability.

Encourage activity.

Maintain a restorative attitude.

It will be helpful to go back and review the chapter on rehabilitation and restorative care at this time.

Body Mechanics and Body Alignment

Body Mechanics. **Body mechanics** refers to the use of the body to produce motion. Always use correct body mechanics when assisting the resident in moving and exercising. Stand with your feet apart for a wide base of support. Keep your spine straight. Bend at your knees, and use the large muscles of your thighs. Turn your body, without twisting, in the direction you are moving the resident.

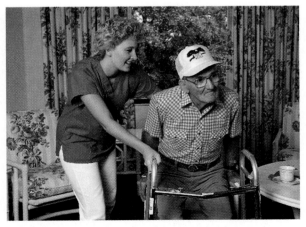

Fig. 17-2 Praise and encouragement are great motivators.

Stand close to the resident and use smooth, coordinated movements. Body mechanics is explained in more detail in Chapter 6.

When positioning the resident or assisting with exercises, bring the bed to a comfortable working height for you. The bed should be as flat as the resident can tolerate. Keep the side rail up on the opposite side. Use a turning sheet (draw sheet), and get help when necessary.

Body Alignment. It is important that the resident is positioned in correct body alignment. Correct **body alignment** means maintaining a normal or correct anatomical position. When the resident is lying down, the trunk of the body should be in a straight line. The extremities should be positioned for comfort and supported as necessary (Fig. 17-3A). Correct body alignment prevents stress on the musculoskeletal system and promotes comfort. Stand back and look at the resident when you are finished. The resident who doesn't look straight is probably not comfortable or in correct body alignment. This increases the risk for complications.

Body alignment is also important when sitting in a chair. The resident should sit straight, with the back against the back of the chair. Feet should either touch the floor or be propped on a stool (see Fig. 17-3B). A person who is slumped over in a chair or leaning to the side is not in proper body alignment and will soon become tired and uncomfortable.

Restorative Equipment. Equipment designed to help the resident maintain correct body alignment includes footboards, foot supports, bed cradles, trochanter rolls, hand rolls, splints, and armboards (see Fig. 17-4). Footboards and foot supports are used to keep the feet and ankles in alignment and prevent foot drop. A bed cradle keeps the top linen from pressing on the toes. Trochanter rolls prevent the hips and legs from rolling inward or outward. They should extend from the knee to the top of the hip. A trochanter roll can be made by rolling up a blanket.

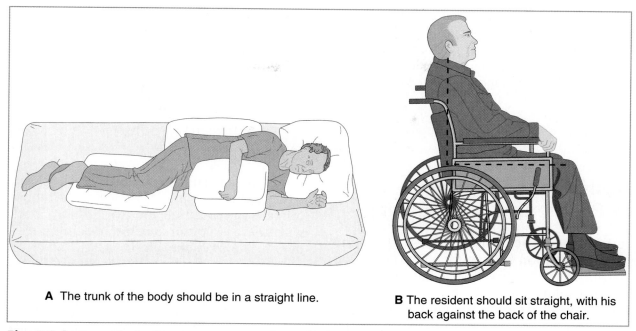

A The trunk of the body should be in a straight line.

B The resident should sit straight, with his back against the back of the chair.

Fig. 17-3 Correct body alignment promotes comfort and helps to prevent complications.

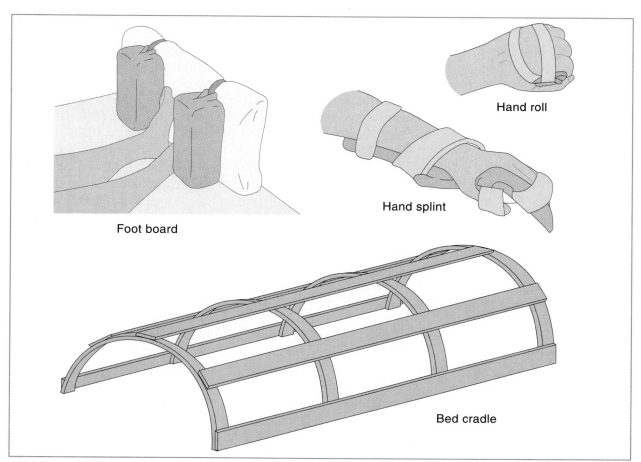

Foot board

Hand splint

Hand roll

Bed cradle

Fig. 17-4 Special equipment used to help the resident maintain correct body alignment.

Handrolls are used to keep the hand slightly flexed and prevent the fingers from curling into the palm. Hand and wrist splints are individually designed for the person who needs them. Armboards can be used to support the arm when a person is sitting in a chair. Pillows and linens are commonly used as positioning devices to help maintain correct body alignment.

SECTION II: MOVING AND POSITIONING RESIDENTS

Assisting the Resident in Positioning and Turning

It is very important that the resident changes position frequently when in bed or sitting for any length of time. Although some residents will be able to do this for themselves, others will need your assistance. A person who is very ill or comatose (unconscious) needs to be turned at least every two hours. Changing positions promotes comfort, stimulates circulation, and helps to prevent complications.

Basic Body Positions. Although there are many ways of positioning the body, there are four basic positions: supine, prone, lateral, and Fowler's. Semiprone and semisupine positions may be used because there is less pressure on bony prominences (see Figs. 17-5E and 5F).

A person in a **supine position** is lying on the back. (Clue: The spine is in the back. Add a "u" to the word "spine" and it becomes "supine.") (See Fig. 17-5A.) This position is sometimes called "horizontal recumbent." In this position the person is flat on the back. For correct body alignment, the resident's head and shoulders are supported on a pillow. The arms are at the sides, and may also be supported by pillows. A weak or paralyzed arm should be positioned on a pillow to prevent edema. If needed, a hand roll may be used to support the hand in a natural position. The feet should be braced with pillows or a footboard to keep them positioned correctly.

In the **prone position**, the resident is lying on the abdomen. The arms may be at the sides or flexed upward by the head. The head is turned to the side and may be supported by a small pillow. The bed should be flat (see Fig. 17-5B). Most residents cannot tolerate this position for two hours. Check with the charge nurse before placing a resident in the prone position.

A person in **lateral position** is lying on the side. There are many types of lateral positions. The upper arm and upper leg are supported on pillows. A pillow against the back helps the resident to maintain correct body alignment. If possible, bring the upper leg forward and support it with a pillow. If the resident cannot assume this position comfortably, pillows must be placed between the calves and thighs to prevent pressure on the knees (see Fig. 17-5C).

Fowler's position is a sitting or semisitting position (see Fig. 17-5D). The head of the bed is elevated, and sometimes the foot of the bed is raised slightly. To maintain correct body alignment, the resident should sit with the spine straight. The head and arms may be supported by pillows. You might be asked to place the resident in a high-Fowler's or a semi-Fowler's position. These terms refer to the degree of elevation of the head of the bed. Residents with respiratory problems and those with feeding tubes may need to be in a Fowler's position.

There are other positions that may be used occasionally. Sims' position is a lateral position, in which the lower arm is behind the resident and the upper leg is bent or flexed in a knee-chest position (see Fig. 17-6A). Elderly residents with limited mobility may have difficulty assuming this position.

The orthopneic position is often used by residents who have respiratory problems. The person sits straight up in bed, or on the side of the bed, and leans forward in an

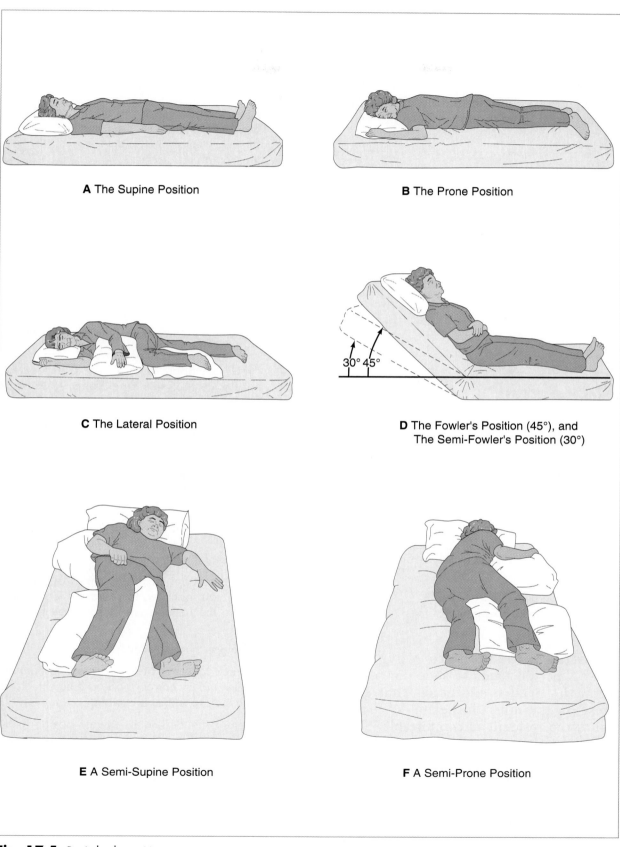

A The Supine Position

B The Prone Position

C The Lateral Position

D The Fowler's Position (45°), and
The Semi-Fowler's Position (30°)

30° 45°

E A Semi-Supine Position

F A Semi-Prone Position

Fig. 17-5 Basic body positions.

attempt to breathe easier. The arms are raised and supported by an overbed table (see Fig. 17-6B). A pillow placed on the table helps to cushion and support the body. If the resident is sitting on the side of the bed, a stool or chair should be placed under the feet to support the lower extremities.

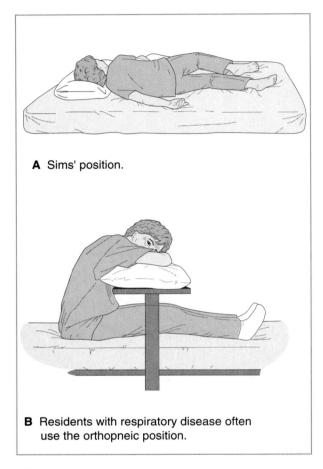

A Sims' position.

B Residents with respiratory disease often use the orthopneic position.

Fig. 17-6 Special body positions.

Assisting a Resident to Move Up in Bed. A person tends to slide down in bed when the head is elevated. That causes stress on the musculoskeletal system and makes the resident uncomfortable. Sliding also causes friction and leads to skin damage. It may be necessary to assist the resident up in bed several times during a shift. Encourage the resident to help as much as possible. To protect yourself and the resident, get help when necessary.

Assisting the Resident to Move Up in Bed

Before any procedure you must always follow the five basic steps: wash your hands, collect the equipment, identify the resident, explain the procedure, and protect privacy.

Follow universal precautions and wear gloves when appropriate.

1. Raise the bed to a comfortable working height and lock the brakes.

2. Adjust the bed to as flat a position as possible.

3. Raise the side rail on the opposite side and lower the side rail on your working side.

4. Place the pillow against the headboard.

5. Facing the head of the bed, stand with your feet apart (one in front of the other), bend your knees and keep your back straight.

6. Place one arm under the resident's shoulders and the other under the thighs.

7. Ask the resident to bend the knees and brace the feet against the bed. The arms may be at the side, elbows bent and hands braced against the bed (see Fig. 17-7A).

8. Explain that on the count of three, the resident should push with the hands and feet at the same time that you lift.

9. On the count of three, shift your weight from your back leg to your front leg, as you move the resident up in bed (see Fig. 17-7B).

10. Replace the pillow and straighten the linen.

11. Check to see that the resident is comfortable and in correct body alignment. Raise the side rails if appropriate.

12. Return the bed to its lowest position and place the call signal within the resident's reach.

13. Wash your hands.

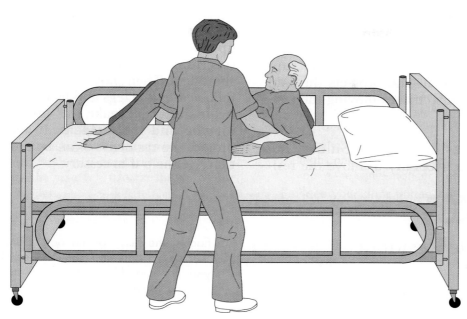

A Ask the resident to bend his knees and brace his feet;
he should also bend his elbows and brace his hands, if possible.

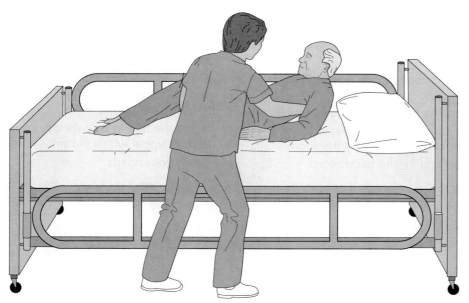

B Shift your weight from your back leg to your front leg as you move
the resident up in bed.

Fig. 17-7 Assisting the resident up in bed.

221

Assisting the Resident to Turn. You may assist the resident to turn to either side. The lateral (side-lying) position is a comfortable position and helps to relieve pressure on the bony areas of the back. A lift sheet will make the procedure easier to turn the resident. Get help if necessary.

Assisting the Resident to a Sitting Position. There are times when you will assist the resident to sit up in bed. This procedure can be used for personal care, for positioning, as a comfort measure, or to assist a resident out of bed. Sometimes, you will only need to raise the resident's head and shoulders to straighten linens or a pillow. This procedure is located on page 227.

Assisting the Resident to Sit on the Side of the Bed (Dangle). Dangling means sitting on the side of the bed. Dangling may be used as a form of restorative exercise, or it may be a part of the procedure to assist the resident to get out of bed. Provide a footstool if the resident's feet do not reach the floor. *Never* leave a resident alone while dangling.

You should always allow the resident to dangle for a few minutes before standing. The resident may feel dizzy while sitting upright. Dangling for a few minutes helps prevent the resident from losing balance or fainting. Observe the resident carefully while dangling. Observe the color of the skin for paleness or perspiration. Take the pulse and respirations. The resident who complains of pain or dizziness should be returned to a supine position immediately. Notify the nurse.

Report to the nurse after you have completed the procedure. Include the following in your report: the length of time the resident was dangling, how well the procedure was tolerated, vital signs, and any other observations you made. This procedure is located on page 228.

PROCEDURE

Assisting the Resident to Turn Away from You

Before any procedure you must always follow the five basic steps: wash your hands, collect the equipment, identify the resident, explain the procedure, and provide privacy.

Follow universal precautions and wear gloves when appropriate.

1. Raise the bed to a comfortable working height, and lock the brakes.
2. Adjust the bed as flat as possible.
3. Raise the side rail on the opposite side and lower the side rail on your working side.
4. Move the resident to the side of the bed nearest you, following the correct procedure.
5. Flex the resident's farthest arm next to the head, and place the other arm across the chest. Cross the resident's leg that is nearest you over the other leg (see Fig. 17-10A).
6. Place one hand on the resident's near shoulder and the other on the near hip, and turn the resident away from you, onto the side (see Fig. 17-10B).
7. Reposition the pillow under the resident's head.
8. Place a pillow under the upper arm to support the elbow, wrist, and hand. Use a handroll if necessary. Place a pillow under the upper leg, supporting the knee, ankle, and foot (see Fig. 17-10C).
9. Raise the side rail.
10. Go to the other side of the bed, and lower the side rail.
11. Adjust the bottom shoulder and hip for comfort.
12. Place a pillow at the resident's back for comfort and support.
13. Check to see that the resident is comfortable and in correct body alignment.
14. Straighten the linen.
15. Return the bed to its lowest position, and place the call signal within the resident's reach. Raise the side rail if appropriate.
16. Wash your hands.

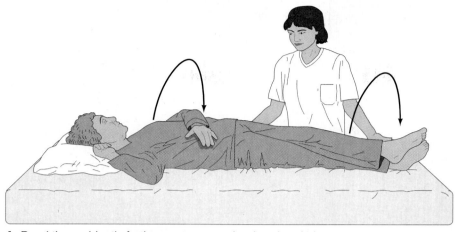

A Bend the resident's farthest arm next to her head and place the other arm across her chest. Cross her near leg over the other leg.

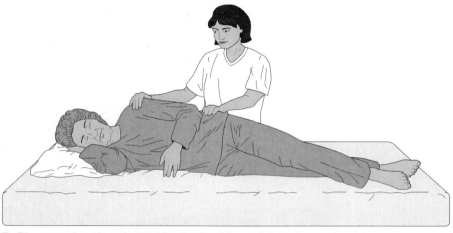

B Place one hand on the resident's shoulder and the other on her hip. Turn her away from you onto her side.

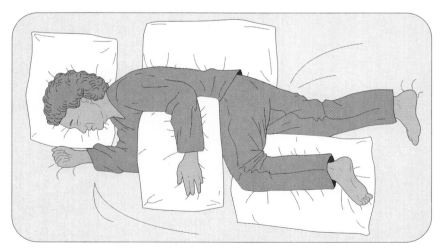

C Place pillows under her upper arm and leg for support.

Figure 17-10 Assisting the resident to turn away from you.

Assisting the Resident to Turn Toward You

Before any procedure you must always follow the five basic steps: wash your hands, collect the equipment, identify the resident, explain the procedure, and protect privacy.

Follow universal precautions and wear gloves when appropriate.

1. Raise the bed to a comfortable working height and lock the brakes.
2. Adjust the bed as flat as possible.
3. Raise the side rail on the opposite side and lower the side rail on your working side.
4. Move the resident to the side of the bed nearest you, following the correct procedure.
6. Raise the side rail that is nearest to you. Go to the other side of the bed, and lower the side rail.
7. Flex the resident's nearest arm next to the head, and place the other arm across the chest. Cross the leg that is farthest from you over the other leg (see Fig. 17-11A).
8. Place one hand on the resident's far shoulder and the other on the far hip, and turn the resident toward you, onto the side (see Fig. 17-11B).
9. Reposition the pillow under the resident's head.
10. Place a pillow under the upper arm to support the elbow, wrist, and hand. Use a handroll if necessary. Place a pillow under the upper leg, supporting the knee, ankle, and foot.
11. Raise the side rail.
12. Check to see that the resident is comfortable and in correct body alignment. Straighten the linen.
13. Return the bed to its lowest position, and place the call signal within the resident's reach. Raise the side rail if appropriate.
14. Wash your hands.

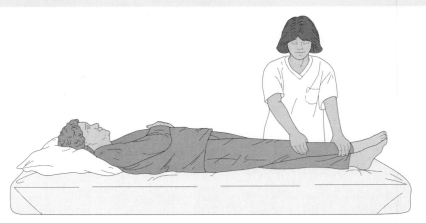

A Place the resident's arm across her chest. Cross the far leg over the near leg.

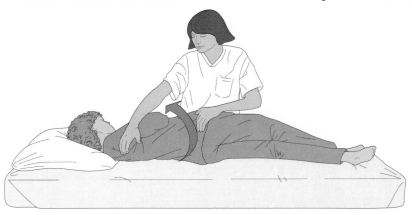

Fig. 17-11
Assisting the resident to turn toward you.

B Place one hand on the resident's shoulder and the other on her hip and turn her toward you onto her side.

Assisting the Resident to a Sitting Position

Before any procedure you must always follow the five basic steps: wash your hands, collect the equipment, identify the resident, explain the procedure, and protect privacy.

Follow universal precautions and wear gloves when appropriate.

1. Raise the bed to a comfortable working height and lock the brakes.

2. Lower the side rail on your working side.

3. Stand facing the head of the bed.

4. Place your arm under the resident's near arm and grasp the shoulder.

5. Ask the resident to grasp your shoulder (see Fig. 17-12A).

6. Place your free arm under the resident's neck and shoulders (see Fig. 17-12B).

7. On the count of three, assist the resident to a sitting position (see Fig. 17-12C).

8. Continuing to lock arms, use the arm that was supporting the resident's neck and shoulders to straighten the linens and pillow. Pull the pillow down so that the shoulders will be supported.

9. Continue the procedure:

   a. If the resident wants to remain in this position for a while, assure comfort and support.

   b. If the resident wants to return to the supine position, use the locked arm procedure to assist.

10. Check for correct body alignment, and place the call signal within reach.

11. Return the bed to its lowest position, and raise the side rails if appropriate.

12. Wash your hands.

   (The first nine steps of this procedure may be used to assist the resident out of bed.)

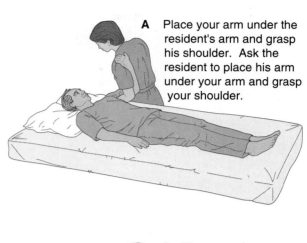

A Place your arm under the resident's arm and grasp his shoulder. Ask the resident to place his arm under your arm and grasp your shoulder.

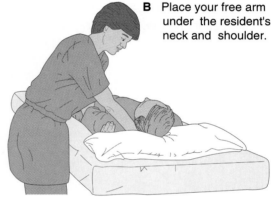

B Place your free arm under the resident's neck and shoulder.

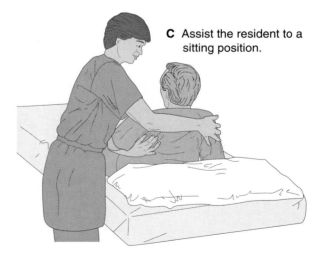

C Assist the resident to a sitting position.

Fig. 17-12 Assisting the resident to a sitting position.

PROCEDURE

Assisting the Resident to Sit on the Side of the Bed (Dangle)

Before any procedure you must always follow the five basic steps: wash your hands, collect the equipment, identify the resident, explain the procedure, and provide privacy.

Follow universal precautions and wear gloves when appropriate.

1. Assist the resident to a sitting position, following correct procedure.
2. Place one arm behind the resident's neck and shoulders, and place your other arm under the resident's knees (see Fig. 17-13A).
3. On the count of three, turn the resident toward you, so that the legs hang over the side of the bed (see Fig. 17-13B).
4. Assist the resident to a position of correct body alignment.

5. Ask the resident to push with hands against the mattress to help to maintain an upright position.
6. Keep your arm behind the neck and shoulders for support until you are sure the resident has regained balance (see Fig. 17-13C).
7. Check the pulse and respirations.
8. Continue the procedure:
   a. Allow the resident to dangle 15–20 minutes while you remain nearby.
   b. Return the resident to bed by reversing the procedure.
9. If you have assisted the resident back to bed, check for correct body alignment and straighten the linens.
10. Place the call signal within the resident's reach.
11. Return the bed to its lowest position, and raise the side rails if appropriate.
12. Wash your hands.
13. Report to the nurse.

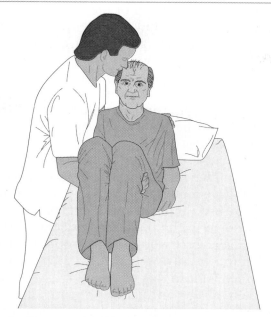

A Place one hand behind the resident's neck and shoulders; place your other arm under his knees.

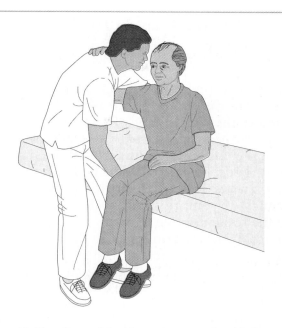

B Turn the resident toward you, so that his legs hang over the bed.

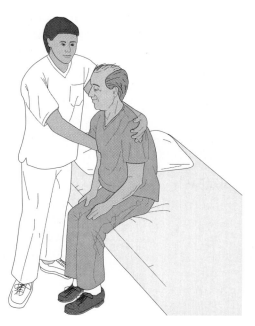

C Keep your hand behind the resident's neck and shoulders to support him until you are sure he has regained his balance.

Fig. 17-13 Assisting the resident to dangle.

Assisting the Resident to Transfer

Assisting the resident to transfer safely (move from one place to another) is an important responsibility of the nursing assistant. To transfer a resident safely, you must have an understanding of basic anatomy, body mechanics, and body alignment. Always follow the rules of body mechanics. If you are not careful, you can injure the resident or yourself.

The resident may transfer from the bed to a chair, a wheelchair, or a stretcher and will also transfer back to the bed. Be sure that the wheels on beds, stretchers, and wheelchairs are locked during a transfer.

Assess the situation before you begin a transfer. Determine how much assistance the resident needs, and if you will be able to perform the procedure alone. Do not attempt to move a helpless resident by yourself. Always get help if you are not sure. Encourage the resident to do as much as possible.

A mechanical lift may be needed. It is particularly useful in transferring paralyzed, comatose, or very heavy residents. The procedure for using the mechanical lift is described later in this chapter.

Determine if the resident has a strong or weak side. The resident should always transfer toward (or in the direction of) the strong side. This means that when the resident stands, weight bearing should be on the strong side first. Think about a person with a weak left arm and leg who wants to get out of a chair. If you assist the resident to push up on the arm of the chair with the strong right hand, and stand with weight on the strong right leg, getting out of the chair will be easier. However, if the weak left arm and weak left leg are used, it will be very difficult, or impossible, to get out of the chair. When the resident gets out of bed, the chair should be positioned by the bed on the strong side.

Decide if any special equipment is needed. The resident who has a walker should be encouraged to use it. If you are going to use the mechanical lift, prepare it, and arrange for help. You may decide that a gait/transfer belt would be appropriate. The procedure for using a gait/transfer belt is described later in this chapter.

Much of the information you need to assist the resident to transfer will be found on your assignment sheet, in the kardex, or on the care plan. However, the circumstances may vary from time to time. For example, a resident who is not feeling well may need more assistance than usual. If you are still not sure what to do after you have made your assessment, check with the charge nurse.

Assisting the Resident to Transfer from the Bed to a Chair. It is better for the resident to sit up in a chair when possible. This helps to prevent the complications of bedrest. Body organs are in natural alignment and function more effectively in an upright position. The resident may be using a regular chair or a wheelchair. If the chair has wheels, be sure they are locked before beginning the procedure.

PROCEDURE

Assisting the Resident to Transfer from the Bed to a Chair

Before any procedure you must always follow the five basic steps: wash your hands, collect the equipment, identify the resident, explain the procedure, and protect privacy.

Follow universal precautions and wear gloves when appropriate.

1. Position the chair at the head of the bed on the resident's strong side. Place a pad or blanket on the seat of the wheelchair (see Fig. 17-14A).
2. Lock the wheels and fold up the footrest of the wheelchair.
3. Place the bed in its lowest position and lock the wheels.
4. Be sure the resident is wearing non-skid shoes.
5. Assist the resident to sit on the side of the bed and dangle for a few minutes (see Fig. 17-14B).
6. Assist the resident to put on a robe if not already dressed.
7. Assist the resident to a standing position using the following steps:
   a. Stand facing the resident, bend your knees, and keep your back straight.
   b. Place your arms under the resident's arms, with your hand supporting the back.
   c. Brace your knees against the resident's knees and block the feet with yours (see Fig. 17-14C).
   d. If possible, the resident should brace with hands against the mattress and push up as you lift.
   e. On the count of three, straighten your knees as you bring the resident to a standing position (see Fig. 17-14D).
8. Ask the resident to take small steps as both of you turn toward the chair.
9. Ask the resident to back up until the back of the knees touch the front of the chair.
10. Ask the resident to grasp the arms of the chair, if able. If not, the resident can place hands on your forearms (see Fig. 17-14E).
11. On the count of three, bend your knees, as you lower the resident into the chair (see Fig. 17-14F).
12. Check to see that the resident is comfortable and in correct body alignment. Use pillows for support if necessary (see Fig. 17-14G).
13. Cover the resident's legs with a lap robe for warmth and privacy. Be sure the feet touch the floor or are otherwise supported.
14. Place the call signal within reach or position the chair where the resident can be observed by the staff.
15. Wash your hands.

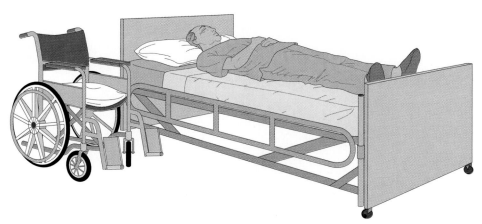

Fig. 17-14

Assisting the resident to transfer from the bed to a chair.

A Position the chair with the back even with the head of the bed.

Fig. 17-14 (cont.)
Assisting the resident to transfer from the bed to a chair.

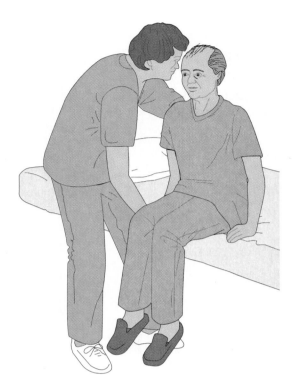

B Assist the resident to dangle.

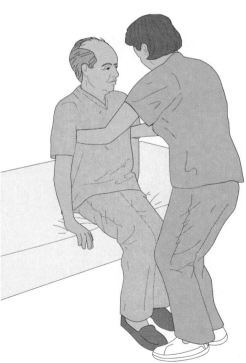

C Brace your knees against the resident's knees and block his feet with your feet.

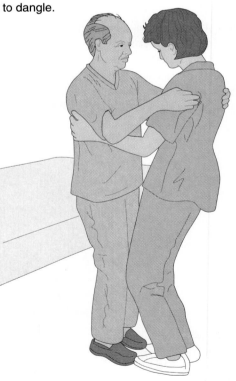

D Bring the resident to a standing position.

Fig. 17-14 (cont.)
Assisting the resident to transfer
from the bed to a chair.

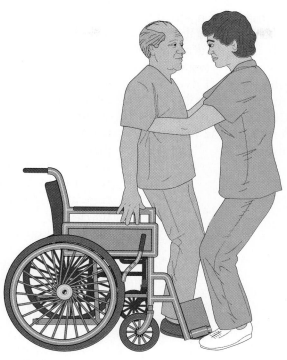

E Ask the resident to grasp the chair as you
support him.

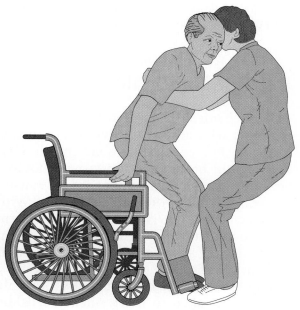

F Bend your knees as you lower the resident to the
chair.

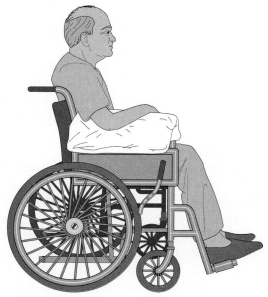

G Use pillows as necessary to position the
resident in correct body alignment.

Using a Gait/Transfer Belt. A gait/transfer belt is used to assist unsteady residents to transfer or walk. It is made of a strong, washable material and has a safety buckle (see Fig. 17-15). The belt is applied around the resident's waist, over soft tissue. It should fit snugly and not slide up over the ribs or down over the hips. The belt is applied over the resident's clothing. The buckle is fastened off center, in the front, to prevent discomfort or injury.

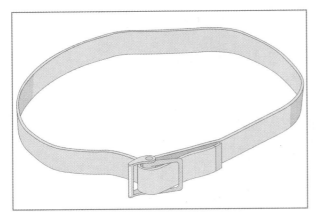

Fig. 17-15 The gait/transfer belt protects the resident and you.

There are several advantages in using a gait/transfer belt. It reduces the chance of injury to either the resident or the nursing assistant. The gait/transfer belt helps prevent falls. Because you have the belt to hold on to, you will feel more in control of the situation. This provides a feeling of security and helps maintain the resident's strength. Using the belt allows you to keep your back straight and practice correct body mechanics.

The gait/transfer belt is used with residents who require assistance in moving. This includes those who are weak, unsteady, or prone to falling. The gait/transfer belt is not used on a resident who has had recent rib fractures or abdominal surgery. It is seldom used with a resident who has a colostomy or a gastrostomy. Sometimes residents who have severe respiratory or heart disease feel suffocated by the belt. It should not be used to totally support a resident who is unable to stand.

Many long-term care facilities have made the use of gait/transfer belts mandatory. This means you must use the belt whenever it is appropriate. Assess the resident physically and mentally to determine if the belt should be used. Consider the resident's mobility, strength, balance, motivation, and limitations. The belt might not always be appropriate. For example, at times, the confused resident might not be able to understand the reason for the belt. It looks much like a restraint. Always explain that the belt is used only for safety reasons and that it will be removed as soon as the procedure is completed.

When you are not using the gait/transfer belt, wear it around your own waist. That way, it will be available whenever you need it. The resident will become used to seeing it on you, and will be reassured that it is not a form of restraint. The gait/transfer belt is a useful tool that will help make your job easier and safer.

Using a Gait/Transfer Belt to Assist the Resident in Transferring from a Bed to a Chair. It is easier and safer to use a gait belt when transferring the resident. This procedure is located on pages 236–237.

Using a Mechanical Lift

The mechanical lift is used to help transfer residents who are very heavy or are unable to move. For example, a quadriplegic resident would be unable to assist in moving. Several people might be required to transfer the resident from the bed to a chair. With the mechanical lift, two people can perform the procedure safely, and with minimum effort. Using a lift protects residents and staff members.

The mechanical lift is usually portable and can be taken to the resident's bedside. Although there are many styles, most lifts are similar to the one in Fig. 17-16.

A sling is positioned under the resident to support the body. Chains or straps secure the sling to the lift. When the handle is pumped, the hydraulic pump raises the sling. When the handle is released, the sling is lowered. (It works much like a jack that is used to change a tire on a car. When you pump the jack handle, it raises the car. When you release the jack handle, the car comes down again.)

The sling is made of a strong, washable material. It may have one piece or two pieces. There may be a commode opening in the sling so that it can be used to position a resident on the toilet. Some slings have a headpiece to support the head and neck (see Fig. 17-16). The sling should be washed regularly.

The sling is placed under the resident's body in the same way that you would position a draw sheet. Because the material is heavy, and there may be metal pieces on the sides, fanfold the sling carefully, so the resident will not be injured when rolling over

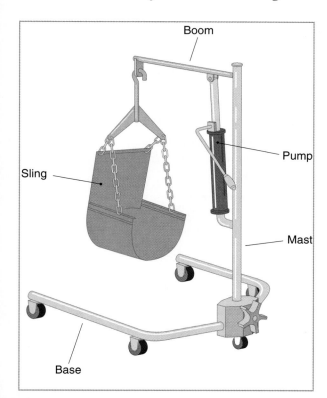

Fig. 17-16 A portable mechanical lift.

it. Be sure to warn that the resident will be rolling over a "hump" when turning.

When the resident is transferred from the bed to a chair or the toilet, the sling is left under the body, so that it will be in position to use in returning the resident to bed. The sling should not be left under the resident who is in bed.

Safety Rules. Important safety rules to remember when using the mechanical lift are as follows:

- Two people are needed when using the lift. One operates the lift, while the other guides the resident's body and the chains or straps.

- Know how to operate the lift. Read the instructions in the procedure book at your facility. The first few times you use the lift, get someone to assist you who is familiar with the equipment.

- Explain the procedure, and reassure the resident frequently. It can be a frightening experience if the resident doesn't know what to expect. When possible, position the resident to face the operator.

- Check to see that the resident is positioned correctly on the sling and that the equipment is working properly *before* moving the lift away from the bed.

- Stabilize the resident and the frame throughout the procedure. Prevent the sling from swinging back and forth.

- Do not transport the resident down the hallway with the lift. It is used for lifting, not transporting. Use a wheelchair for transporting the resident.

- Never leave a resident suspended in a lift. If an emergency occurs, return the resident to the bed, quickly and safely.

Reverse the procedure to transfer the resident from a chair to the bed, using a mechanical lift. The procedure for using a mechanical lift is located on pages 238–240.

PROCEDURE

Using a Gait/Transfer Belt to Assist the Resident in Transferring from the Bed to a Chair

Before any procedure you must always follow the five basic steps: wash your hands, collect the equipment, identify the resident, explain the procedure, and protect privacy.

Follow universal precautions and wear gloves when appropriate.

1. Position the chair at the head of the bed on the resident's strong side. Place a pad or blanket on the seat of the wheelchair.

2. Lock the wheels and fold up the footrest of the wheelchair.

3. Place the bed in its lowest position and lock the wheels.

4. Be sure the resident is wearing non-skid shoes.

5. Assist the resident to sit on the side of the bed and dangle for a few minutes.

6. Assist the resident to put on a robe if not already dressed.

7. Place a gait/transfer belt on the resident, so that it fits snugly. Leave enough room for your fingers to slip under the belt. Fasten the buckle off center, in the front (see Fig. 17-17A).

8. Assist the resident to a standing position using the following steps:

   a. Stand facing the resident, bend your knees, and keep your back straight.

   b. The resident should brace with hands against the mattress and push as you lift. If this is not possible, the resident's hands should be placed on your forearms.

   c. Grasp the gait/transfer belt from underneath, in the front. Your hands should be spaced wide apart for leverage (see Fig. 17-17B).

   d. Brace your knees against the resident's knees and block the feet with your feet.

   e. On the count of three, straighten your knees as you bring the resident to a standing position.

9. Assist the resident to move in front of the chair.

10. On the count of three, bend your knees, as you assist the resident into the chair. Hold onto the gait/transfer belt as you do this (see Fig.17-17C).

11. Remove the gait/transfer belt.

12. Check to see that the resident is comfortable and in correct body alignment. Use pillows for support if necessary.

13. Cover the resident's legs with a lap robe for warmth and privacy. Be sure the feet touch the floor or are otherwise supported.

14. Place the call signal within reach or position the chair where the resident can be observed by the staff.

15. Wash your hands.

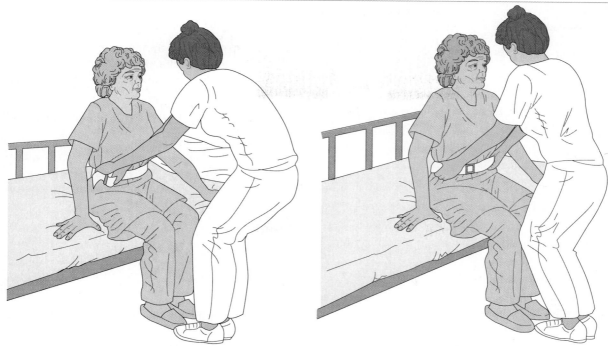

A The gait/transfer belt should fit snugly, and the buckle should be fastened off-center, in the front.

B Grasp the gait/transfer belt from underneath with both hands.

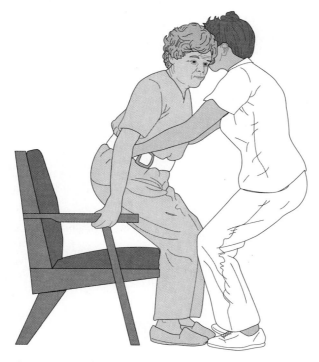

C Holding onto the gait/transfer belt, lower the resident into the chair as you bend your knees.

Fig. 17-17 Using a gait/transfer belt to assist the resident in transferring from the bed to a chair.

PROCEDURE

Using a Mechanical Lift

Before any procedure you must always follow the five basic steps: wash your hands, collect the equipment, identify the resident, explain the procedure, and protect privacy.

Follow universal precautions and wear gloves when appropriate.

1. Position the chair at the head of the bed.

2. Raise the bed to a comfortable working height.

3. Stand on one side, with your assistant on the other.

4. Turn the resident to the side.

5. Center the sling, and fanfold it toward the resident's body, with the lower edge just above the resident's knees (see Fig. 17-18A).

6. Turn the resident across the folded sling.

7. Your assistant will straighten the sling (see Fig. 17-18B).

8. Turn the resident onto the back, and check to see that the resident is centered on the sling (see Fig. 17-18C).

9. Raise the head of the bed.

10. Pump the handle to raise the boom, and with your assistant guiding the chains or straps, position it over the resident (see Fig. 17-18D).

11. Widen the base of the lift and lock the wheels (Fig 17-18E).

12. Attach the sling to the straps or chains. The open end of the hooks should face away from the resident (see Fig. 17-18F).

13. Position the resident's arms over the chest or in the lap.

14. With one hand on the hydraulic pump handle and the other on the steering handle, work the pump handle until the resident clears the bed (see Fig. 17-18G).

15. Check to be sure that the resident is centered on the sling.

16. Unlock the wheels and move the lift away from the bed with the resident facing you. Your assistant will guide the resident's legs off the bed (see Fig. 17-18H).

17. Grasp the steering handle with both hands and move the resident away from the bed toward the chair. Your assistant will stabilize the resident's body and the chains or straps.

18. Position the lift with the resident's back toward the chair. Lock the lift wheels.

19. Lower the resident slowly into the chair. Your assistant will guide the resident's body to a correct position (see Fig. 17-18I). Leave the sling under the resident.

20. Lower the boom enough to detach the chains or straps. Unlock the wheels and move the lift away from the chair, while your assistant guides the chains or straps.

21. Use pillows, if necessary, to support the resident in correct body alignment. Pad the edges of the sling to protect the resident's skin.

22. Cover the resident's knees for privacy and warmth, and place the call signal within reach.

23. Return the mechanical lift to its proper place.

24. Wash your hands.

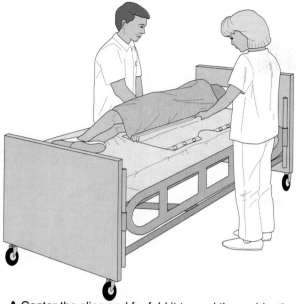

A Center the sling and fanfold it toward the resident's body, with the lower edge just above the resident's knees.

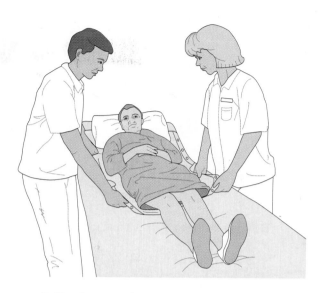

C Check to see that the resident is centered on the sling.

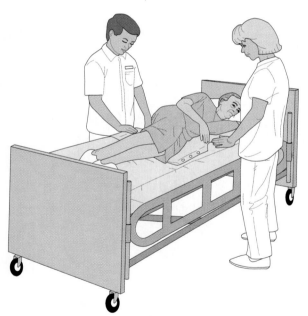

B Your assistant will pull the sling through and straighten it.

D Raise the boom of the lift and position it over the resident.

Fig. 17-18 Using a mechanical lift to transfer a resident.

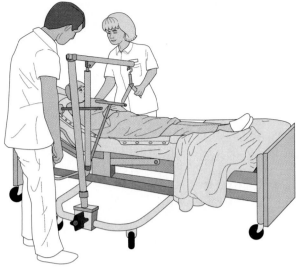

E Widen the base of the lift and lock the wheels.

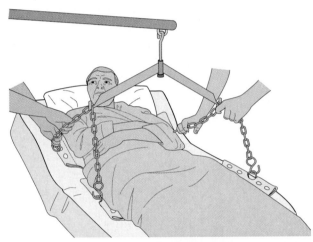

F The open end of the hooks should face away from the resident.

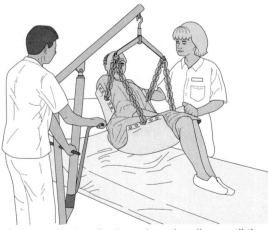

G Pump the handle that raises the sling, until the resident's body clears the bed.

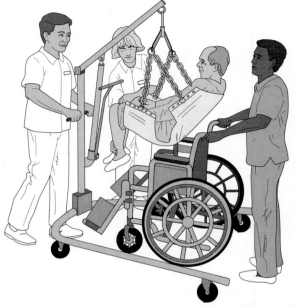

H Your assistant guides the resident's legs off the bed, as you move the lift away.

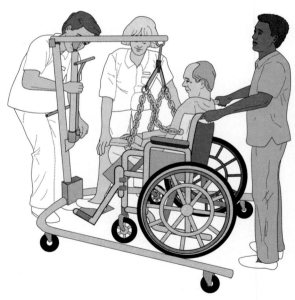

I Your assistant guides the resident's body into the chair as you lower the sling.

Fig. 17-18 (cont.)
Using a mechanical lift to transfer a resident.

Using a Wheelchair

A wheelchair may be used to transport a resident who is unable to walk. The resident may be an amputee, paralyzed, or too weak to stand. A wheelchair may also be ordered for a resident who is recovering from surgery or an illness. This allows the resident to be up and about sooner. A fear of falling may cause the resident to become dependent on the wheelchair. The resident should be encouraged to walk as soon as the doctor allows it. Walking may begin with the nursing assistant pushing a wheelchair behind the resident. The presence of the nursing assistant and the chair provides the resident with a feeling of security.

A wheelchair allows the resident to maintain a normal, sitting position. For the resident who can't walk, a wheelchair increases mobility. It provides opportunities for socializing. A resident in a wheelchair can go outside in the fresh air or out to dinner with a friend. For the resident who has had a stroke, a wheelchair is often a step on the road to recovery. It creates hope and motivation, which leads to increased self-esteem and independence.

A wheelchair may be manual or motorized. A manual chair is moved by turning the wheels by hand, or by someone pushing it. Some residents will need assistance in moving the wheelchair, but many will be able to operate it by themselves. A motorized wheelchair is battery operated and can be moved with little effort on the part of the resident. Wheelchairs come in different styles and sizes to accommodate individual needs. Sometimes a headrest is attached to support the head and neck. Some wheelchairs are lightweight and fold up for easy portability.

One type of wheelchair that is often used in long-term care is a geri-chair (geriatric chair). A **geri-chair** is a recliner on wheels. It has a high back and is well padded and comfortable. A tray fits on the front, which can be used for eating and other activities (see Fig. 17-19). The geri-chair is a form of restraint when it restricts the resident's mobility. Remember, while a resident is in a geri-chair you will be responsible for all basic needs.

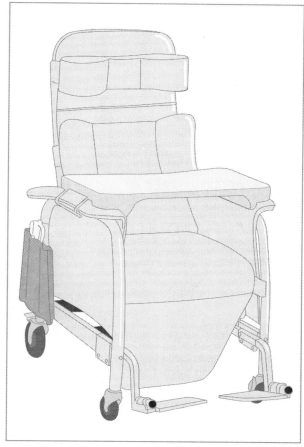

Fig. 17-19 A geri-chair is often used in long-term care.

There are safety measures to be followed when transporting a resident in a wheelchair. Make sure that the chair is in good repair before you use it. Always lock the brakes when the resident is getting in or out of the chair. The brakes should also be locked when the chair is to be stopped for a period of time.

To take a resident down a ramp in a wheelchair correctly, turn the wheelchair around and back down the ramp. In other words, you stand behind the wheelchair and pull it after you (see Fig. 17-20). This allows you to control the chair and also prevents the resident from tipping forward and falling out of the chair. The same procedure is used to enter an elevator or to pass through a doorway. You go in first, and pull the chair in behind you.

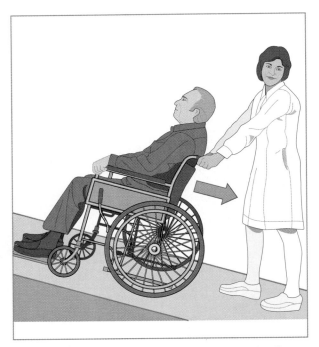

Fig. 17-20 Stand behind the wheelchair and pull it after you when going down a ramp.

Wheelchairs should be cleaned on a regular basis. Always clean a chair that is to be used by another resident. Clean the chair immediately if it is soiled with food or body wastes.

It is important that the resident in a wheelchair is comfortable and in correct body alignment. The chair must be large enough to allow the resident room to shift body position. It must not create pressure. If the chair is too large, pillows will be needed to provide support. A pillow may also be used to support a weak arm. The resident's back, from hip to shoulder, should be positioned against the back of the chair. A pad or folded sheet in the chair seat promotes comfort and skin protection. It can also be used to reposition the resident who has slid down in the chair. Repositioning a resident requires two staff members, one lifting from each side. Lifting a resident by grasping under the arms may cause injury.

Using a Stretcher

A resident who is not able to sit up in a chair, or one who is very ill, may need to be transported by stretcher. Three or four people are needed to perform this procedure safely. The stretcher should be positioned firmly against the side of the resident's bed. The bed is raised to the same level as the stretcher. This provides an even surface for the transfer. Two people stand at either end of the stretcher, pressing it against the bed. At least one person, and preferably two, stand on the opposite side of the bed. A draw sheet makes the transfer easier and safer. If a drawsheet is not available, loosen the bottom sheet all the way around, and use it as a drawsheet.

Safety Rules. Safety rules to remember when transferring a resident to and from a stretcher include:

- At least three people are needed.

- Lock the wheels of the stretcher and the bed.

- Follow rules of correct body mechanics.

- Fasten the safety straps across the resident who is on a stretcher.

- Keep the stretcher side rails up while transporting a resident.

- Two people are needed to transport a resident on a stretcher, one at the resident's head and the other at the feet.

- Move the stretcher feet first. One staff member guides the stretcher, while the other watches the resident.

- When entering an elevator, one staff member should back into the elevator, pulling the stretcher.

- Never leave a resident alone on a stretcher. You are responsible for the resident's safety until someone else takes over.

Reverse the procedure to transfer the resident from the stretcher to a bed.

Moving the Resident from the Bed to a Stretcher

Before any procedure you must always follow the five basic steps: wash your hands, collect the equipment, identify the resident, explain the procedure, and protect privacy.

Follow universal precautions and wear gloves when appropriate.

1. Raise the bed to a comfortable working height and lock the wheels.
2. Remove the top linen after covering the resident with a bath blanket. Loosen the draw sheet.
3. Lower the side rail on your side.
4. Using the draw sheet, move the resident toward you.
5. Your assistant will go to the other side of the bed, lower the rail, and hold the resident, to prevent a fall (see Fig. 17-21A).
6. Position the stretcher against the near side of the bed and lock the wheels. Adjust the height of the bed even with the stretcher (see Fig. 17-21B).
7. Two assistants will stand at the side of the stretcher. You and an assistant will stand beside the bed.
8. Roll the draw sheet close to the sides of the resident's body.
9. On the count of three, move the resident from the bed to the stretcher (see Fig. 17-21C).
10. Center the resident on the stretcher and place a pillow under the head and shoulders, if allowed.
11. Check for correct body alignment and cover the resident with the bath blanket.
12. Fasten the safety straps and raise the side rails (see Fig. 17-21D).
13. Unlock the wheels and transport the resident, with the help of one assistant.
14. Stay with the resident until someone else takes over.
15. Wash your hands.

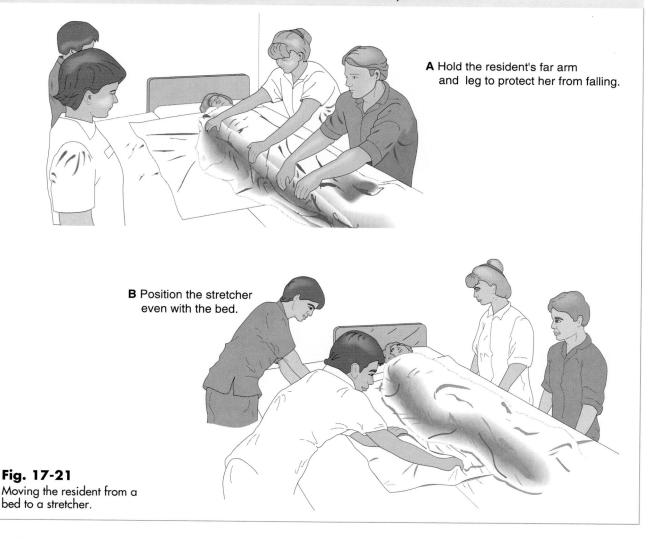

A Hold the resident's far arm and leg to protect her from falling.

B Position the stretcher even with the bed.

Fig. 17-21
Moving the resident from a bed to a stretcher.

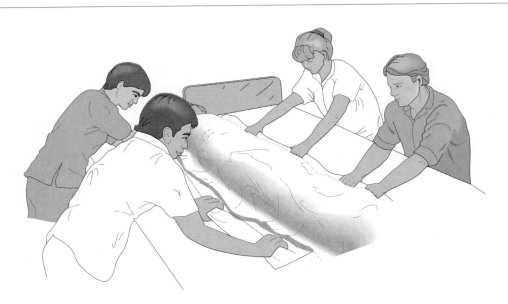

C On the count of three, move the resident from the bed to the stretcher.

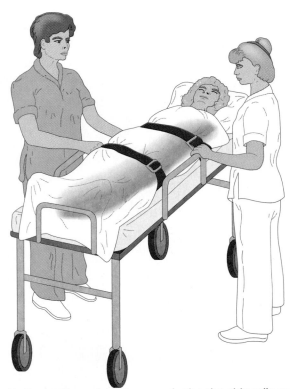

D Fasten the safety straps and raise the side rails as soon as you have the resident properly positioned.

Fig. 17-21 (cont.) Moving the resident from a bed to a stretcher.

SECTION III: AMBULATION AND EXERCISE

Assisting the Resident to Walk

The ability to **ambulate** (walk) allows a person to move about and go from place to place. Ambulation is an excellent form of exercise. It builds strength and stamina. Body functions are more efficient when a person is in an upright position. Ambulation provides independence and leads to increased self-esteem. It is a satisfying feeling to be able to stand up and walk.

Think of the joy that is felt when a young child takes those first, faltering steps. That feeling can be just as strong in the elderly person, particularly for someone who has not been able to walk for awhile. Walking can be fun and can bring much pleasure. The inability to walk is a severe loss to most people. Feelings of frustration, anger, or sadness may cause withdrawal. The isolation that results can lead to depression.

Ambulation opens opportunities to explore the environment, to join in activities, and to make social contacts. It provides a way to communicate one's feelings and personality. For example, what do you communicate when you walk rapidly into the resident's room, turn, and stop abruptly? Your manner of walking (often referred to as gait) indicates that you are in a hurry and may expect the resident to also hurry.

A resident may be unable to walk as a result of disease or injury. An injury to the head or back may result in paralysis which is not always permanent. A broken leg or hip will interfere with ambulation until it heals. A stroke may leave the resident unable to walk. Arthritis may make walking painful and difficult.

Sometimes there is no physical reason why the resident doesn't walk. Confusion or a fear of falling may cause a resident to retreat to the safety of the bed or chair. The person who has had a hip or knee replacement may want to continue to use a wheelchair because of fear of damaging the prosthesis (artificial body part).

A restorative exercise program, ordered by the doctor, helps to prepare the resident for ambulation. These exercises can begin while the resident is still bedbound. The purpose of this program is to increase muscle strength and improve circulation. Dangling (sitting on the side of the bed) can be used as an exercise. It not only helps strengthen, it also helps the resident to regain balance. The resident may need to practice standing. This can be done in physical therapy or at the resident's bedside.

Some residents will need special adaptive equipment to help them ambulate. Braces, crutches, canes, and walkers are used for this purpose. The physical therapist, working with the resident's doctor, will decide what type of equipment is appropriate. The physical therapists will provide the equipment and teach the resident how to use it (see Fig. 17-22). They will evaluate the resident at regular intervals to make any necessary changes or adjustments.

Your role as a nursing assistant is to offer whatever assistance the resident may need to ambulate. An important responsibility is providing the encouragement and opportunity to walk. Use praise frequently, and encourage the resident to do as much as possible. You may need to continually reinforce what the resident has learned in physical therapy. You must know what equipment the resident needs and how that equipment is used. If you are not sure how a device works, check with the physical therapist or the charge nurse.

A gait/transfer belt is very helpful when assisting the resident to ambulate. It will be to your advantage to use it whenever possible.

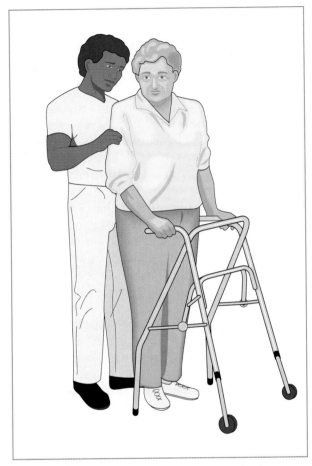

Fig. 17-22 The resident may need special adaptive equipment to assist her in ambulation.

Protecting a Falling Resident. The resident may become weak or dizzy while being assisted to ambulate. If the resident begins to fall, pull the resident close to your body with the gait/transfer belt (see Fig. 17-24A on page 248). Let the resident slide slowly down your leg to the floor (see Fig. 17-24B on page 248). This helps you to control the direction of the fall and to prevent head injuries. Bend your knees as you lower the resident to the floor, and keep your back straight. Do not attempt to prevent the fall by trying to hold the resident off the floor. You could hurt both the resident and yourself.

PROCEDURE

Using a Gait/Transfer Belt to Assist the Resident to Ambulate

Before any procedure you must always follow the five basic steps: wash your hands, collect the equipment, identify the resident, explain the procedure, and provide privacy.

Follow universal precautions and wear gloves when appropriate.

1. Assist the resident in dangling for a few minutes to regain balance.

2. Apply the gait/transfer belt around the waist.

3. Bring the resident to a standing position using the correct procedure (see Fig. 17-23A).

4. Stand at the resident's side until balance is regained. Keep your hands on the gait/transfer belt.

5. While holding onto the gait/transfer belt, change the position of your hands. One hand should be holding the belt at the side and the other hand holding the belt in the back (see Fig. 17-23B).

6. Assist the resident to walk. Walk at the resident's side, and slightly behind, while holding the belt with both hands (see Fig. 17-23C).

7. Encourage the resident to stand straight and walk as normally as possible. If the resident is weak, a coworker can follow behind with a wheelchair.

8. Return the resident to the chair or bed and remove the belt.

9. Position the resident in correct body alignment and place the call signal within reach.

10. Wash your hands.

11. Report the distance the resident has walked and how well the procedure was tolerated.

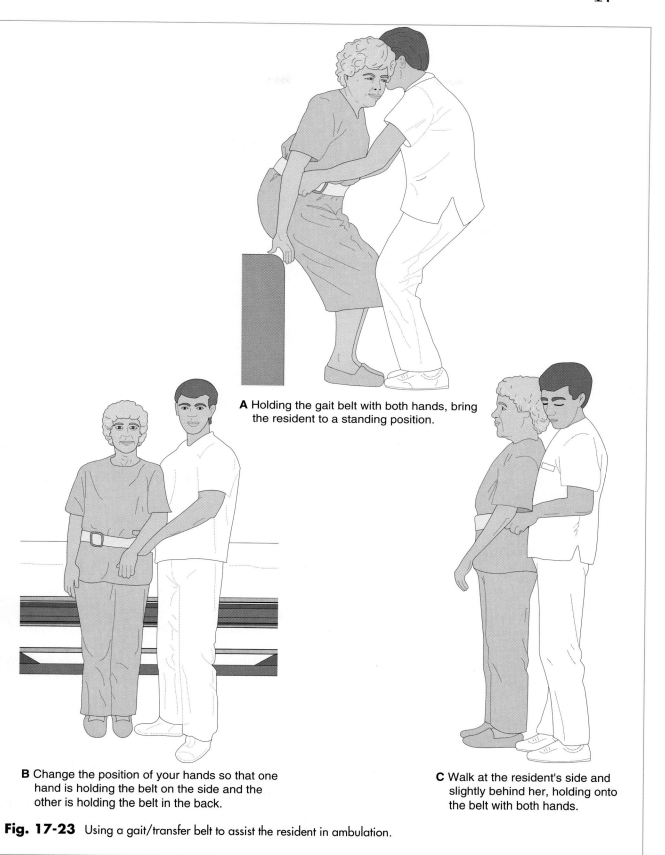

A Holding the gait belt with both hands, bring the resident to a standing position.

B Change the position of your hands so that one hand is holding the belt on the side and the other is holding the belt in the back.

C Walk at the resident's side and slightly behind her, holding onto the belt with both hands.

Fig. 17-23 Using a gait/transfer belt to assist the resident in ambulation.

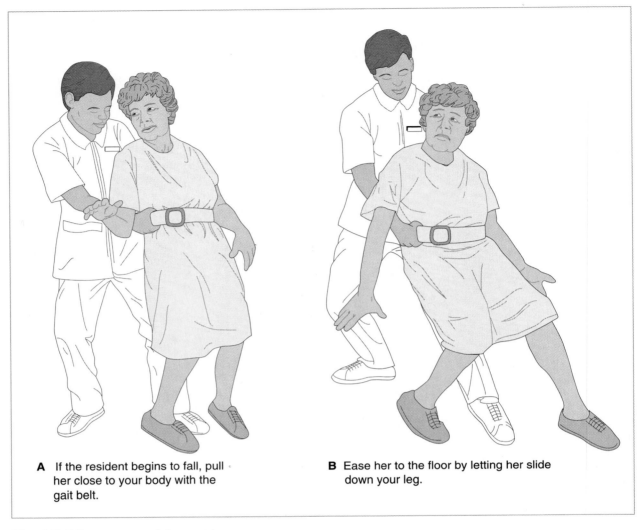

A   If the resident begins to fall, pull her close to your body with the gait belt.

B   Ease her to the floor by letting her slide down your leg.

Fig. 17-24   Protecting a falling resident.

Assisting the Resident to Walk with a Cane, Walker, or Crutches

The use of canes, walkers, and crutches allows independence for residents who are weak, or have poor balance. These devices are recommended by the occupational therapist or physical therapist, who also teaches the residents to use them properly. The therapist teaches staff members about the use of adaptive devices and should be consulted anytime a question arises. Discuss your concern with your charge nurse, who may then contact the therapist.

Canes. Canes provide balance and support when one side of the body is weak. Canes are usually held on the strong side of the body. Single-tip, three-point (tripod), and four-point (quad) canes are available. Although canes with more than one tip are more difficult to move, they provide more support than do canes with only one tip.

When the resident's hand is on the cane grip, the shoulders should be at a normal level. The cane grip should be level with the resident's hip, and the tip is placed 6 to 10 inches to the side of the resident's foot. The arm is flexed slightly, as the cane is moved forward about 12 inches. A step forward is then taken with the opposite (weak) leg. This foot is moved to a position even with the cane. The strong leg is then moved forward beyond the weak leg and cane. This sequence is repeated throughout ambulation.

Walkers. Walkers may have four legs that rest on the floor. They may have wheels on the front legs and tips on the back, or they may have wheels on all four legs. Wheeled walkers are helpful for residents who are unable to lift the walker to move it forward. Baskets, trays, and pouches may be added to allow the resident to carry belongings.

The walker handgrip should be at hip level. As the resident stands erect, the elbows should be flexed approximately at a 20° angle, as the walker is moved forward approximately 6 inches. The resident then steps toward the walker with the affected foot first. The step is completed by bringing the strong foot forward, next to the affected foot. Never allow a resident to use the walker as a support to raise his or her body from a sitting position.

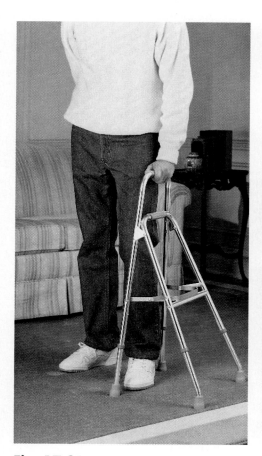
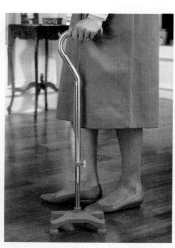
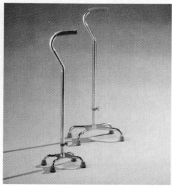
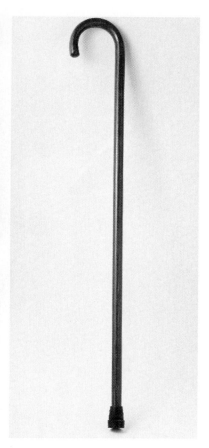

Fig. 17-25
A variety of canes is available to meet individual needs.

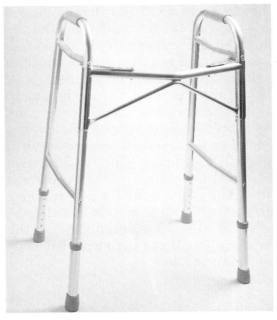
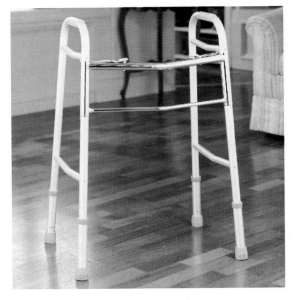
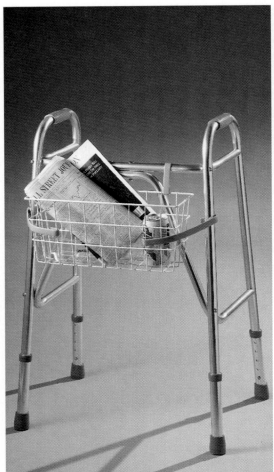
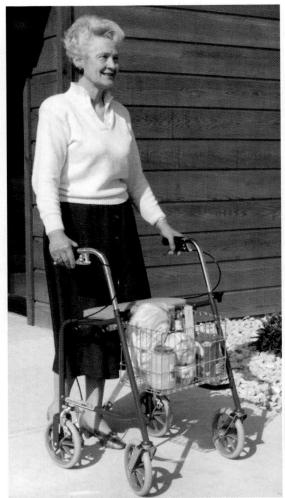

Fig. 17-26 Types of walkers.

Crutches. A resident who is unable to use one leg, or has only one leg, may use crutches. Crutches must be fitted correctly, according to the resident's height. Handgrips and underarm braces must also fit (see Fig. 17-27).

While it is the therapist's responsibility to teach the resident to use walkers, canes, and crutches, you play an important role in observing incorrect use. Make the resident aware of the problem. If incorrect use continues, report this to your charge nurse, so that the therapy department can be notified. Check the tips of canes, walkers, and crutches to ensure that the rubber is intact.

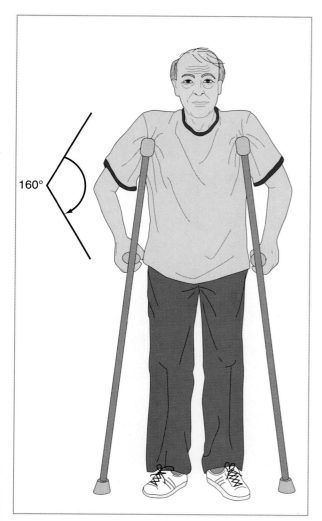

Fig. 17-27 It is important that crutches fit correctly.

Range-of-Motion and Other Restorative Exercises

Restorative Exercises. Restorative exercise programs contribute to the resident's physical and emotional well-being. They help to prevent the complications of inactivity. Aerobic exercise classes and dances may be held in the long-term care facility. Aerobic exercises do not require a lot of strength and stamina. Dancing is an enjoyable exercise for many people.

Walking is an excellent form of exercise. Outdoor nature walks are fun when the weather is nice. Walking in a shopping mall can be comfortable and stimulating. For those who are not strong enough for these activities, a walk in the yard can be helpful. A rocking chair can provide exercise for those who are unable to take part in other physical activities. Rocking is also pleasant and relaxing.

Range-of-Motion Exercises. Range of motion refers to the distance a joint will comfortably move. **Range-of-motion exercises** are exercises that are performed to take each joint through its normal area of movement. These exercises are done to prevent loss of movement or to regain full range of motion after an illness. Range-of-motion exercises are one of the best measures to prevent contractures.

Range-of-motion exercises may be active, assisted, or passive. Active exercises are those that the resident does without assistance. Assisted exercises are performed with residents who need some help. Passive exercises are done by someone else for the resident. The resident's physical and mental condition determines which type of exercise is to be done.

Check with the charge nurse or the care plan to find out which type of exercise the resident needs and which joints should be exercised. The number of times you repeat each exercise will depend on the resident's condition and tolerance. Use slow, rhythmic motions. Stop at the point of resistance, or if the resident complains of pain. Watch the resident's face for signs of pain or discomfort. Use both hands to support the joint you are exercising. Do not be discouraged if the range-of-motion is limited. Exercise within those limitations. A small amount of mobility is better than none.

Plan range-of-motion exercises as a part of self-care or activities of daily living. Brushing the hair, taking a bath, and walking provide opportunities for range of motion. Encourage the resident to do as much as possible. Report any increase or decrease in range of motion to the charge nurse.

You will need to be familiar with some of the terms that are used to describe body movement and direction. Some of the more common terms are found in the following list:

BODY MOVEMENTS AND DIRECTIONS

Extension: straightening and extending

Flexion: bending

Abduction: moving away from the midline of the body

Adduction: moving toward the midline of the body

Pronation: turning down

Supination: turning up

Hyperextension: Extending beyond a straight line

Internal rotation: rolling in toward the body

External rotation: rolling away from the body

Ulnar deviation: moving the hand toward the little finger

Radial deviation: moving the hand toward the thumb

Plantar flexion: bending the foot downward

Dorsiflexion: bending the foot upward

Performing Range-of Motion Exercises

Before any procedure you must always follow the five basic steps: wash your hands, collect the equipment, identify the resident, explain the procedure, and protect privacy.

Follow universal precautions and wear glove when appropriate.

1. Raise the bed to a comfortable working height, lock the wheels, and lower the side rails.
2. Exercise the resident's neck. Support the head with both hands.
   a. Move the head down, up, and back; then straighten the neck and head (see Fig. 17-28A).

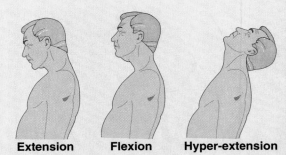

Extension　　**Flexion**　　**Hyper-extension**

Fig 17-28A

　b. Turn the head to the right side, straighten it, turn to the left side, and straighten (see Fig. 17-28B).

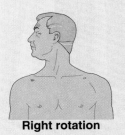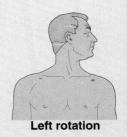

Right rotation　　**Left rotation**

Fig 17-28B

c. Move the head toward the right shoulder, straighten, move the head toward the left shoulder, and straighten the head again (see Fig. 17-28C).

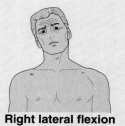 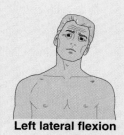

Right lateral flexion **Left lateral flexion**

Fig 17-28C

b. Raise the resident's arm out to the side and bring it back to the side, keeping the elbow straight (see Fig. 17-28E).

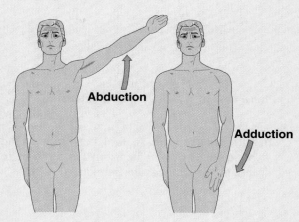

Abduction

Adduction

Fig 17-28E

3. Exercise the shoulder: Place one hand under the resident's elbow. Grasp the resident's hand with your other hand.
   a. Raise the resident's arm over the head and down again while keeping the elbow straight (see Fig. 17-28D).

c. Bring the arm out to the side, bend the elbow and rotate the forearm and hand downward and then upward (see Fig. 17-28F).

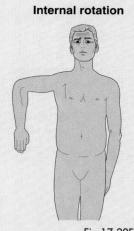

External rotation **Internal rotation**

Fig 17-28F

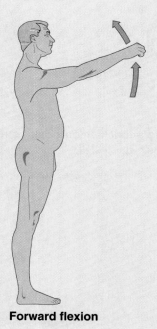 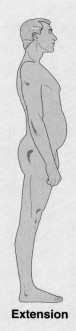

Forward flexion **Extension**

Fig 17-28D

4. Exercise the elbow and the forearm: Place one hand under the elbow and grasp the resident's hand with your other hand.

Performing Range-of-Motion Exercises (cont.)

a. Bend the resident's elbow toward the shoulder and then straighten the elbow (see Fig. 17-28G).

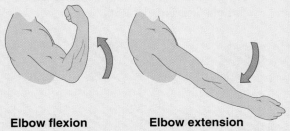

Elbow flexion   **Elbow extension**

Fig 17-28G

b. Turn the forearm so that the palm of the hand faces down, then turn the forearm so that the hand faces up (see Fig. 17-28H).

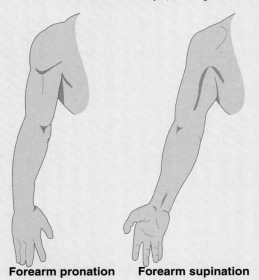

Forearm pronation   **Forearm supination**

Fig 17-28H

5. Exercise the wrist: Both of your hands should support the resident's wrist and hand.
   a. Bend the wrist up and then down (Fig 17-28I).

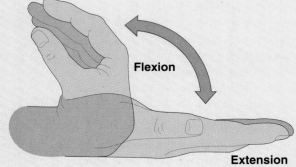

Flexion

Extension

Fig 17-28I

b. Keeping the fingers together, bend the wrist from side to side (see Fig. 17-28J).

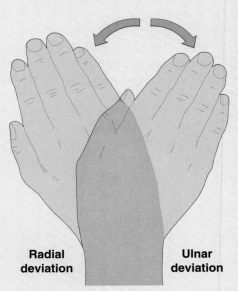

Radial deviation   **Ulnar deviation**

Fig 17-28J

6. Exercise the fingers: Support the hand at the wrist and above each joint that you are exercising.
   a. Bend and straighten each finger separately. Then make a fist and open it with the fingers together (see Fig. 17-28K).

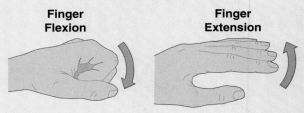

Finger Flexion   **Finger Extension**

Fig 17-28K

b. Bring the fingers together and then spread them apart (see Fig. 17-28L).

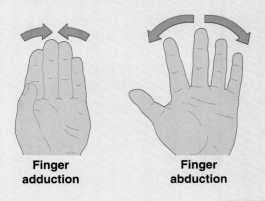

Finger adduction   **Finger abduction**

Fig 17-28L

c. Bring the thumb across the palm of the hand and then bring the thumb away from the hand (Fig 17-28M).

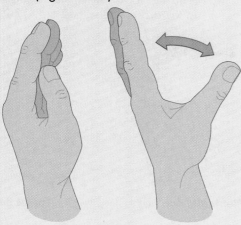

Thumb adduction   **Thumb abduction**

Fig 17-28M

d. Touch the thumb to the tip of each finger (see Fig. 17-28N).

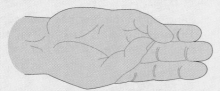

Finger/Thumb opposition

Fig 17-28N

7. Exercise the hip: place one hand below the knee and support the foot with the other hand.
   a. Bend the knee and bring it up toward the chest. Straighten the knee as you lower the leg to the bed (see Fig. 17-28O).

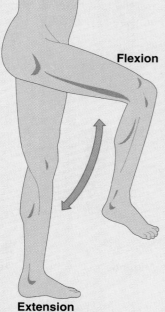

Flexion

Extension   Fig 17-28O

b. Raise the leg up off the bed, keeping the knee straight. Lower the leg to the bed again (see Fig. 17-28P).

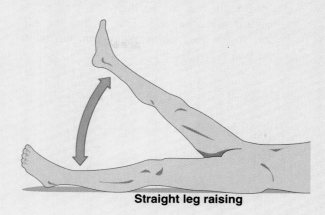

Straight leg raising

Fig 17-28P

c. Keeping the knee straight, bring the leg away from the body, then bring the leg back to the body (see Fig. 17-28Q).

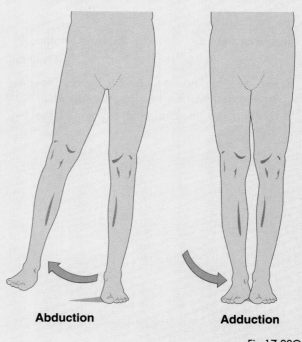

Abduction   **Adduction**

Fig 17-28Q

Performing Range-of-Motion Exercises (cont.)

d. Rotate the hip in, so that the toes point toward the other leg. Then rotate the hip out, so the toes point away from the other leg (see Fig. 17-28R).

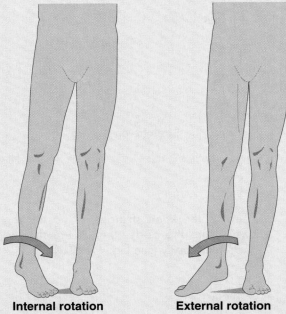

Internal rotation **External rotation**

Fig 17-28R

8. Exercise the knee: Place your hands under the knee and the ankle to support the joints.

   a. Bend the knee; then straighten it (see Fig. 17-28S).

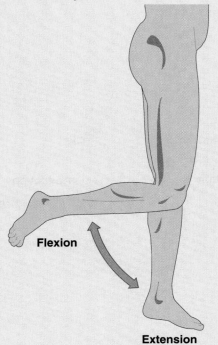

Flexion

Extension Fig 17-28S

9. Exercise the ankle: Place your hands under the foot and ankle to support the joint.

   a. Bend the foot down. Then bend the foot up toward the head (see Fig. 17-28T).

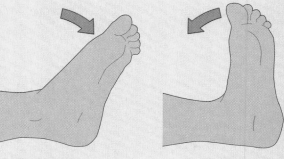

Plantar flexion **Dorsal flexion**

Fig 17-28T

10. Exercise the toes: Support the foot with one hand as you exercise the toes with the other hand.

    a. Bend and straighten the toes separately. Then bend and straighten the toes together (see Fig. 17-28U).

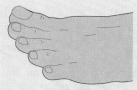

Extension **Flexion**

Fig 17-28U

    b. Bring the toes together and then separate them (see Fig. 17-28V).

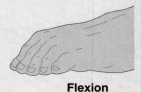

Adduction **Abduction**

Fig 17-28V

Conclusion

Remember these important points:

1. Activity benefits the resident physically and emotionally.

2. Restorative nursing care can prevent most of the complications of inactivity.

3. Encourage the resident to be as independent as possible.

4. Use correct body mechanics when assisting the resident in moving and transferring.

5. Correct body alignment promotes comfort and prevents stress on the musculoskeletal system.

6. Changing body positions promotes comfort, stimulates circulation, and helps to prevent complications.

7. Using a lift sheet makes moving and transferring the resident easier and safer.

8. Keep the side rail up on the opposite side of the bed when you are working with the resident.

9. Return the bed to its lowest position when you are through working with it.

10. Dangling on the side of the bed helps the resident to regain balance.

11. The resident's strong side should lead when moving and transferring.

12. Using a gait/transfer belt reduces the risk of injury to the resident and the nursing assistant.

13. The mechanical lift is used to help transfer residents who are very heavy or are unable to move.

14. Two people are necessary to use a mechanical lift safely.

15. Never leave a resident alone on a stretcher.

16. Ambulation provides exercise that leads to independence and increased self-esteem.

17. Range-of-motion exercises help to prevent loss of joint movement.

Discussion Questions

1. Why is physical activity so important?

2. How would you decide what method and equipment to use in transferring a resident?

3. How can you protect the resident from foot drop if there is no special equipment available?

4. What is meant by the statement, "Using a gait/transfer belt provides you with more control?"

5. Do you like to go for a walk? Why?

6. What might happen if you tried to hold up a falling resident to prevent the fall?

7. Discuss some ways the you could assist the resident with range-of-motion exercises during regular daily care?

Application Exercises

1. The class will divide into groups of three or four. Each group will do a presentation on a transfer procedure. One student will narrate, one or two will perform the procedure, and one will be the "resident." All group members will participate in preparing the presentation. Suggested procedures include the mechanical lift, the gait belt, range-of-motion exercises, and using a wheelchair or stretcher. Narration might include the benefits, important points, and safety factors of the procedure. Each group will be evaluated by other class members and by the instructor.

2. The instructor will demonstrate the procedure for using a mechanical lift. Each student will do a return demonstration, first acting as the "resident," then assisting with, and operating the lift. After the demonstration, the class will discuss their observations about each experience.

Restorative Skin Care: Prevention of Pressure Sores

OBJECTIVES

Upon completing this chapter, you will be able to do the following:

1. List three changes of aging that occur in the skin.

2. Identify three types of injury or skin problems.

3. Explain the need for special foot care of the elderly resident.

4. List two causes of pressure sores.

5. Identify the beginning signs of a pressure sore.

6. Describe the nursing assistant's role in restorative skin care.

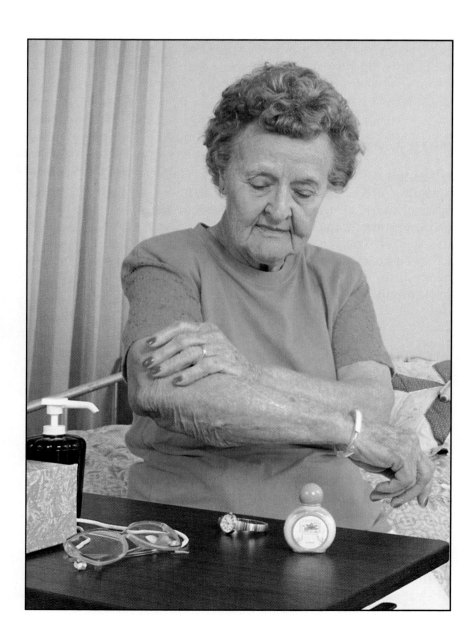

VOCABULARY

The following words or terms will help you to understand this chapter:

Integument	Laceration	Bony prominences
Nutrients	Incision	Hydration
Petechiae	Pressure sore/decubitus ulcer	Sacrum
Bruise	Shearing	Coccyx

Structure and Function of the Skin

The skin is composed of three layers, the epidermis, dermis, and subcutaneous fat. Functions of the skin include protection, regulation of body temperature, sensory reception, and awareness of the environment. A review of the integumentary system in Chapter 11 will be helpful.

Skin Conditions

Changes of Aging. The first visible signs of aging often occur in the integumentary system. Many of the changes that occur in the **integument** (skin) with aging increase the risk of injury and skin damage for the elderly person. These changes include dryness, thinning, loss of padding and insulation, fragility, and decreased sensitivity. Not only can damage occur more easily, there is an increased risk of infection, and healing slows.

To be healthy, the cells of the skin must receive a constant and adequate supply of **nutrients** (food elements) and oxygen. Poor circulation may decrease the delivery of nutrients and oxygen to the skin. Decreased circulation also prevents the removal of waste products and toxins. Healing slows and infection may result.

Aging skin may develop liver spots, moles, and other signs of aging. Some of these are believed to be due to the environment. Any changes in the skin must be reported immediately. Bleeding or a change in the size or color of a mole may be a sign of skin cancer. **Petechiae** (patches of surface bleeding due to fragile blood vessels) are covered with extremely fragile skin. Although they are not uncommon in the skin of the elderly resident, they should be reported. Dryness and skin sensitivity may lead to rashes and skin breakdown.

Injuries. The skin is the body's first line of defense against the environment. Injured skin cannot protect the body from the invasion of microorganisms. Slight injuries may lead to major problems. A **bruise** is an injury that discolors, but does not break the skin. A **laceration** is a rough tear, and an **incision** is a clean, smooth cut.

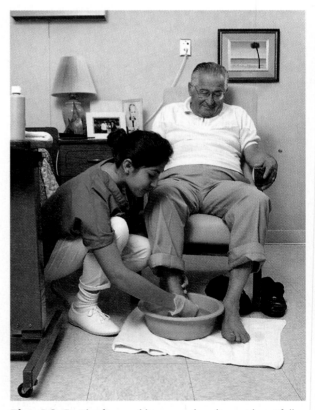

Fig. 18-1 The feet and legs must be observed carefully.

Foot Care. Because the feet and legs are especially at risk, due to poor circulation, they must be protected from injury. This is especially true for diabetics who develop circulatory complications. Washing the feet and drying well between the toes helps to prevent infection and skin breakdown. Shoes must fit well. Socks help to cushion and absorb moisture. Careful observation and prompt reporting of corns, callouses, and other skin changes are necessary. In some states, nursing assistants are not allowed to cut or trim toenails.

Causes and Prevention of Pressure Sores/Decubitus Ulcers

A **pressure sore/decubitus ulcer** is a breakdown of skin tissue that occurs when blood flow is interrupted. When blood flow cannot deliver nutrients and oxygen, or remove waste products and toxins, tissue dies and an ulcer forms. Pressure sores are also called bedsores. Pressure and shearing cause pressure sores. **Shearing** is a force upon the skin that stretches it between the bone inside and a surface outside the body.

Pressure. You may see how pressure stops blood flow by pressing your thumbs against a plate of clear plastic or glass. Observe, through the glass, the skin color that results during this pressure. As soon as you have released the pressure, the color will return to normal.

Pressure causes problems over **bony prominences** (places where bones are near the surface of the skin). Figure 18-2 indicates the bony prominences of the body where decubiti are likely to develop. The skin in these areas is thin enough that the blood vessels can be pinched closed. The vessels are pinched between the bony prominence and the surface upon which it rests (see Fig. 18-3).

Pressure sores are the most challenging of skin problems that may affect the elderly, paralyzed, comatose, malnourished, or obese resident. Obese residents may develop pressure sores in skin folds. Pressure from casts, braces, or traction can also cause

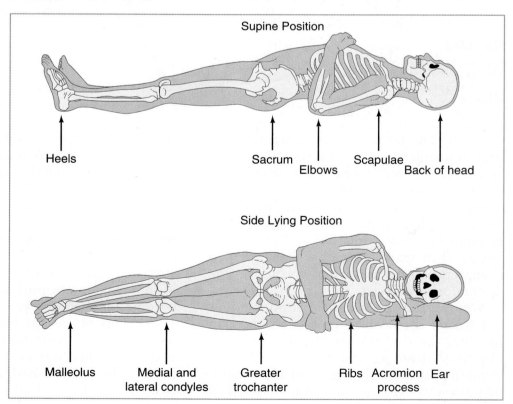

Fig. 18-2
Pressure sores form, most often, over bony prominences.

Supine Position

Heels   Sacrum   Scapulae
         Elbows   Back of head

Side Lying Position

Malleolus   Medial and lateral condyles   Greater trochanter   Ribs   Acromion process   Ear

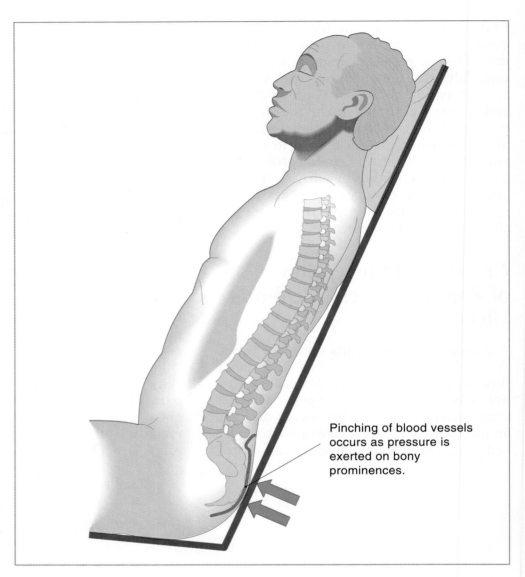

Pinching of blood vessels occurs as pressure is exerted on bony prominences.

Fig. 18-3
Pressure sores form when pressure against a bone stops the flow of blood.

decubiti. The paralyzed or comatose resident is unable to move in a normal manner and does not experience skin sensations that encourage movement.

You can understand this better by thinking about what happens when you sit in one position for a long time. What do you feel? You're skin warns you that you need to change positions, and when you move, the discomfort is relieved.

A paralyzed or comatose resident does not realize the need to reposition and will not feel the discomfort of pressure from objects that are against the skin. Without frequent position changes and movement, pressure sores will develop. A malnourished

resident has less subcutaneous fat and, therefore, is at increased risk of pressure sore formation. The skin must be well nourished and have adequate **hydration** (supply of fluids) to be healthy.

Shearing. In addition to pressure, shearing can also cause pressure sores. As the skin is stretched under pressure, the small surface blood vessels are pulled at an angle and become pinched or twisted closed (see Fig. 18-4). This blocks the blood flow and skin tissue dies. Shearing takes place when the body slides on a surface, as it does when the head of the bed is raised. As the body slides toward the foot of the bed, the skin is

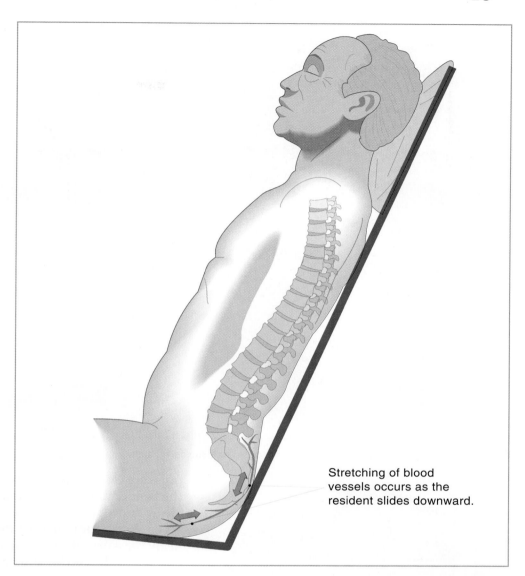

Stretching of blood vessels occurs as the resident slides downward.

Fig. 18-4
When the skin is stretched by shearing, blood vessels are pulled at an angle.

stretched, and the blood vessels over the sacrum and coccyx are pinched. The **sacrum** and **coccyx** are bones at the base of the spine. The coccyx is often referred to as the "tail bone." This is the most common location for pressure sores to occur.

Factors that may cause the pressure sores to become worse include excessive perspiration, incontinence, continued pressure, friction, poor nutrition and hydration, poor skin care, and disease. Most of these factors can be avoided or corrected.

Signs of Pressure Sores. Beginning signs of pressure sores may include skin that is pale, red, dark in color, or unusually warm. The resident may complain of pain, numbness, and tingling. This is the first stage of pressure sore development. The second stage will occur with blisters and possible broken skin on the surface (the epidermis). If the pressure sore continues to develop, the ulcer will open into the deeper tissues and may become deep enough to expose muscle or bone. Infection may occur in the broken skin. The resident may experience pain, and treatment is lengthy and very expensive. Pressure sores progress rapidly and are much easier to prevent than to treat. Early reporting of signs of pressure sores may prevent the progress of a stage I to a stage IV. Stages of pressure sore development may be seen in Fig. 18-5.

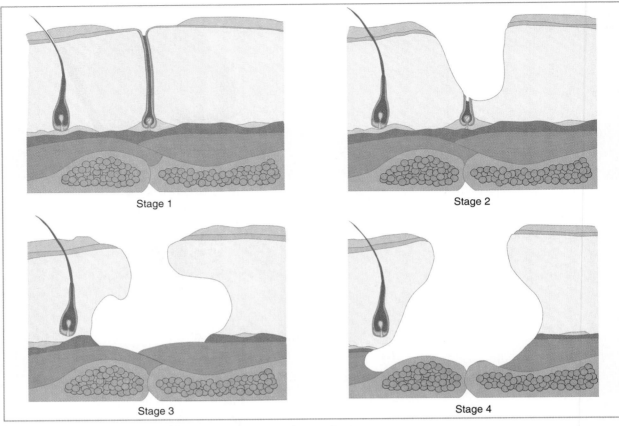

Stage 1

Stage 2

Stage 3

Stage 4

Fig. 18-5 Pressure sores are classified by the depth of tissue destruction.

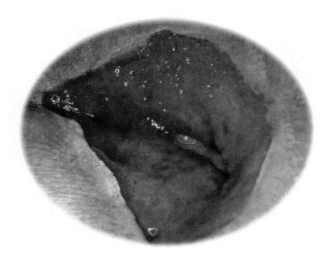

Fig. 18-6 A pressure sore can result in pain and infection.

Restorative Skin Care

As a nursing assistant, you will play an important role in the prevention of pressure sores. While prevention requires much attention and time, curing a pressure sore is much more time consuming and stressful. Most pressure sores can be prevented. Changing the resident's position, while keeping the skin clean and dry, are the basic preventive concerns. Reposition at least every two hours to keep pressure off areas at risk. Immediately cleanse and dry the skin of urine and feces which contain chemicals and bacteria that will cause skin breakdown. Proper repositioning prevents pressure from remaining on any area long enough to cause a problem. Shearing force is also prevented. Correct positioning is discussed in Chapter 17.

Massage around a reddened area with lotion. Massaging over the reddened area can cause additional tissue breakdown. Massage gently because rubbing or scrubbing briskly can cause injury. Lotion keeps skin moist and healthy. Keeping linen clean, dry, and free of wrinkles will help prevent skin problems. Be sure that the bed is free of small objects that might injure the skin. Maintain good nutrition and hydration. Tubes must always be positioned so they will not press upon skin. Observe carefully

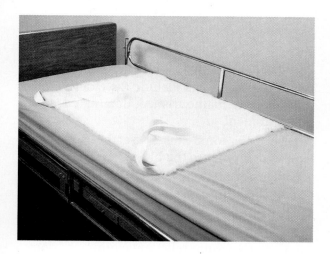

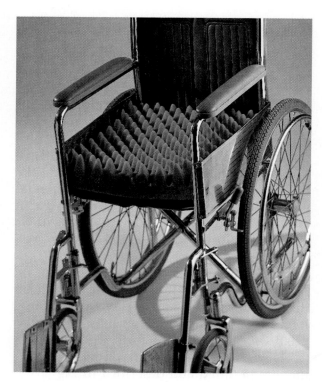

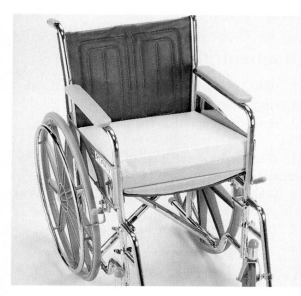

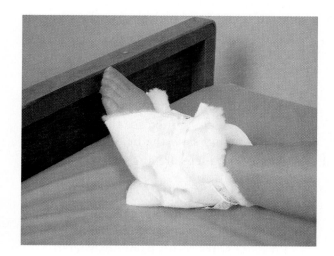

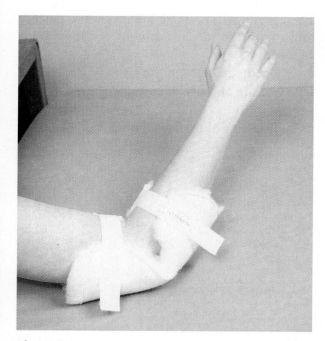

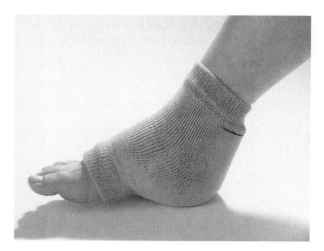

Fig. 18-7 Pressure-relieving devices help to protect the skin.

for pressure that may be caused by braces, splints, casts, traction, or shoes. Clean and trim fingernails to prevent scratching.

Preventing long-lasting, painful, and costly skin problems depends upon your careful observation and commitment to preventative care. Immediately report skin changes to the nurse. The care plan may include special medications, equipment, and treatments that are ordered by the physician. You will be responsible for proper use and care of pressure relieving devices (equipment).

This equipment includes devices that are designed to relieve pressure and friction on the resident's skin and to prevent shearing. Items as ordinary as pillows may be used to position the body in a way that relieves pressure. Other pressure-relieving equipment is pictured and described in Fig. 18-7. Remember that this equipment only provides additional protection for the skin. It does not replace skin care.

Conclusion

Remember these important points:

1. Changes of aging increase the risk of injury to skin and slow the healing process.

2. The feet and legs are at greatest risk, due to poor circulation.

3. Thorough and careful observation, and immediate reporting of skin changes, are necessary to prevent severe skin problems.

4. Pressure sores result from obstructed blood flow which causes tissue death.

5. Bony prominences of the body are common pressure points where pressure sores develop.

6. Residents who are at higher risk of developing pressure sores include the elderly, immobilized, malnourished, debilitated, and obese resident.

7. Shearing force causes stretching of the skin which pinches the blood vessels.

8. Signs of pressure sores include pale or darkened skin, redness, and warmth.

9. The nursing assistant plays an important role in the prevention of pressure sores.

10. Use of pressure relieving equipment does not replace proper positioning and skin care.

Discussion Questions

1. Why are elderly residents at increased risk for skin problems.

2. How does impaired circulation affect the skin?

3. What areas of the body are most affected by pressure?

4. What can be done for the resident to prevent skin problems.

5. Describe the development of a decubitus.

Application Exercise

1. The class will divide into small groups. Each group will research and present a poster and a report to the class on one of the following subjects:

    a. Skin changes in the elderly

    b. Care and use of equipment to relieve pressure

    c. Effects of the environment upon skin

    d. Functions of the skin

Personal Care and Hygiene

OBJECTIVES

Upon completing this chapter, you will be able to do the following:

1. Describe the effect of personal care on self-esteem.

2. Describe three daily care routines.

3. Identify four important observations to make during oral hygiene.

4. List three steps to be taken to protect dentures during denture care.

5. Identify general guidelines for bathing.

6. Identify two aseptic principles of perineal care.

7. Identify four safety measures to be taken when giving a shower or tub bath.

8. List four important guidelines for nail care.

9. Identify four guidelines for changing the resident's clothing.

10. Describe the effect that independence in personal care and dressing has upon the resident's self-esteem.

11. Perform the procedures described in this chapter.

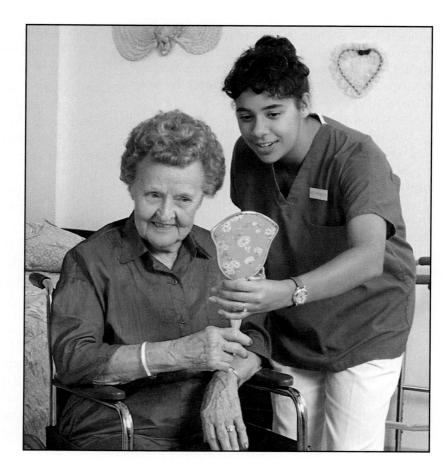

VOCABULARY

The following words or terms will help you to understand this chapter:

Personal hygiene	Expectorate	Axillae
Incontinence	Toothettes	Perineal care (peri-care)
Oral hygiene	Comatose	Defecation
Nasogastric tube	Dentures	Intravenous (IV)
Emesis basin		

Personal Care Choices

Personal care includes bathing; care of the mouth, nails, and hair; shaving; dressing; and applying makeup. This care is provided whenever it is needed. Care of one's body is a very personal choice. Health and self-esteem affect personal care choices. Attending to personal care helps to improve the resident's self-esteem and maintain health. Grooming and **personal hygiene** (cleanliness and care of health) are influenced by culture and religion. Choices that the resident may make regarding hygiene include whether to bathe in the tub or shower, when and how often to perform hygiene, and what products to use. Think about your own preferences for bathing and shampooing.

Many residents depend upon the nursing assistant for assistance with personal hygiene. Some are totally dependent for maintaining healthy skin, cleanliness, and grooming. **Incontinence** (inability to control urine or feces), immobility, illness, and confusion increase the time and effort required for maintaining hygiene. Encourage the resident to be involved and to do as much as possible. If you are not sure what personal care is required for each resident, check the care plan, or ask the nurse.

Daily Care Routines

In the long-term care facility there are usually some routines that are followed for daily hygiene of residents.

Early A.M. Care. Most residents are awakened before breakfast. Care performed before breakfast includes offering **oral hygiene** (mouth care), washing the face and hands, toileting, preparing for breakfast, and straightening the unit and linens. Some residents may go to the dining room to eat, while others may eat in their rooms, in bed, or in a chair. Awakening the resident and assuring comfort may improve the appetite. A freshly washed face and clean mouth will make breakfast more pleasant. The activity of performing this self-care will help provide exercise, improve the appetite, and maintain independence.

A.M. Care After Breakfast. If the resident hasn't bathed before breakfast, this may be done after the meal is finished. Other personal care that may be accomplished after breakfast includes toileting, peri-care, oral hygiene, care of hair and nails, shaving, backrubs, and dressing. After A.M. care is provided, the bed is made and the room tidied.

H.S. Care. H.S. care is performed at bedtime when the resident is preparing to go to sleep. The purpose of this care is to help the resident relax. At bedtime the resident should toilet and perform peri-care. Oral hygiene is also performed, and the face and hands should be washed. Linen should be changed or straightened. Night clothes are provided and the unit is tidied at this time. A backrub at bedtime is very helpful to promote relaxation and a good night's sleep.

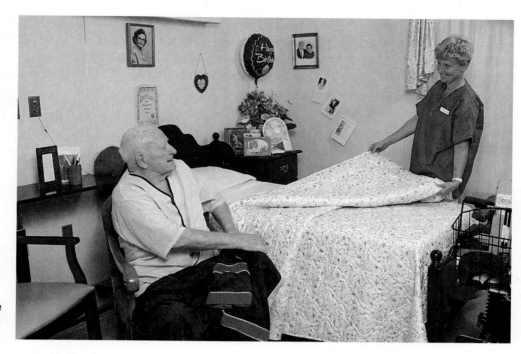

Fig. 19-1
H.S. care refreshes the resident and promotes relaxation for sleep.

Oral Hygiene

Oral care includes brushing the teeth, gums and tongue. Observation of all areas of the mouth and lips are important. Observations of the mouth that should be reported include the following:

- Cracked, blistered, or swollen lips
- Unpleasant mouth odor
- Swelling, redness, sores, bleeding, white patches, or coating of the mouth
- Loose, broken, or chipped teeth
- Resident complaints

A nasogastric (NG) tube (a tube that is inserted through the nose into the stomach), oxygen, illness, and some medications can cause the mouth to become dry and sore or develop a bad taste. Mouth care may be necessary every two hours. An uncomfortable mouth or bad taste can lead to a poor appetite and inadequate fluid intake. Oral hygiene improves the resident's health and self-esteem.

Some residents will perform oral hygiene independently and may only need your assistance to gather supplies. Others, who are weak, paralyzed, bedridden, or con-fused, may need you to perform oral care for them. Comatose residents must also depend on you to perform oral hygiene. Disoriented or forgetful residents may be able to provide their own oral care if reminded and assisted to do so each time. As with all activities of daily living (ADLs), encourage the resident to be as independent as possible. Be sure that the care is completed satisfactorily. Remember that poor oral health can cause discomfort, loss of appetite, low self-esteem, and a decline in general health.

Equipment and Supplies. The basic equipment and supplies needed for oral hygiene may include a toothbrush or denture brush, toothpaste, glass of water, towel, and gloves. Check the care plan to determine if adaptive equipment is to be used to assist in self-care. If the resident will receive oral care in bed, it will be necessary to provide a straw and an **emesis basin** (a small curved basin). The resident may use the emesis basin to **expectorate** (spit). Mouthwash, dental floss, and **Toothettes**® (sticks with small sponges to be used for oral care) may be used. Remember that gloves should be worn for any contact with body fluids, including saliva.

You will assist the resident who cannot perform oral hygiene independently. Some principles for thorough tooth brushing include

- Wear gloves.
- Use a soft- to medium-bristled brush.
- Brush in a circular motion while holding the brush at a 45° angle.

- Brush the gums as well as the teeth.
- Brush inner, outer, and then chewing surfaces of upper teeth.
- Brush lower teeth in the same manner.

Oral Care for the Comatose Resident. If the resident is **comatose** (unconscious or unresponsive), communication remains as important as it is for conscious residents.

PROCEDURE

Assisting with Oral Hygiene

Before any procedure you must always follow the five basic steps: wash your hands, collect the equipment, identify the resident, explain the procedure, and protect privacy.

Follow universal precautions and wear gloves when appropriate

1. Place equipment and supplies on paper towels on the overbed table.
2. Raise the bed to a comfortable working height and lock the wheels.
3. Raise the head of the bed if allowed.
4. Place a bath towel across the resident's chest.
5. Place the overbed table across the bed in front of the resident.
6. Put on gloves.

7. Allow the resident to rinse the mouth with water or diluted mouthwash. You may hold the emesis basin to the chin for expectoration (see Fig. 19-2).
8. Place toothpaste on the wet toothbrush and encourage the resident to do the brushing.
9. Assist the resident to rinse the mouth and expectorate into the emesis basin.
10. Clean and put away equipment; discard disposables.
11. Wipe off the overbed table.
12. Remove your gloves and wash your hands.
13. Return the resident to a comfortable position. Be sure the call signal is in reach.
14. Open the privacy curtain and assure the resident's safety.
15. Record assistance and report observations.

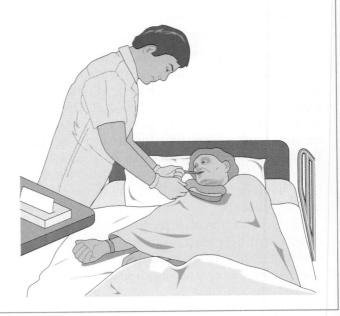

Fig. 19-2
The emesis basin may be used for expectoration.

Explain the procedure and talk to the resident. When the resident is unable to swallow, oral care is provided with the resident turned to the side. Toothpaste and water are not used. Special oral care supplies, such as lemon-glycerine swabs and Toothettes (see Fig. 19-4) are used in performing oral care for the comatose resident. If these items are not available, use applicators moistened with diluted mouthwash. Oral care should be provided every two hours and more often if needed.

Equipment and Supplies. The basic equipment and supplies needed for oral hygiene of the comatose resident may include a towel, emesis basin, mouthwash, cup, padded tongue depressor, Toothettes, lemon-glycerine swabs or applicators, and gloves.

PROCEDURE

Giving Oral Care to the Comatose Resident

Before any procedure you must always follow the five basic steps: wash your hands, collect the equipment, identify the resident, explain the procedure, and protect privacy.

Follow universal precautions and wear gloves when appropriate.

1. Place equipment and supplies on paper towels on the overbed table.
2. Raise the bed to a comfortable working height, lock the wheels, and lower the side rail.
3. Place the resident in a side-lying position.
4. Place a bath towel under the resident's head and face and the emesis basin under the side of the chin.
5. Put on gloves.
6. Use a padded tongue depressor to separate the teeth and open the mouth (see Fig. 19-3).
7. Clean the mouth using Toothettes or lemon-glycerine swabs or applicators with diluted mouthwash (see Fig. 19-4). Clean all surfaces of the mouth (tongue, cheeks, roof, and teeth).
8. Apply petroleum jelly to the lips for lubrication.
9. Reposition the resident.
10. Raise the side rail.
11. Clean and put away equipment and discard disposables.
12. Wipe off the overbed table.
13. Remove your gloves and wash your hands.
14. Place the call signal within reach.
15. Record the procedure and report observations.

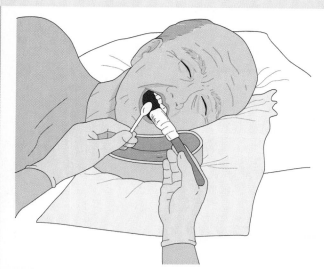

Fig. 19-3
A padded tongue blade may be used to hold the mouth open during oral hygiene of the comatose resident.

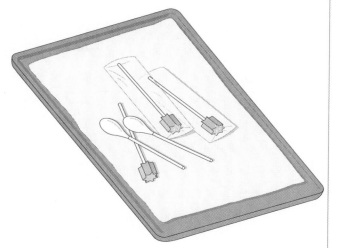

Fig. 19-4
Lemon-glycerine swabs and toothettes are commercial products for oral care.

Denture Care. **Dentures** (false teeth) should be cleaned as often as natural teeth. The mouth should also be rinsed while the dentures are out. Food, bacteria, and seeds that collect on mouth surfaces should be rinsed out. Because dentures are slippery, and can be easily broken, they should be held firmly over a basin when being carried. While brushing them, hold them over a basin filled with water or lined with a towel (see Fig. 19-5).

Dentures are expensive to replace, and replacement may be extremely difficult or impossible for some elderly residents. Nutrition may become a major problem if dentures are broken or missing. Think about the limited variety of foods that can be eaten without teeth. Without the ability to chew food, an already poor appetite may become worse. Weight loss and declining health may result. Protect the resident's dentures. You may become negligent if you fail to use precautions.

Protecting Dentures. Dentures must be cleaned and stored in cool water. Hot water can cause them to fit improperly. Because drying can warp dentures, they must be stored in cool water when they are not being worn. Be sure the denture container is labeled with the resident's name, because sets of dentures look very much alike. When stripping the bed, remember to look for dentures that may have been placed in the linen. Search the pillowcase carefully.

People who wear dentures usually prefer to clean the dentures themselves. Self-care should always be encouraged. Provide assistance and check the care plan for use of adaptive equipment. You may assist some residents to the bathroom to clean their own dentures, while it may be necessary for you to clean the dentures for others. The procedure for care of dentures is located on page 273.

Equipment and Supplies. The basic equipment and supplies needed for denture care include gloves, denture brush or toothbrush, toothpaste, mouthwash, denture cup, glass of water, emesis basin, and towel.

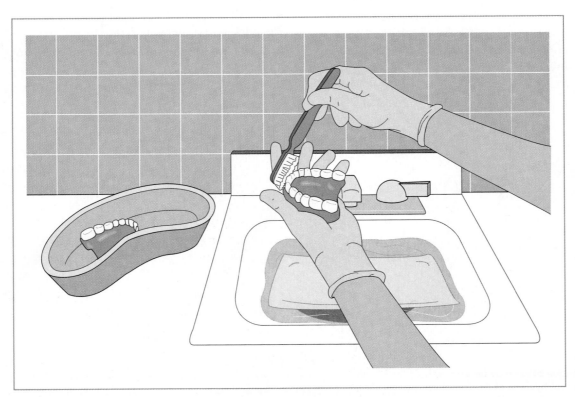

Fig. 19-5 Brushing dentures over a sinkful of water will protect them.

Care of Dentures

Before any procedure you must always follow the five basic steps: wash your hands, collect the equipment, identify the resident, explain the procedure, and protect privacy.

Follow universal precautions and wear gloves when appropriate.

1. Place the necessary equipment at the sink.
2. Take the denture cup, emesis basin, mouthwash, glass of water, and gloves to the bedside.
3. Place the towel over the resident's chest.
4. Put on the gloves.
5. Ask the resident to remove the dentures and place them in the emesis basin.
6. If the resident cannot remove the dentures you may do so as follows:
   a. Move the upper denture up and down slightly by grasping it with your thumb and index finger at the front. This breaks the seal (see Fig. 19-6A).
   b. When loose, remove the denture, and place it into the emesis basin.
   c. Grasp the lower denture at the front with your thumb and index finger.
   d. Remove it gently, turning it if necessary to bring the end of one side out before the other (see Fig. 19-6B). Place the lower denture into the emesis basin.
7. Take the dentures, denture cup and emesis basin to the sink.
8. Place a paper towel in the sink or fill the sink with water to cushion the dentures in case they slip from your hands (see Fig. 19-5).
9. Place toothpaste or denture cleaner on each denture in the emesis basin.
10. Holding one denture in your palm, brush all surfaces thoroughly. Return it to the emesis basin while you brush the other denture in the same manner.

11. Rinse each denture thoroughly, one at a time, under cool running water.
12. Place the dentures in the denture cup with fresh cool water.
13. Rinse the emesis basin.
14. Bring the emesis basin and dentures (in the cup) to the resident.
15. Dilute the mouthwash with water, and assist the resident to rinse out the mouth. You may hold the emesis basin to one side of the resident's chin for expectoration (see Fig. 19-2).
16. Have the resident replace the dentures in the mouth.
17. If the resident is unable to replace dentures proceed as follows:
    a. With your thumb and finger at the front of the upper denture, insert it into the resident's mouth. You may lift the upper lip with your other hand.
    b. If necessary, you may turn the denture slightly to the side to insert one side, and then turn it gently against the inner cheek to insert the other side.
    c. Secure it by pressing it into place lightly.
    d. With your thumb and index finger at the front of the lower denture, insert it. You may lower the bottom lip with your free hand. You may also turn the denture as described in step 17b to insert it. Gently press downward to secure it.
18. Leave the denture cup with clean water at the resident's bedside. If dentures are not to be replaced in the resident's mouth, leave them in the labeled denture cup at the bedside.
19. Return equipment and supplies to proper storage.
20. Remove the gloves and wash your hands.
21. Make the resident comfortable.
22. Place the call signal in reach and assure the resident's safety.
23. Record the procedure and report observations.

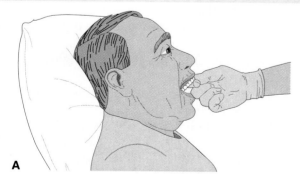
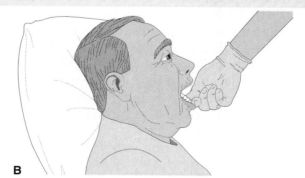

A **B**

Fig. 19-6 Dentures are removed for denture care.

Bathing and Personal Hygiene

Although many residents will be able to bathe themselves, others will need your assistance. If the bath must be given by the nursing assistant, this is usually one of the lengthiest procedures performed. A bath cleanses the skin and prevents odor. It also provides exercise and allows for thorough observation of the resident.

You have an excellent opportunity to observe for skin problems while assisting with bathing. Areas that are prone to skin problems are bony prominences and skin creases and folds, such as breasts, knees, and **axillae** (underarms). Report any unusual skin problems to the nurse.

Bath time observation also includes the opportunity to listen to the resident and allows the nursing assistant to observe physical complaints as well as mental, emotional, and speech changes. Questions may be asked to encourage conversation. Bath time provides an excellent opportunity for reality orientation and validation therapy. The movement that is required for bathing exercises the limbs and allows observation of limitations of movement.

How does bathing affect you? When you step from the tub or shower, do you feel refreshed and relaxed? Does your skin feel good? How is your self-esteem after a bath? The skin and circulation are stimulated by bathing. It is a very nurturing process that often results in an improved sense of well-being.

Methods of bathing include the complete bed bath, partial bath, tub bath, shower, and specialty bath. In long-term care, showers or specialty baths are most frequently used because of their restorative value. The resident's personal preference, physical condition, and level of independence will determine the method of bathing required. Bath time should be chosen according to the resident's preference.

Frequency of bathing varies for individuals. Some bathe daily, and others may choose to do so once or twice a week. Illness, activity, and aging affect the need to bathe. Daily partial baths are usually adequate for the elderly who receive a complete bath or shower twice a week. Bathing may tend to dry the skin. The use of soap may be limited to prevent drying and irritation.

GENERAL GUIDELINES FOR BATHING

- Check the care plan or your assignment sheet to determine the type of bath required for the resident.
- Allow the resident to use the toilet before bathing, as water stimulates the urge to void.
- Provide for privacy by pulling the privacy curtain, closing the door, and closing window coverings.
- Provide for warmth by checking room temperature, preventing drafts and using a bath blanket.
- Protect the resident from falls. Never leave a resident unattended in the tub or shower.
- Check the water temperature before bathing.
- Use correct body mechanics, standing with your feet apart and your back straight.
- Raise the bed to a comfortable working height when giving a bed bath.
- Wear gloves for washing the genital area or if there will be contact with any body fluids. Gloves may be worn for the entire bath.
- Make a mitt out of the washcloth when bathing the resident (see Fig. 19-7).
- Change water as frequently as needed for temperature, or when it becomes soapy.
- Wash from the cleanest to the dirtiest areas, beginning with the face and finishing with the genital area.
- Uncover, wash, rinse, and dry only one part at a time.
- Rinse soap from the skin thoroughly.
- Apply deodorant.
- Check pockets of clothing for valuables before placing in the laundry hamper.
- If the resident is incontinent, the skin must be cleansed and linen must be changed before continuing with the bath.

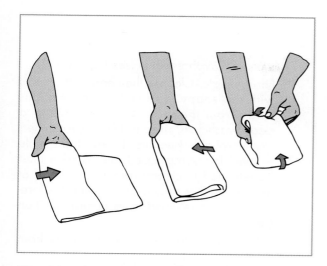

Fig. 19-7 Using the washcloth as a mitt will prevent water from dripping.

Perineal Care

Perineal care (peri-care) is the cleansing of the genital and rectal areas of the body. This procedure prevents infection and odor in an area that is susceptible to bacterial growth. You will recall that bacteria grow best in a moist, dark, warm environment. Perineal care is an important part of daily care for all residents. Residents who are incontinent, and those who have catheters, must receive peri-care frequently. A procedure for caring for residents with catheters will appear later. Peri-care is provided every day, usually at bath time, and as often as necessary.

The resident should be allowed to perform peri-care if able to do so. When speaking of the procedure, use words that are familiar to the resident such as "your private parts" or "the area between your legs." The resident probably will not be familiar with the medical term for this procedure.

Aseptic Principles. In performing peri-care the principles of asepsis must be followed. The area is cleansed from the cleanest to the dirtiest. It is important to cleanse away from the urinary meatus. This helps to prevent urinary infections by removing germs from the entrance to the urinary system. The rectal area contains bacteria that can cause infection in the vaginal and urinary areas. A buildup of ammonia and bacteria causes severe skin breakdown. Incontinent residents must receive peri-care immediately after urination or defecation. **Defecation** is the elimination of solid wastes from the body. Remind the resident to follow aseptic practices.

Solutions are available for peri-care. The solution should be warmed to body temperature before spraying it directly onto the genitalia. Thorough cleansing with soap and water is necessary to remove urine and feces. A kit may be used for peri-care. These kits contain antiseptic wipes or swabs and disposable gloves. The most common method for providing peri-care is washing with soap and water. Follow the policy and procedure at your facility. Although peri-care procedures vary, the principles remain the same. The procedure for perineal care is located on pages 276–277.

Equipment and Supplies. The basic equipment and supplies needed for perineal care include a protective pad, towel, wash cloths, soap, bath basin, gloves, peri-care kit (optional), and solution (optional).

The Complete Bed Bath

The resident who requires a bed bath may be able to participate in bathing. If necessary, place the wet washcloth in the resident's hands and give step-by-step instructions. Encourage self-care. Give praise for the slightest effort, while preventing frustration. The procedure for giving a complete bed bath is located on pages 278–280.

Equipment and Supplies. Equipment and supplies needed for giving a complete bed bath include bath blanket, bath basin, washcloths, towels, soap, water, deodorant, lotion, and clean clothing.

PROCEDURE

Perineal Care

Before any procedure you must always follow the five basic steps: wash your hands, collect the equipment, identify the resident, explain the procedure, and protect privacy.

Follow universal precautions and wear gloves when appropriate.

1. Raise the head of the bed to a comfortable working height and lock the wheels.
2. Raise the side rail on the opposite side, and lower the side rail on the side nearest you.
3. Assist the resident to a supine position with legs separated and knees bent (see Fig. 19-8).
4. Place a protective pad or towel under the buttocks.
5. Cover the resident with a bath blanket. Fold top linens to the foot of the bed. Raise the side rail when you leave the bedside.
6. Fill a wash basin with water at a comfortable temperature (approximately 105°F or 40.5°C) and place it on paper towels on the overbed table.
7. Put on gloves.
8. Provide peri-care for the male and female as follows:
   a. For the female: Separate the labia and wash from front to back (away from the urinary meatus) with the soapy washcloth. Use a different area of the cloth for each stroke. With a clean washcloth, rinse in the same manner. Dry thoroughly (see Fig. 19-9A).
   b. For the male: Cleanse the head of the penis with the soapy washcloth using motions away from the urinary meatus. Using a clean washcloth, rinse in the same manner. Dry thoroughly (see Fig. 19-9B). If the male resident is uncircumcised, the foreskin must be retracted to cleanse around the head of the penis. After rinsing and drying, the foreskin must be returned to its natural position (see Fig. 19-10)
9. Turn the resident to the side facing away from you.
10. Cleanse with soapy washcloth from the vagina or scrotum to the rectal area. Use a different area of the cloth for each stroke. Rinse in the same manner. Dry thoroughly.
11. Remove the protective pad and dispose of it.
12. Raise the side rail.
13. Empty, rinse, and dry the basin.
14. Remove the gloves and wash your hands.
15. Return equipment and supplies to their proper location.
16. Lower the side rail on the side of the bed nearest you.
17. Remove the bath blanket after covering the resident with the top linen.
18. Lower the bed and raise the side rail if required.
19. Be sure the resident is comfortable.
20. Place the call signal in reach.
21. Wash your hands.

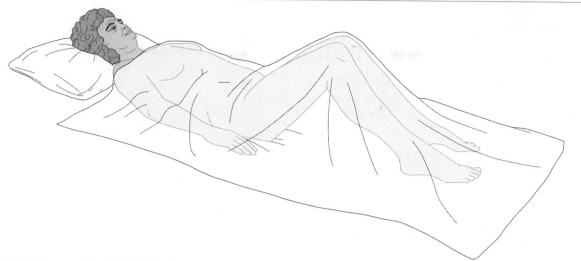

Fig. 19-8 Position the resident for peri-care.

A

Urethra area
(wipe downward
never upward)

Perineum

Anus

B

Urethra (start
here and wipe
downward)

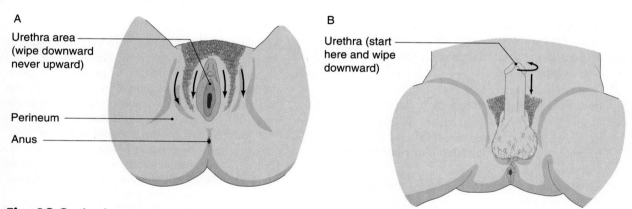

Fig. 19-9 The cleansing motion for peri-care should be away from the urinary meatus.

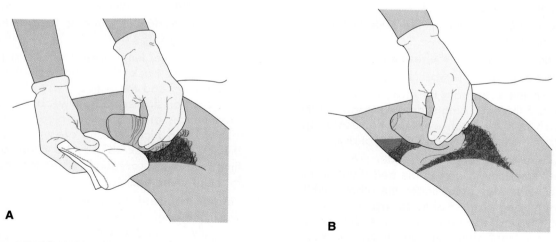

A

B

Fig. 19-10 After the foreskin is retracted for peri-care, it must be returned to its natural position.

PROCEDURE

Giving a Complete Bed Bath

Before any procedure you must always follow the five basic steps: wash your hands, collect the equipment, identify the resident, explain the procedure, and protect privacy.

Follow universal precautions and wear gloves when appropriate.

1. Raise the bed to a comfortable working height, lock the wheels, and raise the side rail on the farthest side of the bed.
2. Offer the bedpan to the resident. Raise the side rail nearest you.
3. Adjust the bed to as flat a position as possible.
4. Check for drafts and proper room temperature.
5. Arrange the equipment on the overbed table. Place the bath basin upon clean paper towels.
6. Be sure the resident is lying on the side of the bed nearest to you.
7. Remove the bedspread and blanket from the bed. Fold them over the back of the chair.
8. Place the bath blanket over the top sheet. Remove the top sheet from under the bath blanket without uncovering the resident (see Fig. 19-11).
9. Remove any clothes and jewelry that the resident is wearing.
10. Fill the bath basin, two-thirds full, with water that is a comfortable temperature (approximately 105°F or 40.5°C).
11. Lower the side rail on the side of the bed nearest you.
12. Place the towel over the resident's chest.
13. Make a mitt with the washcloth (see Fig. 19-7).
14. Wash the eyes from the nose (inner aspect) toward the ear, using a different corner of the wash mitt for each eye. Do not use soap. Wash the face, ears, and neck. Pat dry.
15. Place a towel lengthwise under the arm farthest from you to protect the bed. Support the arm with your palm under the elbow, while using long firm strokes to wash the arm, axilla, and shoulder. Observe the axilla, elbows, and shoulders carefully. The hand may be soaked in the basin of water (see Fig. 19-12). Rinse, pat dry, and cover the arm.

16. Repeat step 15 for the arm nearest you.
17. While the fingernails are damp, clean under them with an orange stick.
18. Place the bath towel across the resident's chest. Fold the bath blanket to the waist. Lifting the towel partially, wash and rinse the chest. Observe the breast creases carefully for the female resident. Rinse and dry thoroughly (see Fig. 19-13A).
19. With the towel covering the chest, fold the bath blanket to the pubic area. Wash the abdomen and navel. Observe any abdominal folds for irritation. Rinse and pat dry. Cover the chest and abdomen with the bath blanket and remove the towel (see Fig. 19-13B).
20. Change the water, if needed, and rinse the basin. Raise the side rail when you leave the bedside.
21. Uncover the leg farthest from you and place a towel under it lengthwise. Have the resident flex the knee if possible or place your palm under the knee to support the leg. Wash the leg and foot carefully, observing for skin problems at the knee, ankle, and heel and between the toes. Wash thoroughly between the toes. The foot may be soaked in the basin of water. Pat dry, taking special care to dry thoroughly between the toes. Observe the toenails. Cover the leg and foot with the bath blanket.
22. Repeat step 21 for the leg nearest you. Raise the side rail when you leave the bedside.
23. Change the bath water and rinse the basin.
24. Assist the resident to turn onto the side facing away from you.
25. Place the towel lengthwise on the bed along the resident's back. Wash the back, the back of the neck, and the buttocks with firm, long, and circular strokes. Carefully observe bony prominences at the shoulder blades, sacrum, coccyx, and hips. Dry the area and remove the towel. A backrub may be given at this time (see next procedure). Assist the resident to return to the back.
26. Perform peri-care if the resident is unable to wash the genital area. Pat dry and observe carefully for skin problems.
27. Assist the resident to dress and complete grooming.

28. Raise the side rail when you leave the bedside.
29. Empty, rinse, and dry the bath basin and return equipment and supplies to their proper place. Place soiled linen in the hamper.
30. Wipe off the overbed table with a paper towel.
31. If the resident is to remain in bed, make an occupied bed. Lower the bed and make the resident comfortable. Raise the side rail if required.

32. Assist the resident out of bed, when possible, and make the bed.
33. Open the window covering if the resident desires it. Open the privacy curtain and place the call signal in reach.
34. Wash your hands.
35. Record the procedure and report unusual observations to the nurse.

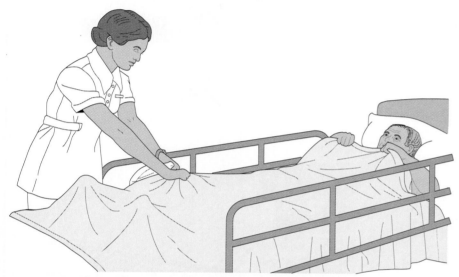

A Remove the top sheet from under the bath blanket by working from the side.

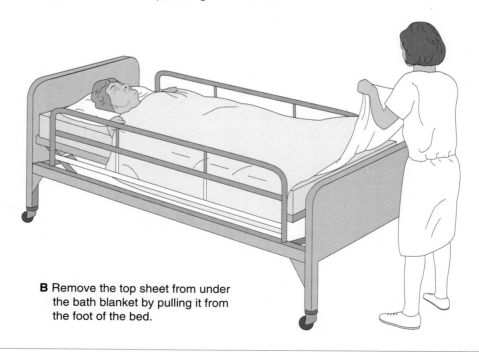

Fig. 19-11
Remove the top sheet without uncovering the resident.

B Remove the top sheet from under the bath blanket by pulling it from the foot of the bed.

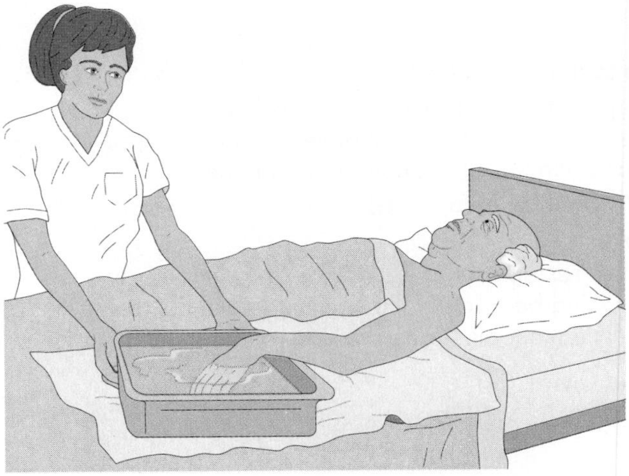

Fig. 19-12
Soaking the hands and feet may be enjoyable, and it makes the nails easier to clean and trim.

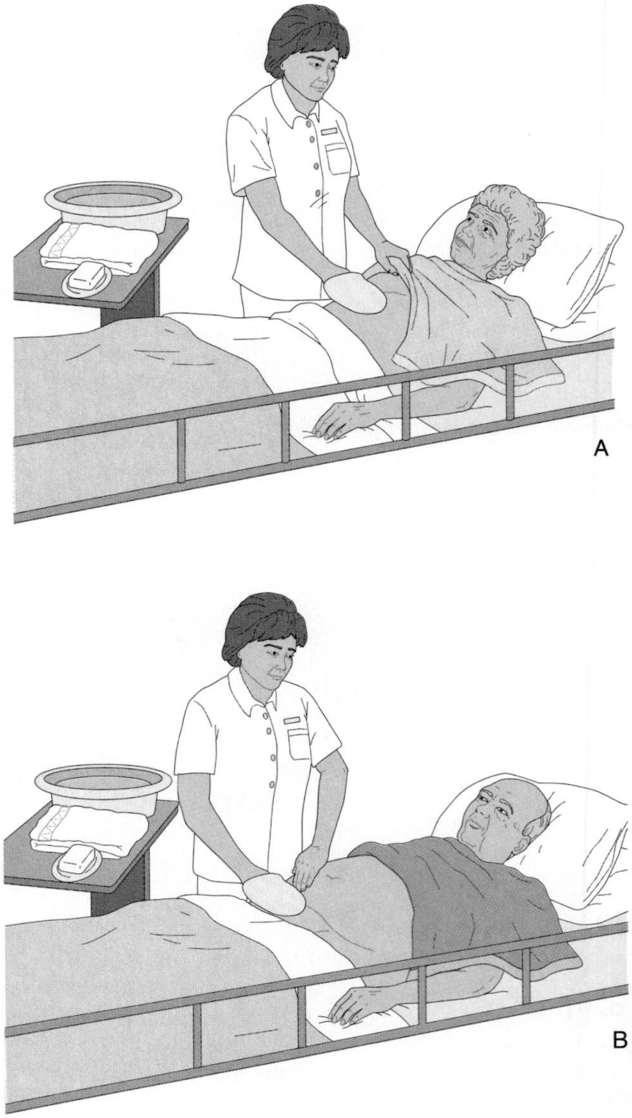

A

B

Fig. 19-13
While washing the chest and abdomen, observe skin creases.

The Partial Bath

Although residents may receive a shower, tub bath, or bed bath only twice a week, a partial bath is completed every day. The areas of the body that require daily hygiene include the face, hands, axilla, perineal area, all creases, and skin folds. Excessive perspiration, vomitus, and incontinence may increase the need for bathing.

Many residents may be able to take a partial bath with minimal assistance. Getting equipment and supplies together and assisting the resident to the bathroom can help promote independence. Stay near by and be prepared to help as needed. Bathing may be done in the bed or chair, or at the sink. It may be necessary for the nursing assistant to provide the partial bath for the resident. The guidelines for a complete bed bath also apply to the partial bath.

Giving a Backrub

The backrub is an enjoyable part of personal care. Besides producing a refreshing feeling and sense of well-being, the backrub relaxes muscles and stimulates circulation. Backrubs are routinely given during A.M. care, at H.S., and every time that a bedridden resident is turned and repositioned. This is a good time to observe for skin problems related to pressure and poor circulation.

The resident may be in a lateral or prone position for the backrub. Lotion should be warmed to body temperature in one of the following ways, before being applied:

- Rub a small amount between your hands.
- Hold the bottle under warm running water.
- Place the bottle in warm water for a few minutes.

After warming the lotion, apply it to the resident's back. Use long, firm, upward strokes to the shoulders and down over the upper arms. Stroke upward to the shoulders and then, with gentler strokes, move downward to the buttocks. Use circular motions to promote circulation to pressure areas over bony prominences.

The Shower and Tub Bath

Showers and tub baths are additional ways of bathing. The choice is a matter of personal preference and mobility. The use of showers and tubs increase the need for safety precautions.

Safety in the Shower and Tub. Residents must always be attended when taking a shower or tub bath. They may *never* be left alone in the tub, shower, or shower chair.

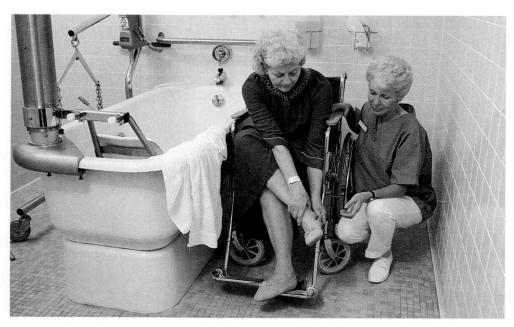

Fig. 19-14
Hands-on assistance prevents falls in the tub area.

PROCEDURE

Assisting the Resident to Shower

Before any procedure you must always follow the five basic steps: wash your hands, collect the equipment, identify the resident, explain the procedure, and protect privacy.

Follow universal precautions and wear gloves when appropriate.

1. Arrange supplies and equipment on a chair near the shower.

2. Assist the resident to the shower. Use a shower chair if necessary.

3. Turn the water on, and adjust the temperature and pressure.

4. Assist the resident to undress.

5. Assist the resident into the shower. If a shower chair is used, lock the wheels.

6. Provide the resident with soap and a washcloth. Encourage self-care and stand by to assist as needed (see Fig. 19-15).

7. After the resident has finished bathing and rinsing, turn off the water.

8. Provide towels for drying. Assist as necessary to be sure the resident is completely dry.

9. Remove the gloves, if used, and wash your hands.

10. Assist the resident to dress and leave the shower area.

11. Apply gloves to clean the shower. Place soiled linen in the hamper.

12. Remove gloves and wash your hands.

13. Return equipment and supplies to their proper place.

14. Wash your hands.

15. Assist the resident to complete grooming.

16. Wash your hands.

17. Record the procedure and report observations.

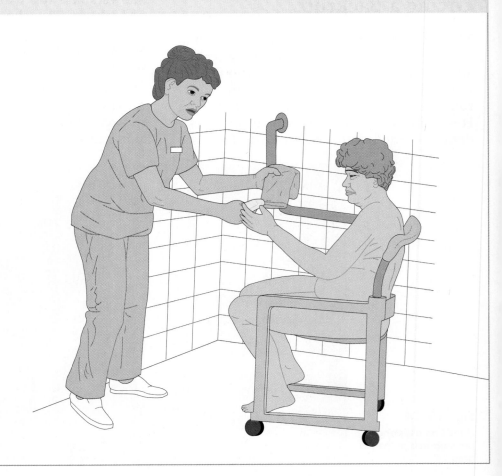

Fig. 19-15
A shower chair may be used for weak or paralyzed residents.

Chilling must be prevented. Tubs and showers must be properly cleaned before and after use. These are dangerous areas, which require additional precautions to protect the resident's safety. Surfaces are slippery when wet. Assist the resident into and out of the tub. Drain the tub before assisting the resident to get out. Water temperature must be carefully guarded and should be set before the resident enters.

The Shower. Weak or paralyzed residents may be wheeled in a shower chair to and from the shower. They may sit in the shower chair throughout the shower. The shower chair is a plastic or metal wheeled chair, with a seat similar to a toilet seat (see Fig. 19-15 located on page 282). Because the chair is lightweight and easily upset, always stay with the resident. The chair may be used to transport the resident for showers, or the resident may be seated in the shower chair upon beginning the shower.

Maintaining the resident's privacy is important. The resident should be taken to the shower in clothes, changed in the shower, and returned from the shower, fully clothed. Although it is not practical to cover the body during a shower, privacy should be assured by closing doors or curtains. Towels should be used to cover the resident while a shampoo or foot care is performed.

Equipment and Supplies. Equipment and supplies needed for assisting the resident to shower may include a chair, shower chair, towels, washcloth, soap, deodorant, and clean clothing.

The Tub Bath. Getting in and out of the tub requires balance and strength. Upon leaving a tub of warm water, the resident may become weak or faint. The tub should be drained before the resident gets out. Always provide hands on assistance as the resident enters and leaves the tub.

Equipment and Supplies. Equipment and supplies needed for assisting the resident with a tub bath may include a chair, towels, washcloth, soap, tub cleaning solution, bath thermometer, and clean clothing.

PROCEDURE

Assisting with a Tub Bath

Before any procedure you must always follow the five basic steps: wash your hands, collect the equipment, identify the resident, explain the procedure, and protect privacy.

Follow universal precautions and wear gloves when appropriate.

1. Arrange supplies and equipment on a chair near the bath tub.
2. Assist the resident to the bathroom or tub room.
3. Wear gloves to clean the tub according to facility policy.
4. Remove gloves and wash your hands.
5. Fill the tub half-full of water at 105°F (40.5°C). Test the temperature with a bath thermometer.
6. Place a towel or bath mat on the floor beside the tub.
7. Assist the resident to undress.
8. Assist the resident into the bathtub.
9. Provide the resident with soap and a washcloth. Encourage self-care.
10. Stay with the resident and prepare to help. Wear gloves if assistance is necessary.
11. Place a towel on the chair and drain the tub.
12. Assist the resident out of the tub and into the chair.
13. Provide towels for drying. Assist as necessary to be sure the resident is completely dry.
14. Remove gloves and wash your hands.
15. Assist the resident to dress and leave the tub area.
16. Wear gloves to clean the tub. Place soiled linen in the hamper.
17. Remove the gloves and wash your hands.
18. Return supplies and equipment to their proper place.
19. Wash your hands.
20. Record the procedure and report observations.

The Specialty Bath

There are several types of specialty tubs that are used for bathing. Many of these combine bathing with whirlpool action. Whirlpool action stimulates circulation and relaxes muscles. These tubs must be cleaned before and after use. Always check the water temperature before the resident enters the tub. Some tubs have special transport chairs, and many use a hydraulic lift. If a seat belt is available, it should always be used. Because procedures may vary between types of tubs and chairs, it is your responsibility to learn the correct procedure for each tub that you use. Never leave the resident alone in the tub. Prevent chilling and protect privacy.

The procedure for assisting with a tub bath may be followed when using a specialty tub. The steps for assisting the resident in and out of the tub will vary, according to the type of specialty tub you are using. Follow the policies and procedures of your facility.

Care of the Hair and Nails

Care of the hair and nails affects health, as well as appearance and self-esteem. Hair combing and brushing are done at bath time every day, and more often as desired. Residents should be encouraged to comb and brush their own hair. Nursing assistants should not cut residents' hair. Matted hair or knots are best removed by beginning to comb them out from the ends, working toward the scalp.

Most facilities have professional beauticians with whom residents can make appointments for hair care. Appointments should not be made without the permission of the resident or legal guardian. If the resident has regularly scheduled appointments with the beautician, the hair should not be washed in the shower.

Shampooing the Hair. Shampooing is usually done one to three times a week. Shampooing may be done in the bed or shower if it is not to be done by a beautician. Special equipment such as a shampoo tray and bucket make bed shampooing more manageable (see Fig. 19-17). Shampoos should be done as indicated on the assignment. The hair should be dried as quickly as possible after a shampoo. Allow the resident to choose a hairstyle.

GUIDELINES FOR ASSISTING WITH A SHAMPOO

- Use a hand-held shower nozzle if available.
- Encourage the resident to perform self-care.

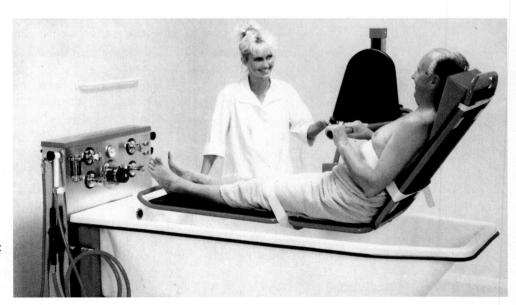

Fig. 19-16
The whirlpool action of specialty tubs stimulates circulation and relaxes muscles.

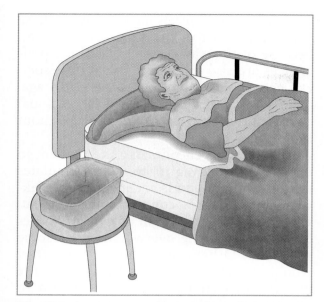

Fig. 19-17 A shampoo tray may be used to shampoo the resident's hair while she is in bed.

- Prevent shampoo from getting in the resident's eyes.
- Massage the scalp while washing the hair.
- Clean the hair thoroughly.
- Rinse shampoo out completely.
- Dry as quickly as possible.
- Style the hair according to the resident's preference.

Nail Care. Proper care and observation of fingernails and toenails is very important. Infection or injury can cause serious problems. Fingernails must be kept clean and at a reasonable length. Nails are cleaned and trimmed easily while damp. Scissors are not used to cut fingernails. Usually, nursing assistants may not trim the resident's toenails and should never trim fingernails or toenails for diabetic residents. Observing the condition of nails and reporting to the nurse when care is needed is very important.

GUIDELINES FOR NAIL CARE

- Soak the hands or feet in warm water 105°F (40.5°C).
- Use an orange stick to clean under the nails.
- Dry the hands or feet thoroughly before trimming the nails.
- Use clippers to trim the nails.
- File rough nail edges with an emery board.

- Apply lotion to the hands or feet, and massage well.
- Report observations to the charge nurse.

An attractive hairstyle, makeup, and manicured, polished nails can change a poor self-image into one of beauty. Male residents also require nail cleaning and trimming. Remember that appearance is important to both men and women.

Shaving the Resident

Many men shave daily. This is usually done in the morning or at bath time. Residents should be encouraged to shave themselves if possible. Shaving affects the self-image of many male residents in the same way that makeup improves the female's self-image. The male resident has a right to make decisions concerning shaving and to choose the shape and length of a beard, moustache, or side burns. Some female residents may wish to shave their legs and underarms. Female residents may also choose to remove facial hair. Personal electric razors, brought from home, or safety razors may be used for shaving. Safety rules for electrical equipment should be followed.

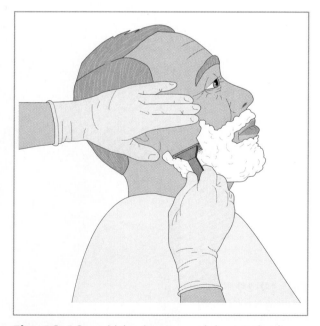

Fig. 19-18 Hold the skin taut, and shave in the direction that the hair grows.

Before shaving with a safety razor, the beard must be softened by applying a warm damp washcloth for a few minutes. Soap and water or shaving cream is then applied.

GUIDELINES FOR SHAVING THE RESIDENT

- Wear gloves and follow universal precautions.
- Place a towel across the resident's chest.
- Soften the beard with warm water before shaving.
- Dentures in the mouth make shaving easier.
- Hold the skin taut with the fingers of one hand while shaving away from your fingers in the direction the hair grows (see Fig. 19-18 located on page 285).
- Rinse the razor after each stroke.

Dressing the Resident

Assisting the Resident to Dress. In the long-term care facility, residents usually are able to get out of bed, so they are dressed in street clothes. Clothing is part of an individual's identity. The choice of clothing a person wears reflects and affects mood and self-esteem. Can you recall days that you chose particular colors or types of clothing because of the way you felt? Clothing preferences are also influenced by culture, society, body image, comfort, climate, and age. A person's choice of dress is very personal and continues to be important throughout life.

Allowing and encouraging the resident to choose the clothing to be worn stimulates thinking and supports independence. Making choices returns control to the resident. Choosing from more than one or two pieces of clothing may be overwhelming to some residents. Others may choose what they would like to wear by considering the entire wardrobe. If it is necessary for you to choose the clothing that will be worn, be sure to pick color-coordinated, well-fitting clothes that are appropriate for the weather and activities of the day. Offer sweaters or jackets even though it may seem warm to you. The elderly are more sensitive to temperature changes.

After the resident has decided what to wear, organize the undergarments and outer clothing within reach. The clothing should be placed in the order in which it will be

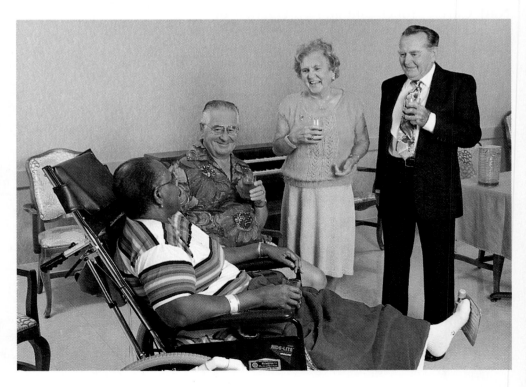

Fig. 19-19
Clothing is a personal choice that reflects a person's mood and personality.

put on. The resident should be sitting on the side of the bed or in a chair. Adaptive equipment, if needed, should be in reach.

Do not rush the resident. Relearning to dress oneself can be time consuming. Have you ever tried to dress yourself with one hand? Think of the effect that dizziness or pain would have upon you. Praise the resident's small accomplishments as well as the major ones and emphasize how nice the resident looks. Help the resident to regain a positive self-image.

Dressing the Resident. Some residents may be unable to dress and undress themselves. If the resident is dependent upon you, it is easier and safer to change the clothing while the resident is lying in bed.

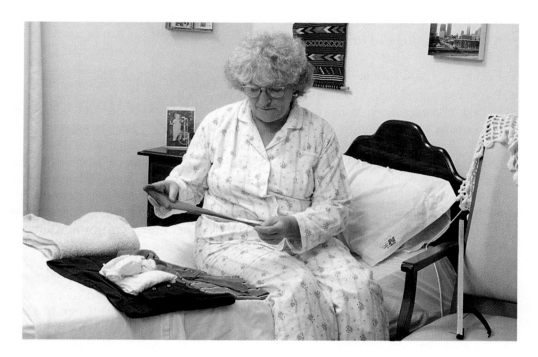

Fig. 19-20
The resident may dress herself if clothing is organized within her reach.

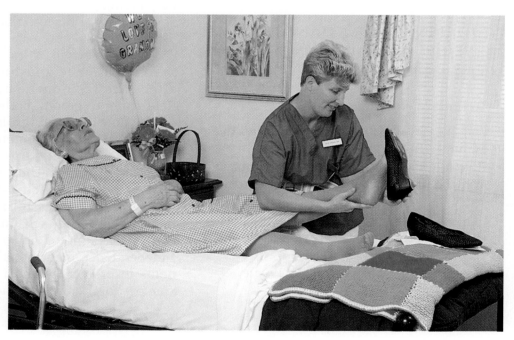

Fig. 19-21
It is easier to put on the resident's shoes while she is in bed.

GUIDELINES FOR CHANGING CLOTHES

- Allow choices whenever possible.
- Provide privacy.
- Remove clothing from unaffected limbs first.
- Place clothing on the affected limbs first.
- Support weak or paralyzed limbs.
- Gather sleeves and pant legs before inserting arms or legs.
- Assist the resident to turn from side to side as needed.
- Residents should wear undergarments.
- Put socks and shoes on while the resident is in bed. (Protect linen from shoes with a paper towel under them.)

Dressing the Resident with an IV. Some residents may be receiving fluids by intravenous. **Intravenous (IV)** is a needle into the vein. The presence of an IV requires special assistance in dressing and undressing. Common locations for an IV are the arm, wrist, or hand. Care must be taken to prevent tension and pressure on the tubing or needle. Allow for slack in the tubing when moving the resident. Clothing should be loose and short sleeved so the IV site is visible for frequent observation.

GUIDELINES FOR CHANGING CLOTHES OF A RESIDENT WITH AN IV

To remove clothing,

- Remove clothing from the arm without the IV, first.
- Carefully slide the sleeve down the arm, over the site of the IV, and then off of the arm.
- Remove the IV bag or bottle from the pole and slide it through the sleeve (see Fig. 19-22A).
- Do not lower the bag below the IV site.
- Return the bag to the pole.

To place the clean clothing on the resident,

- Gather the sleeve to be placed on the arm with the IV.
- Remove the bag from the pole and slip it through the sleeve as if the bottle was the resident's hand.
- Slide the sleeve over the tubing, hand, arm, and IV site and onto the shoulder (see Fig. 19-22B).
- Ask the nurse to check the IV as soon as you have finished dressing the resident.

Restorative Personal Care and Dressing

A restorative approach must be taken in all personal care, bathing, grooming, and dressing. Always encourage the resident to do as much as possible. Be sure that you have arranged equipment, supplies, and personal items so they will be within easy reach of the resident.

The nurse and occupational therapist will establish a plan of care to assist the resident with ADLs and personal care. You will need to be familiar with the plan for your resident and follow it consistently. The plan of care may include the use of adaptive equipment. Some adaptive devices that are designed for use in personal care can be seen in Fig. 19-23 located on page 290.

Your patience and understanding can affect the resident's success or failure. Relearning to groom, bathe, or dress oneself can be time consuming and frustrating. Your praise and encouragement will relieve the resident's anxiety and frustration.

Being able to bathe, groom, and dress oneself is vital to self-esteem. Each small effort that is successful increases the resident's confidence, self-image, and sense of control over his or her own body and life. Independence in personal care allows residents to protect the most personal and private part of themselves, their own bodies.

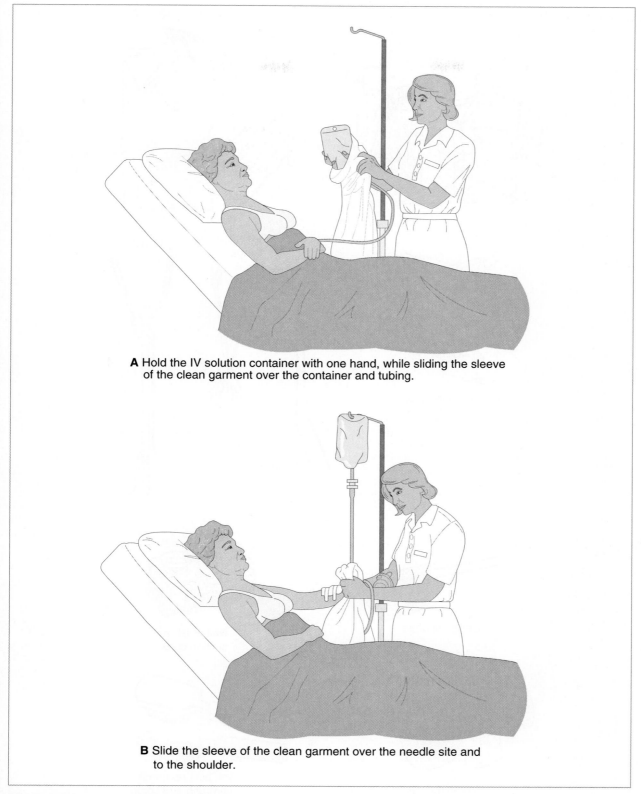

A Hold the IV solution container with one hand, while sliding the sleeve of the clean garment over the container and tubing.

B Slide the sleeve of the clean garment over the needle site and to the shoulder.

Fig. 19-22 Dressing the resident with an IV.

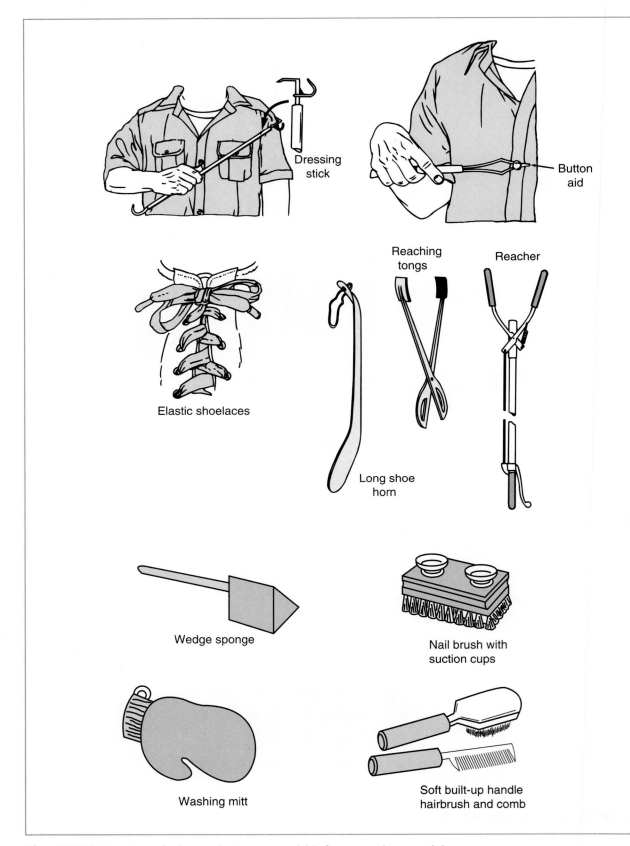

Fig. 19-23 A variety of adaptive devices are available for personal care and dressing.

Conclusion

Remember these important points:

1. Attending to personal care helps to improve self-esteem and maintain health.

2. Residents have the right to make choices about personal care.

3. H.S. care helps the resident to relax and sleep well.

4. N.G. tubes, oxygen, illness, and some medications increase the need for more frequent mouth care.

5. Steps must be taken to protect dentures from breaking.

6. Bath time is an excellent time for thorough observation of the skin, movement and mental, emotional, and speech changes.

7. Bathing is a very nurturing process that results in an improved sense of well-being.

8. Never leave a resident unattended in the tub or shower.

9. Always wash from the cleanest to the dirtiest area.

10. Perineal care should be provided immediately after urinary or fecal incontinence.

11. During the bath all skin creases, folds, and pressure areas should be observed carefully.

12. Protect the resident's privacy during bathing by uncovering only the part of the body that is being bathed.

13. Backrubs stimulate circulation and relax muscles.

14. Water temperature should be set before the resident enters the tub or shower.

15. Remove clothing from the unaffected limb first. Place it on the affected limb first.

16. Clothing is part of an individual's identity and reflects personality and self-esteem.

17. Regaining independence in personal care improves the resident's confidence, self-image, and sense of control over his or her life.

Discussion Questions

1. Why is it important to do early A.M. care before breakfast?

2. What are some precautions to follow when you are performing denture care?

3. Why is bath time the best time for a thorough observation of the resident's condition? What kind of observations should you make?

4. What must you do if the resident is incontinent of urine when you are part way through the bath?

5. How is peri-care different on an uncircumcised male than on a male resident who is circumcised?

6. What would you do if a resident wanted to select her own clothes, but was unable to reach a decision?

Application Exercises

1. The instructor will have the students divide into two groups. One group will play the role of residents, and the other will assume the role of nursing assistants. Each "resident" will pretend to have an affected arm. Each "nursing assistant" will assist a "resident" to put on and remove a jacket or other piece of clothing. The "nursing assistants" will share their observations and experience with the class. The "residents" will share their feelings about needing assistance.

2. The students will massage each others back. After completing the backrubs, students will discuss their experiences of both, giving and receiving.

Measuring Vital Signs

OBJECTIVES

Upon completing this chapter, you will be able to do the following:

1. List five factors that affect vital signs.

2. Identify the normal range of body temperature.

3. List four guidelines for reading a glass thermometer.

4. Record vital signs accurately.

5. List five guidelines for counting the radial pulse.

6. List five guidelines for counting respirations.

7. Explain the meaning of systolic and diastolic pressure.

8. List six guidelines for measuring a blood pressure.

9. Perform the procedures described in this chapter.

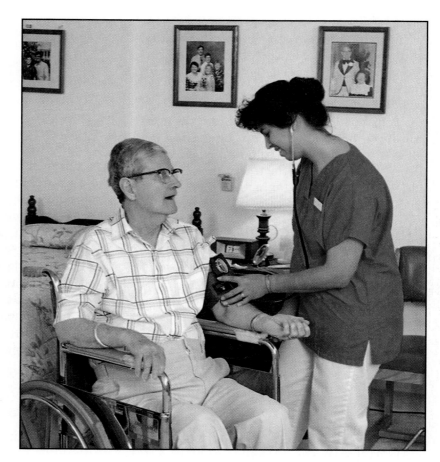

VOCABULARY

The following words or terms will help you to understand this chapter:

Vital signs	Respirations	Hypotension
Body temperature	Dyspnea	Systolic pressure
Pulse	Blood pressure (BP)	Diastolic pressure
Apical pulse	Hypertension	Sphygmomanometer
Stethoscope		

The temperature, pulse, respirations, and blood pressure are **vital signs**. These are measurements of body functions (heart, breathing, and temperature regulation which are vital to life. Changes in any of these may indicate illness or a life-threatening condition. Since the early days of medicine, physicians have measured vital signs to evaluate a person's condition.

Vital signs are taken when a resident is admitted to a health care facility. They are also measured at regular intervals (as ordered by the doctor, or as required by facility policy) and anytime there is an unusual occurrence or suspected change in the resident's condition. For example, vital signs should be taken if a resident falls or complains of chest pain. The progress of treatment may be determined by these measurements.

The Importance of Accuracy

A person's vital signs may normally vary slightly. Factors that may affect vital signs include

- Illness
- Emotions
- Exercise and activity
- Age
- Weather
- Caffeine
- Medications

Accuracy in the measurement of vital signs is extremely important to the well-being of the resident. If they vary from the normal range report it immediately to the charge nurse. If you are unsure of the measurement you have taken, tell the nurse. All vital signs are recorded according to facility policy. Respond to resident and visitor questions about vital signs measurements, according to the policy of your facility.

Measuring Body Temperature

A thermometer is used to measure **body temperature** (the amount of heat in the body). Body heat is produced when food is used for energy. Heat is lost from the body through breath, urine, feces, and the skin. The same factors affect body temperature that affect all other vital signs. Body temperature normally remains fairly constant, although it is usually slightly lower in the morning and slightly higher in the evening.

The normal body temperature is determined by the site of measurement. Temperatures are commonly measured in the rectum, mouth, and axilla (underarm). The mouth is most often used for measurement, and the axilla is least often used because it is considered to be the least accurate. Fahrenheit and centigrade are two types of temperature measurement systems. Celsius is the same as centigrade. Normal adult temperature ranges for both systems are

Axillary	96.6° to 98.6°F (36° to 37°C)
Oral	97.6° to 99.6°F (36.5° to 37.5°C)
Rectal	98.6° to 100.6°F (37° to 38.1°C)

Temperatures outside of the normal range should be reported to the nurse.

There are many types of thermometers available, including glass and electronic thermometers, disposable oral thermometers, temperature-sensitive tape, and ear thermometers (see Fig. 20-1).

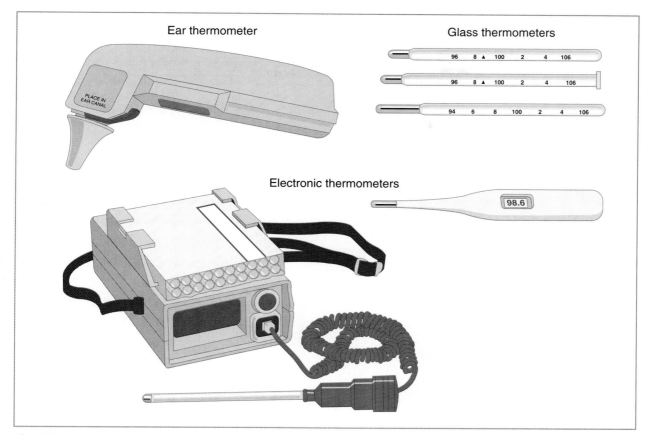

Fig. 20-1 Types of thermometers.

Glass Thermometers. The glass thermometer is a small glass tube, that is marked with measurements and contains mercury in a bulb at one end. Heat expands the mercury causing it to rise in the tube. Oral, axillary, and rectal thermometers may be identified by shape and color markings (see Fig. 20-2). These thermometers must never be switched for use. Oral and axillary thermometers usually have slender bulbs of mercury and may be color coded with blue. Rectal thermometers have round or stubby bulbs of mercury and may be color coded with red. It may be helpful to associate the three "R's" (round, red, and rectal).

Reading a Glass Thermometer. The glass thermometer may be marked with a Fahrenheit or centigrade scale (see Fig. 20-3). On both scales, the long lines represent one degree of temperature. The Fahrenheit scale usually extends from 94° to 108° F and the centigrade scale from 34° to 42° C. The short lines are read differently for the two types of measurement scales. On a thermometer with a Fahrenheit scale, each short line represents

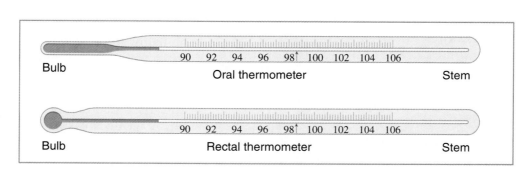

Fig. 20-2
Glass oral and rectal thermometers with Fahrenheit scales.

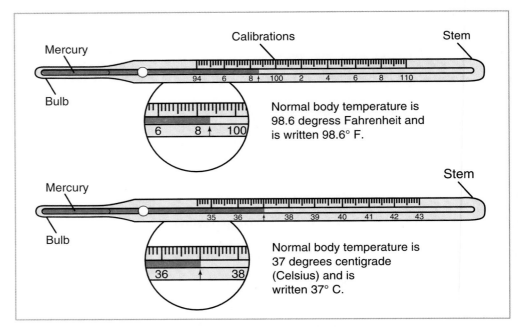

Fig. 20-3
Thermometers may be calibrated with a Fahrenheit or centigrade scale.

two-tenths (0.2) of a degree. The short lines of the centigrade thermometer represent one-tenth (0.1) of a degree (see Fig. 20-3).

GUIDELINES FOR READING A GLASS THERMOMETER

- Hold the thermometer by the stem (the end opposite the mercury bulb) in a horizontal position at eye level (see Fig. 20-4).
- Light should shine on the thermometer from behind you.
- Holding the thermometer with your thumb and index finger, rotate it slowly until you can see both the numbers and lines (see Fig. 20-4).
- Read the temperature to the nearest degree (long line) and then to the nearest tenth of a degree (short line).
- Record the temperature and report any abnormality immediately.

Recording Temperatures. It is important that you record temperatures accurately. Temperatures are usually recorded in decimals; for example, an oral temperature might be recorded 98.2°F, 99.4°F, or 100.6°F. It is usually not necessary to designate Fahrenheit or centigrade. Most facilities use only one scale.

Care and Use of a Glass Thermometer. Glass thermometers must be shaken down

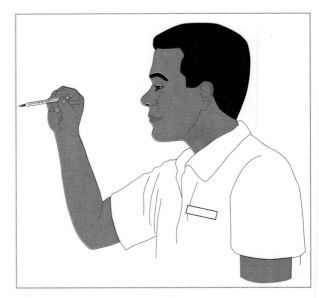

Fig. 20-4 Reading a glass thermometer.

before and after use. This is done by holding the thermometer stem firmly with your thumb and index finger, while snapping your wrist (see Fig. 20-5). The mercury will be below 96°F when it is shaken sufficiently. After the glass thermometer is checked for chips or breaks, a plastic shield or cover may be placed over it. These are removed and discarded before reading the thermometer. A tissue must be used to wipe off saliva or lubricant from stem to bulb before reading the thermometer.

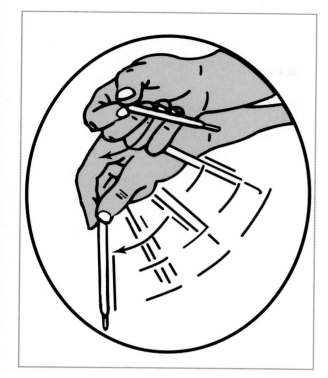

Fig. 20-5 Use a snapping action of the wrist to shake down a glass thermometer.

Oral and rectal glass thermometers are soaked in disinfectant solution and stored in separate containers. They may be washed in cool, soapy water before placing them in disinfectant. Follow the procedure of your facility for cleansing and storing thermometers. Always rinse the thermometer with cool water when removing it from the disinfectant solution.

Taking an Oral Temperature. There are some residents for whom you may not take an oral temperature. These include residents who

- Have tubes in the nose or mouth
- Are receiving oxygen
- Are unconscious
- Breath through the mouth
- Have seizures
- Are confused or disoriented
- Have had recent surgery of the mouth, nose or face

The thermometer must be placed on the unaffected side of the mouth for residents who are paralyzed on one side (hemiplegics).

The normal oral temperature is 98.6°F or 37°C. Temperatures are measured most often by the oral method. Drinking, eating, smoking, or chewing gum can change the oral temperature. It is necessary to wait 15 minutes to take the temperature, after the resident has participated in any of these activities. The resident should be sitting or lying down when the temperature is being taken. Stay with the resident until the procedure is completed.

Equipment and Supplies. Equipment needed for taking an oral temperature includes a pen, paper, oral glass thermometer with cover and tissues, or an electric thermometer, oral probe, and probe cover. This procedure is located on page 298.

Taking a Rectal Temperature. A rectal temperature is taken when the nurse instructs you to do so. The normal rectal temperature is 99.6°F or 37.5°C. This is the most accurate method of temperature measurement. A rectal temperature cannot be taken if there has been rectal injury or surgery.

Lubricant must be applied to the thermometer cover or probe tip before inserting it into the rectum. Lubrication promotes comfort and prevents injury. The tip is lubricated by dipping it into a small amount of water-soluble lubricant that has been placed on a tissue.

The resident must be lying down while a rectal temperature is being measured. It is very important to hold the thermometer in place until measurement is complete. This prevents the thermometer from being drawn into the rectum, and it also assures that the resident will not turn onto the thermometer. Glass thermometers are fragile. Injury could result from a broken thermometer. The procedure for taking a rectal temperature is located on page 299.

Equipment and Supplies. Equipment needed for taking a rectal temperature includes a pen, paper, tissue, water-soluble lubricant, gloves, and a glass rectal thermometer with a plastic cover, or an electronic thermometer with a rectal probe and probe cover.

PROCEDURE

Taking an Oral Temperature Using a Glass or Electronic Thermometer

Before any procedure you must always follow the five basic steps: wash your hands, collect the equipment, identify the resident, explain the procedure, and protect privacy.

Follow universal precautions and wear gloves when appropriate.

1. After rinsing and drying the glass thermometer, check it for cracks, shake it down, and place a cover on it.

or

   Insert the electronic probe into the probe cover (see Fig. 20-6A).

2. Place the bulb or probe under the resident's tongue, on one side of the mouth.
3. Ask the resident to lower the tongue, and close the lips around the thermometer.
4. Leave the glass thermometer in place three to five minutes.

or

   Wait for the electronic thermometer to signal.

5. Remove the cover from the glass thermometer, or wipe it from stem to bulb with a tissue, and read the temperature.

or

   Read the temperature on the digital display; then press the eject button to discard the cover, and return the probe to its holder (see Figs. 20-6B and 20-6C).

6. Record the resident's name and temperature.
7. Assure the resident's comfort and safety.
8. Shake down and prepare the glass thermometer for disinfection and storage, according to facility policy.

or

   Return the electronic thermometer to the charging unit.

9. Wash your hands.
10. Report any abnormal temperature immediately to the charge nurse, and record the measurement in the chart.

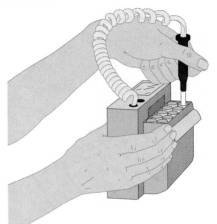

A Insert the probe into a probe cover.

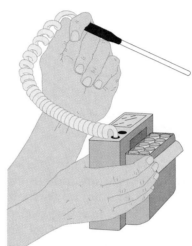

B After measuring the temperature, press to eject the probe cover.

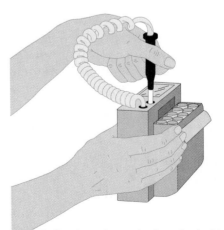

C Replace the probe into the holder.

Fig. 20-6
Using the electronic thermometer.

PROCEDURE

Taking a Rectal Temperature Using a Glass or Electronic Thermometer

Before any procedure you must always follow the five basic steps: wash your hands, collect the equipment, identify the resident, explain the procedure, and protect privacy.

Follow universal precautions and wear gloves when appropriate.

1. After rinsing and drying the glass rectal thermometer, check it for damage, shake it down, and place a cover on it.

or

   Insert the rectal probe of the electronic thermometer into a probe cover.

2. Flatten the bed and place the resident into a Sims' position, if possible.
3. Put on disposable gloves.
4. Lubricate the tip of the thermometer cover or probe with a small amount of lubricant that has been placed on a tissue.
5. Fold the top linens back to expose the rectal area.
6. Raise the upper buttock with one hand so you can see the anus.
7. Gently insert the tip of the glass thermometer, one inch, into the rectum (see Fig. 20-7).

or

Gently insert the tip of the electronic probe, one-half inch, into the rectum.

8. Hold the glass thermometer for three to five minutes before removing it.

or

Hold the electronic probe in place until the thermometer signals.

9. Remove the cover from the glass thermometer or wipe it from stem to bulb with a tissue, and read the temperature.

or

Read the temperature on the digital display of the electronic thermometer; then press the eject button to dispose of the probe cover. Return the probe to its holder.

10. Wipe the anal area with toilet tissue to remove excess lubricant and feces.
11. Discard the tissue into the toilet.
12. Remove the gloves and wash your hands.
13. Record the resident's name and temperature.
14. Assure the resident's comfort and safety.
15. Prepare the glass thermometer for disinfection and storage, according to the facility policy.

or

Return the electronic thermometer to the charging unit.

16. Wash your hands.
17. Report any abnormal temperature immediately to the charge nurse and record the temperature in the chart. Indicate that a rectal temperature was taken by recording an "R."

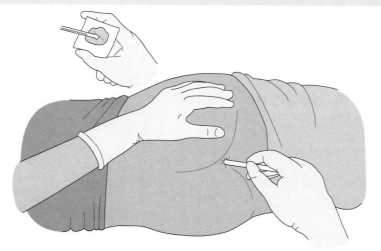

Fig. 20-7 Insert the tip of the rectal thermometer one inch into the rectum.

Taking an Axillary Temperature. An axillary temperature is taken only when no other temperature measurement can be used. Axillary temperatures are the least accurate. The normal axillary temperature is 97.6°F (36.5°C). The glass thermometer must be held in place for ten minutes. The resident must be sitting or lying down during the measurement of an axillary temperature. An oral glass thermometer or oral probe for the electronic thermometer is used to measure the axillary temperature. Stay with the resident during the procedure and hold the thermometer, if necessary. The resident should be sitting or lying down for this procedure. The procedure is located on page 301.

Equipment and Supplies. Equipment needed for taking an axillary temperature includes a pen, paper, oral glass thermometer with cover, and tissue or an electronic thermometer with an oral probe and probe cover.

The Pulse

The most basic indicator of heart function is the pulse. The **pulse** is the heartbeat. Each pulse beat is a wave of blood passing through the artery. Each time the heart contracts, a wave of blood is forced into circulation. The pulse can be counted at several points on the body by pressing an artery against a bone, near the surface of the skin (see Fig. 20-8).

The adult normal pulse range is between 60 and 100 beats per minute. Any pulse above or below the range should be reported to the charge nurse immediately. The factors that affect all other vital signs also affect the pulse.

When the rate of the pulse is counted, the rhythm (regularity) and force (strength) should also be noted. An irregular pattern or rhythm should be reported to the nurse. If the pulse force is weak or thready (changeable), this should also be reported.

Counting the Radial Pulse. The radial pulse is the pulse that you will usually count. This pulse is located on the inner aspect of the wrist, at the base of the thumb (see Fig. 20-8). With the resident sitting or lying down, place the first three fingers against the radial artery, until you have located the pulse.

GUIDELINES FOR COUNTING THE RADIAL PULSE

- Do not use your thumb to count the pulse because you will feel your own pulse.
- Count the pulse for 30 seconds, and multiply that number by two, to determine the pulse rate
- The pulse rate is the number of heartbeats per minute.
- An irregular pulse must be counted for one full minute, in order to be accurate.
- Record the pulse for each resident as soon as you have counted it.
- Report any unusual observations immediately to the charge nurse.
- If you are asked about the pulse rate by the resident or visitors, respond according to facility policy.

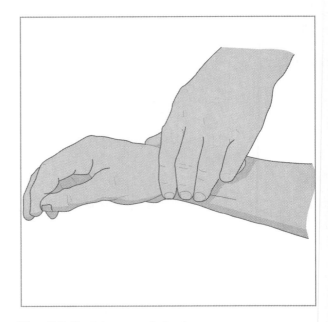

Fig. 20-8 Taking a radial pulse.

PROCEDURE

Procedure for Taking an Axillary Temperature Using a Glass or Electronic Thermometer

Before any procedure you must always follow the five basic steps: wash your hands, collect the equipment, identify the resident, explain the procedure, and protect privacy.

Follow universal precautions and wear gloves when appropriate.

1. After rinsing and drying the glass thermometer, check it for cracks, shake it down, and place a cover on it.

or

Insert the electronic probe into the probe cover.

2. Expose the axilla.
3. Place the bulb of the glass thermometer, or the probe tip of the electronic thermometer, into the center of the axilla. Place the resident's arm over the chest (see Fig. 20-9).
4. Hold the glass thermometer in place for ten minutes before removing it from the axilla.

or

Hold the electronic thermometer probe in place until the thermometer signals that the measurement is complete.

5. Remove the plastic cover from the glass thermometer, or wipe it from stem to bulb with a tissue and read the temperature.

or

Read the temperature on the digital display of the electronic thermometer and press the eject button to discard the probe cover. Return the probe to its holder.

6. Record the resident's name and temperature.
7. Assure the resident's comfort and safety.
8. Shake down and prepare the glass thermometer for disinfection and storage, according to facility policy.

or

Return the electronic thermometer to the charging unit.

9. Wash your hands.
10. Report any abnormal temperature to the charge nurse immediately, and record the temperature in the chart. Record an "A" to indicate an axillary temperature.

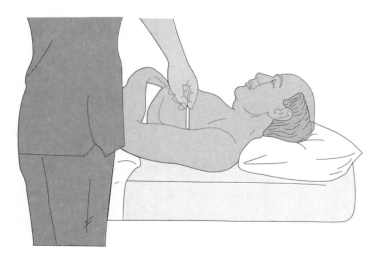

Fig. 20-9 Taking an axillary temperature.

The Apical and Apical-Radial Pulses.
The doctor may order that pulses be taken at sites other than the radial pulse. In most long-term care facilities these procedures are done by a licensed nurse. The **apical pulse** is taken by listening to the heartbeat over the apex of the heart. This position is located two to three inches to the left of the sternum (breast bone) and slightly below the nipple (see Fig. 20-10).

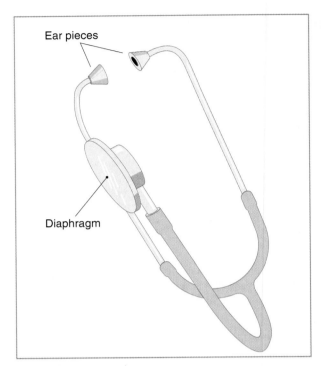

Fig. 20-11 A stethoscope.

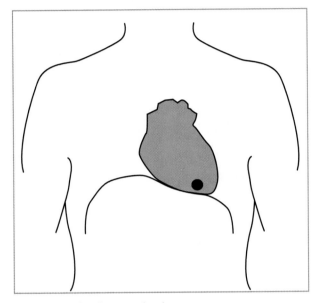

Fig. 20-10 The apical pulse site.

To hear the apical pulse, a stethoscope must be used. A **stethoscope** is an instrument used for listening to body sounds (see Fig. 20-11). The earpieces of the stethoscope should be turned slightly forward to fit snugly into the ear. The diaphragm (flat part) is placed against the chest over the apex of the heart. The earpieces and diaphragm should be cleaned with alcohol before and after use. The heartbeat will be heard as two sounds ("lub-dub"). Only one of these sounds (the "lub") is counted for each pulse beat. The apical pulse is counted for a full minute. It is recorded with an "AP" after the measurement (76 AP). "AP" indicates that the recorded pulse was an apical pulse.

The apical-radial pulse procedure is performed by two individuals. One person counts the apical pulse, while the other counts the radial pulse, during the same period of time. The pulse is taken for one full minute, using one watch. Only one person watches the time (see Fig. 20-12). If heart contractions are not strong enough to create pulses in the radial artery, the radial count will be less than the apical count. In recording, indicate that an apical-radial pulse was taken with an "A-R." The apical pulse is recorded before the radial.

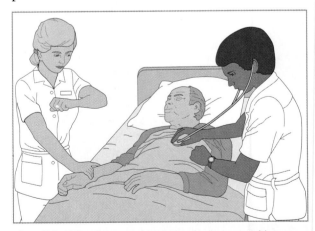

Fig. 20-12 The apical-radial pulse is counted by two people.

Respirations

Counting **respirations** (breathing) is another routine vital sign measurement. Each respiration that is counted includes one inhalation (the chest rises) and one exhalation (the chest falls). The adult normal range is 12 to 20 respirations per minute. This rate is influenced by the factors that affect all other vital signs. While counting the rate of respirations, you should also note the depth and rhythm of breathing. **Dyspnea** (difficult, labored, or painful breathing) should be reported immediately. Normal breathing is regular, comfortable, effortless, and quiet. Any breathing sounds such as wheezes, coughs, gurgles, or rattles should also be reported.

Counting Respirations. The resident should not be aware that respirations are being counted because the breathing pattern may unintentionally change. Breathing can be voluntarily or involuntarily changed by conscious thought. What happens when you think about your breathing? Do you find that you suddenly draw a deep breath, or breathe differently? This is an involuntary change due to conscious awareness. To avoid the resident's awareness, you may begin counting respirations immediately following the pulse. Continue to hold the wrist, as if continuing to count the pulse. After making a mental note of the pulse, begin to count respirations. The resident will think that you are still counting the pulse (see Fig. 20-13).

GUIDELINES FOR COUNTING RESPIRATIONS

- Watch the chest rise and fall.
- Count one each time the chest rises (each rise of the chest counts as one respiration).
- Count the respirations for 30 seconds, and multiply the number by two, to determine the rate of respirations.
- The rate is the number of respirations per minute.

- If the respirations are irregular, count for one full minute.
- Record the respirations for each resident as you finish counting them.
- Report any unusual findings to the charge nurse.
- If you are asked about the rate of respirations by the resident or visitors, respond according to facility policy.

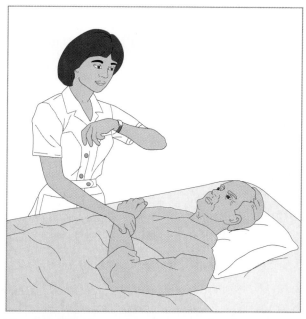

Fig. 20-13 The resident must not realize that you are counting respirations.

Blood Pressure

Blood pressure (BP) is the force of blood against the artery walls, as it is circulated by the heart. Blood pressure is affected by internal factors. These include the strength of the heart contractions, the amount of blood flowing, and the resistance or elasticity of the blood vessels. As with all other vital signs, there are many factors that affect blood pressure. Blood pressure that is abnormally high is called **hypertension** ("hyper"—above normal or high; "tension"—pressure). **Hypotension** ("hypo"—low or below normal; "tension"—pressure) is abnormally low blood pressure.

Systolic and Diastolic Pressures. Two pressures are measured while taking the blood pressure. The higher pressure is the **systolic pressure**, which measures the pressure of the blood flowing during the heart's contraction (systole). The **diastolic pressure**, the lower measurement, is the pressure of the blood flowing during the heart's relaxation (diastole). The blood pressure is recorded as a fraction, with the systolic pressure as the top number and the diastolic as the bottom number (120/70). Blood pressures are measured in millimeters (mm) of mercury (Hg).

The adult normal systolic pressure range is 100–140. The adult diastolic pressure normally ranges from 60–90. Therefore, a systolic measurement below 100 or above 140 and a diastolic measurement below 60 or above 90 should be reported to the charge nurse immediately (see Fig. 20-14).

```
SYSTOLIC      100    —    140

DIASTOLIC      60    —     90
```

Fig. 20-14 Normal ranges for adult blood pressures.

Using Blood Pressure Equipment. Measuring the blood pressure requires the use of a stethoscope, a sphygmomanometer, and alcohol wipes. The stethoscope is used to listen to pulse sounds (this instrument, and its care, were discussed earlier). The alcohol wipes are used to clean the earpieces and the diaphragm of the stethoscope, before and after use.

The blood pressure cuff is called a **sphygmomanometer**. The four main parts of the sphygmomanometer are the cuff, bulb, valve, and measuring device (manometer or gauge). Many manometers are designed with a column of mercury that is calibrated (marked). These may be attached to a stand on wheels, folded into a case, or fastened to a wall. Another type, aneroid manometers, uses a calibrated circular dial and a pointer. These are smaller and are more easily transported.

The cuff is wrapped around the arm and fastened. The cuff is a bladder, which is inflated with air, to apply pressure on the artery. When the valve is closed (clockwise), the bulb can be pumped by hand, to inflate the cuff. The valve is then turned counterclockwise, to open it and deflate the cuff, by allowing air to escape. The valve and bulb are connected to the bladder and cuff by a tube. A tube also connects the bladder to the manometer, which indicates the pressure (see Fig. 20-15).

Blood pressure cuffs are available in a variety of sizes. The cuff must fit the resident's arm snugly, and must stay fastened when inflated. If the resident is very thin, so that the cuff slides, or if a larger size is needed, tell the nurse.

A sphygmomanometer is fragile, expensive equipment, so handle it with care. Do not drop it. Accuracy of this instrument is very important. If you feel that the instrument is not functioning properly, do not use it. Follow your facility policy regarding broken equipment.

Reading the Manometer (Gauge). Manometers are calibrated with long lines, which represent 10 mm Hg (millimeters of mercury), and short lines, which represent 2 mm Hg. When reading the manometer, you will see that the pressure is dropping. Read the systolic (upper) pressure first and the diastolic (lower) pressure last. Practice reading the calibrations so that you will be able to take a blood pressure accurately (see Fig. 20-16).

Measuring a Blood Pressure. After you have learned how to read the manometer, you will be ready to take a blood pressure. This is a complicated procedure, because you must read the gauge, listen for pulse sounds, and use your hands. Be patient with yourself and practice, so that you will be accurate.

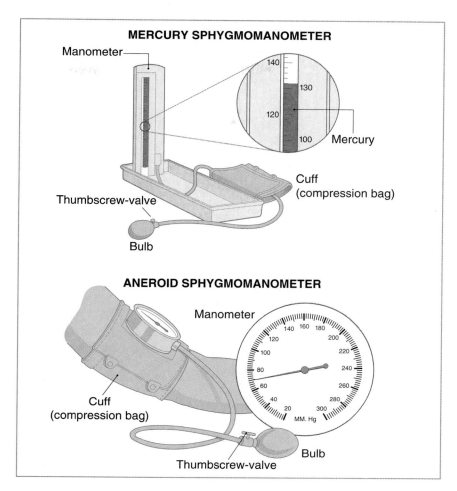

Fig. 20-15
A sphygmomanometer is the blood pressure instrument.

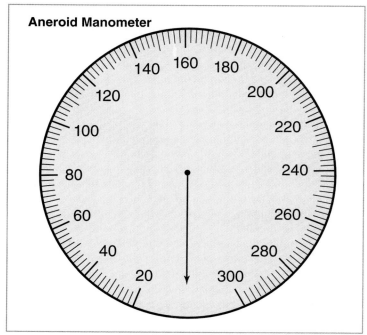

Fig. 20-16 Accuracy of measurement depends on reading the gauge correctly.

Taking the Blood Pressure

Before any procedure you must always follow the five basic steps: wash your hands, collect the equipment, identify the resident, explain the procedure, and protect privacy.

Follow universal precautions and wear gloves when appropriate.

1. Clean the stethoscope earpieces and diaphragm with alcohol wipes.
2. Have the resident sitting or lying down with the arm extended at heart level. The palm of the hand should be turned up.
3. Remove clothing over the area of the arm where the cuff will be placed.
4. With the valve open, squeeze the cuff to be sure it is completely deflated.
5. Wrap the cuff comfortably around the arm one inch above the elbow, with the arrow on the cuff pointing to the brachial pulse site.
6. The gauge should be clearly visible.
7. Place the stethoscope earpieces (turned slightly forward) snugly into your ears.
8. Locate the brachial pulse with your fingertips.
9. Place the bell or diaphragm of the stethoscope flat on the pulse site, holding it firmly in place with the index and middle fingers of one hand. The stethoscope should not touch the cuff.
10. Close the valve (clockwise) until it stops. Do not tighten it.
11. Inflate the cuff to 160 mm Hg (or 30 mm Hg above the resident's usual systolic pressure). You will no longer hear a pulse.
12. With your thumb and index finger, open the valve slightly (counterclockwise). Allow the air to escape slowly, while listening for a pulse sound. (If you hear it immediately, you will have to begin again after deflating the cuff for one minute, and reinflating it to 30 mm Hg higher than the first time.)
13. Remember the reading at which you hear the first clear pulse sound. This is the systolic pressure.
14. Continue listening for a change or muffling of the pulse sound. The reading at the point of change is the diastolic pressure. (If no change of pulse sound is detectable, the point at which the sound disappears is the diastolic pressure.) Remember this reading.
15. Open the valve to deflate the cuff completely and remove it from the resident's arm.
16. Record your reading.
17. Wipe the stethoscope earpieces and diaphragm with alcohol.
18. Assure the resident's comfort and safety.
19. Return the stethoscope and sphygmomanometer to storage.
21. Wash your hands.
21. Report any abnormality to the charge nurse and record the measurement on the chart.

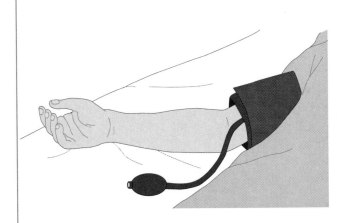
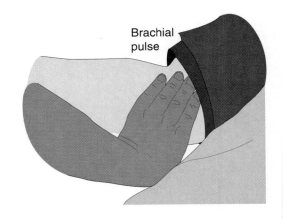

Brachial pulse

Figure 20-17 Taking the blood pressure.

GUIDELINES FOR MEASURING A BLOOD PRESSURE

- Do not take a blood pressure on an arm that is paralyzed, or has a wound, cast, or IV.
- Place the cuff on bare skin, not over clothing.
- The entire surface of the stethoscope diaphragm should be held firmly and flat against the bend of the elbow, over the brachial artery.
- Repeating the procedure will change the pressure. If you are not sure of the reading, do not reinflate the cuff until you have completely deflated it for one minute.
- Deflate the cuff slowly so that you can accurately read the pressure.
- Inflate the cuff to 160 mm Hg, or inflate the cuff to 30 mm Hg above the resident's usual systolic pressure.
- If you are not sure of a resident's pressure after two attempts, tell the nurse.
- Deflate the cuff immediately, when the reading is complete. The needle will be on zero when all the air is out of the cuff.
- If you are asked about the blood pressure reading by the resident or visitors, respond according to facility policy.

Equipment and Supplies. Equipment and supplies needed for taking a blood pressure include a pen and paper, a stethoscope, a sphygmomanometer, and alcohol wipes.

5. Do not use your thumb when taking a pulse, or you will count your own pulse as well.

6. Observe the depth and rhythm, as well as the respiratory rate.

7. The respiratory pattern may change if the resident is aware that you are counting respirations.

8. The blood pressure cuff must fit the resident's arm snugly and stay fastened when inflated.

9. Wrap the cuff one inch above the elbow, with the arrow pointing to the brachial pulse site.

10. The first clear sound you hear when taking a blood pressure is the systolic pressure. The last clear sound is the diastolic pressure.

11. Deflate the cuff slowly, so you can accurately read the gauge.

12. Clean the earpieces and diaphragm of the stethoscope between uses.

13. The resident should be sitting or lying down, with the arm resting at heart level, while a blood pressure is being taken.

14. If you are unsure of the vital signs that you have taken, notify the nurse.

15. Follow facility policy regarding information that you may give the resident or family about vital signs.

16. Report abnormalities to the nurse immediately.

Conclusion

Remember these important points:

1. The temperature, pulse, respirations and blood pressure are measurements of body functions that are vital to life.

2. Wait 15 minutes before taking an oral temperature if the resident has been eating, drinking, smoking, or chewing gum.

3. Lubricate the rectal thermometer and hold it in place until measurement is complete.

4. When counting the pulse, also observe the rhythm and strength.

Discussion Questions

1. How do you decide whether to take an oral, rectal or axillary temperature?

2. Why is an axillary temperature the least accurate measurement of body heat?

3. You have pumped the blood pressure cuff to 160 mm Hg. When you open the valve, you immediately hear a sound. What does that indicate, and what actions should you take?

4. Why is it important to release the valve of the sphygmomanometer slowly?

5. Why shouldn't you take a blood pressure on the arm that has an IV infusing?

Application Exercise

1. The instructor will divide the class into pairs of students who will take each other's vital signs and record them. After all are finished, the instructor will lead the class in a 10- to 15-minute exercise routine. The same pairs of students will take vital signs again.

The students will share their findings with the class, and discuss the results. The discussion will include

- the difference in vital signs in the same person, before and after exercise
- which vital signs are most affected
- individual observations

Nutrition and Dining

OBJECTIVES

Upon completing this chapter, you will be able to do the following:

1. Explain how dining meets the needs of the whole person.

2. Explain what is meant by proper nutrition.

3. Describe the digestive process.

4. List three factors that affect nutrition in the elderly.

5. Identify two residents' rights related to nutrition.

6. Identify adaptive equipment and methods to assist the resident with dining.

7. Describe the clock method used in assisting the visually impaired resident at mealtime.

8. List four guidelines to follow when feeding the resident who is unable to eat independently.

9. List four restorative guidelines to assist the resident to eat independently.

10. Identify two types of supplemental nutrition.

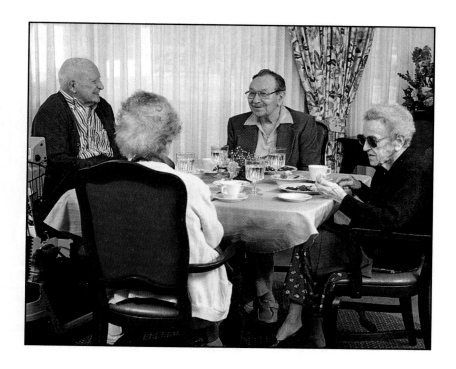

- Iron is necessary for hemoglobin in the blood, and for other body processes. The best sources of iron are meat, eggs, dry beans, whole-grain cereals, and green, leafy vegetables.

Vitamins. Vitamins that are needed by the body include vitamin A, B-complex, vitamin C, vitamin D, vitamin K, and vitamin E. Vitamins A, D, E, and K are stored by the body; the other vitamins are used and eliminated daily. A discussion of important vitamins follows.

- Vitamin A is needed for healthy skin, vision, and mucous membranes and to help fight infection. Foods containing vitamin A include yellow fruits and vegetables, milk, cheese, liver, and green, leafy vegetables.
- B-complex vitamins include B_1, B_2, B_6, and B_{12} and niacin. These vitamins are used for digestion, muscle tone, and growth and to help maintain a healthy nervous system. They also help form red blood cells. Foods that contain the B-complex vitamins include meat (especially organ meats like liver), fish, milk, eggs, cereals, bread, and green, leafy vegetables.
- Vitamin C is necessary for many metabolic functions including tissue formation, mineral absorption, and healthy skin and mucous membranes. It also helps to fight infection. Citrus fruits, tomatoes, strawberries, and many other fresh fruits and vegetables contain vitamin C.
- Vitamin D is needed by the body to build healthy bones and teeth. Foods containing vitamin D include milk, butter, eggs, and liver. Many foods, such as bread, have vitamin D added.
- Vitamin K is necessary for blood clotting. Vitamin K is found in liver, eggs, and green, leafy vegetables.

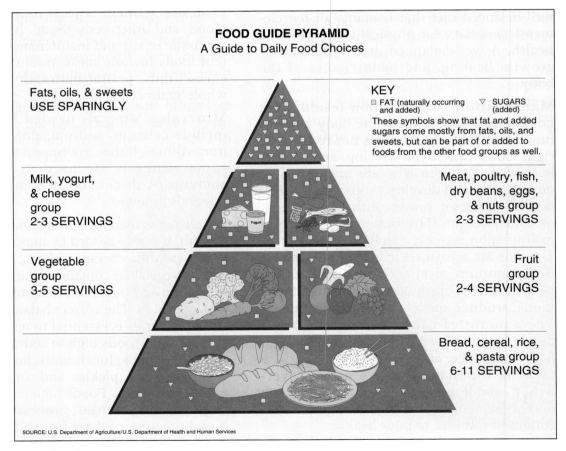

FOOD GUIDE PYRAMID
A Guide to Daily Food Choices

Fats, oils, & sweets
USE SPARINGLY

KEY
☐ FAT (naturally occurring and added)   ▽ SUGARS (added)
These symbols show that fat and added sugars come mostly from fats, oils, and sweets, but can be part of or added to foods from the other food groups as well.

Milk, yogurt, & cheese group
2-3 SERVINGS

Meat, poultry, fish, dry beans, eggs, & nuts group
2-3 SERVINGS

Vegetable group
3-5 SERVINGS

Fruit group
2-4 SERVINGS

Bread, cereal, rice, & pasta group
6-11 SERVINGS

SOURCE: U.S. Department of Agriculture/U.S. Department of Health and Human Services

Fig. 21-2 Food guide pyramid.

- Vitamin E is used for the formation of red blood cells and for healthy muscle function. Vitamin E is found in green, leafy vegetables, liver, eggs, and vegetable oils.

Although a particular food may be high in a specific nutrient, remember that no food contains only one nutrient. Spinach, for example, is a good source of calcium, potassium, and vitamins A, B, and C. It also supplies some protein, carbohydrate, and iron.

Water. The body needs water for proper nutrition. Water is as essential to life as food and oxygen. It is found in many foods and beverages. In fact, some fruits and vegetables are mostly water. The importance of water is discussed in detail in the next chapter.

Food Groups. Foods can be divided into basic groups: meats, poultry, and fish; milk and dairy products; breads and cereals; and fruits and vegetables.

All foods can be classified in one or more of these groups. A well-balanced diet contains a variety of foods from each group every day.

The Food Guide Pyramid. In 1992 the U.S. Department of Agriculture developed the food guide pyramid. Following these guidelines will help you to eat a well-balanced diet daily (see Fig. 21-2 on page 312).

Types of Diets

The doctor orders the type of diet that a resident will have. The order is given before or upon admission to the facility. Any change in the diet also requires a doctor's order.

DIET	DESCRIPTION	FOODS
Diabetic	Used to treat diabetes mellitus. Carbohydrates, fat, protein & calories are controlled.	A variety is allowed as long as the calorie & nutrient count is maintained. Candy & desserts should be avoided.
Bland	Used to treat ulcers, gallbladder & colon problems. Foods should be non-irritating & easily digested.	Restricted: Fried foods, beans, cabbage & other gas-forming foods, highly seasoned & high fiber foods, fresh fruit.
Clear Liquid	Liquids that have no residue. Used after surgery, for nausea & vomiting, for acute illness.	Water, broth, apple juice, tea, coffee, carbonated beverages & jello.
Full Liquid	All liquid foods & solids that will melt at room temperature. May be used for residents who have problems swallowing. Next diet after clear liquids.	Clear liquid, plus: milk, custard, pudding, cream soup & ice cream.
Low Sodium	Used for residents who have heart problems, hypertension or kidney disease. Restricts all salty foods & those with a high sodium content. Usually no salt is added to food. Doctor orders amount of salt allowed.	Restricted: Salt, ham, bacon, luncheon meat, hot dogs, pickles, mustard, canned soups & vegetables that are not low-sodium.
Low Cholesterol	Used for residents with heart disease, gallbladder problems, or a high cholesterol count.	Restricted: Eggs, cheese, whole milk, butter, beef & pork.
High Residue/Fiber	Used for constipation & other bowel problems. Increases peristalsis & adds bulk.	Whole grain bread, cereal, cheese, fruits & vegetables, especially green, leafy vegetables.

Fig. 21-3 Therapeutic diets.

ITEM	CALORIES	TOTAL FAT (g)	CHOLESTEROL (mg)	SODIUM (mg)
BREAKFAST				
Scrambled Eggs	140	10	399	290
Sausage	160	15	43	310
Egg McMuffin®	280	11	224	710
Sausage McMuffin® (with egg)	415	25	256	915
Hotcakes (with margarine and syrup)	410	9	8	640
Breakfast Burrito	280	17	135	580
Oat Bran Muffin (plain)	330	11	0	450
Danish (cinnamon raisin)	440	21	34	430
LUNCH/DINNER				
Cheese Pizza (2 slices, 16 in. thin crust)	376	10	19	483
Double Cheese/ Pepperoni Pizza (2 slices 16 in. thin crust)	545	25	48	1042
Big Mac®	500	26	100	890
French Fries, Large	400	22	0	200
Chicken McNuggets (6 pieces)	270	15	56	580
Personal Pan Pizza, Pepperoni	675	29	53	1335
Fried Chicken Wings (6 pieces)	376	24	148	677
Beef Burrito, with Red Sauce	493	21	57	1311
Nachos	346	18	9	399
Baked Potato, Stuffed Bacon & Cheese	520	18	20	1460
Cheeseburger	410	21	80	760
Chicken Club Sandwich	506	25	70	930
Roast Beef Sandwich	353	15	39	588
Chicken Fajita Pita	256	9	33	787
DESSERTS				
Chocolate Glazed Donut	324	21	2	383
Jelly Filled Donut	220	9	0	330
Apple Pie, 3 oz.	300	19	–*	–
Chocolate Shake, Large	472	15	45	286
Chocolate Ice Cream, 1 scoop	270	14	37	160
French Vanilla Ice Cream, 1 scoop	280	18	90	90
BREADS, CEREALS, PASTAS				
Bagel (3" diameter)	296	2.6	–*	360
English Muffin (plain)	138	1.2	–	370
Bran Muffin (plain)	104	3.9	–	179
40% Bran Flakes (1 oz)	93	0.5	0	264
Corn Flakes (1 oz)	110	0.1	0	351
Shredded Wheat (1 biscuit)	83	0.3	0	0
Oatmeal (instant, regular)	145	2.4	0	1
Spaghetti (1 cup)	155	0.6	–	1
Rice, White, Brown, or Wild (1 cup)	223	0.2	0	4
Bread Sticks (5)	96	0.8	0	175
Graham Crackers (4 squares)	110	2.6	–	190

ITEM	CALORIES	TOTAL FAT (g)	CHOLESTEROL (mg)	SODIUM (mg)
VEGETABLES				
Starchy Vegetables– Corn, Lima Bean, Peas, Potato, Yams, Winter or Acorn Squash (1/2 cup)	80	0	0	0
Other Vegetables (on average, 1/2-1 cup)	25	0.2	0	0
FRUIT				
Apple (2 3/4" diameter)	81	0.5	0	1
Banana (9")	106	0.6	0	1
Cantaloupe (1 cup, cubes)	57	0.4	0	14
Fruit Cocktail (canned in juice, 1/2 cup)	56	0.1	0	4
Grapefruit (half)	37	0.1	0	0
Kiwi (1 large)	55	0.4	0	4
Peach (2 1/2: diameter)	37	0.1	0	0
Strawberries (whole, 1 1/4 cup)	56	0.7	0	3
Raisins (2 tablespoons)	62	0.1	0	2
Orange juice (1/2 cup)	55	0.3	0	1
DAIRY PRODUCTS				
Milk–Skim (1 cup)	86	0.4	4	126
Milk–1% Fat (1 cup)	102	2.6	10	123
Milk–2% Fat (1 cup)	121	4.7	18	122
Frozen Yogurt (1/2 cup)	123	2.3	9	60
Ice Milk	92	2.8	9	53
Cottage Cheese–2% Fat (1/2 cup)	101	2.2	9	459
Mozzarella, Part Skim (1 oz)	72	4.5	16	132
MEAT, POULTRY, AND SEAFOOD				
Flank Steak–Lean, broiled (4 oz)	276	16.8	80	76
Ground Beef–Lean, broiled (4 oz)	316	20	116	100
Pork Tenderloin– Lean, roasted (4 oz)	188	5.6	104	76
Chicken–Light meat without skin (4 oz)	180	4.4	88	76
Chicken–Dark meat without skin (4 oz)	216	10	100	84
Lobster–Cooked (4 oz)	112	0.8	80	432
Clams–Cooked (4 oz)	168	2.4	76	128
Tuna–White, canned in water (4 oz)	156	2.8	48	444
Trout–Rainbox (4 oz)	172	4.8	84	40
Swordfish (4 oz)	176	6.0	56	132
Flounder (4 oz)	132	1.6	76	120

* A dash means that the value is not available.

Fig. 21-4 The ADA exchange list makes it easier for a person to follow a diabetic diet.

Regular Diets. A regular diet is one in which a person may eat whatever he likes. There are no restrictions. This is sometimes called a house diet or general diet.

Therapeutic Diets. A therapeutic diet is used to treat a disease condition. It is often called a special diet. In a therapeutic diet, the amount and type of food may be controlled. Examples of therapeutic diets are shown in Fig. 21-3 on page 313.

The Diabetic Diet: The purpose of the diabetic diet is to maintain correct blood sugar levels and prevent complications. It is based on the resident's age, sex, height, weight, and activity level. The doctor will also consider the resident's current diet, cultural background, and food preferences. The amount of each of the major nutrients (protein, carbohydrate, and fat) is controlled. Foods that contain simple sugars, which go quickly to the bloodstream, are usually not allowed. Examples of this kind of food include sugar, candy, jelly, syrup, soft drinks, and desserts. Weight control may be a part of the diet, when necessary.

The diabetic diet is often referred to as an ADA diet. The American Diabetes Association, the American Dietetic Organization, and the Public Health Department work together to establish food exchange lists to help with meal planning. Any food on the list may be exchanged with any other food that contains the same food value. This allows the resident to choose foods of preference.

There has been a change in recent years concerning diabetic diets. In earlier diets, carbohydrates (which include foods containing sugar and starch) were severely restricted. This meant that most of the calories came from protein and fat. Studies have shown that fatty foods contribute to cardiovascular disease, which is a common problem in diabetes. Today's diabetic diet increases the amount of carbohydrates allowed and decreases the amount of protein and fat. Long-term diabetics, who are accustomed to the previous diet, may not understand why they are allowed more carbohydrates. If the resident questions you concerning the diet, let the charge nurse know. Either the nurse or the dietitian can reassure the resident and explain the changes.

Mechanical Diets. A mechanical diet is one in which the texture of the food is changed. A regular or therapeutic diet may be ordered as mechanical. For example, the doctor might order a regular, mechanical diet or a low-sodium, mechanical diet. This type of diet may be ordered for the person who has difficulty chewing or swallowing. The food may be chopped, pureed, or blended.

The Digestive Process

The Digestive System. The major organs of the digestive system are the mouth, esophagus, stomach, small intestine, and large intestine (see Fig. 21-5). Accessory organs include the teeth, tongue, liver and gallbladder. The digestive system is also called the gastrointestinal or GI system. It is basically a long, continuous tube that begins at the mouth and ends at the anus (the opening to the rectum). The function of the digestive system is to prepare food for the body's use. A review of the digestive system in Chapter 11 will be helpful.

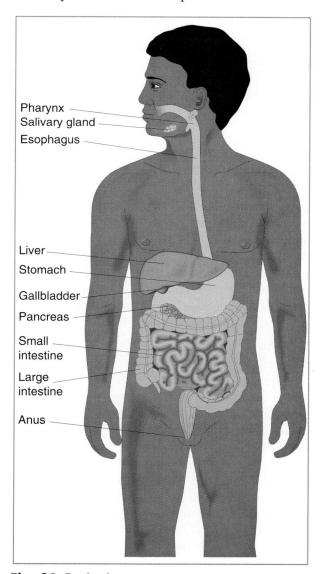

Fig. 21-5 The digestive system.

Digestion. Food is taken in through the mouth, where it is moistened by saliva, and chewed by the teeth. The tongue pushes it to the back of the throat and it is swallowed. From there it enters the esophagus and moves by peristalsis into the stomach. **Peristalsis** is the muscular contractions that move food through the digestive system. The stomach stores and mixes the food. It secretes digestive juices that help to break down the food. The liver and gallbladder also contribute digestive juices. Most of digestion takes place in the small intestine, where nutrients from food are absorbed into the bloodstream, through the villi. By the time food enters the large intestine, very little is left except water and waste material called feces. The colon (large intestine) removes fluid from the waste material for the body's use. Feces enters the rectum at the end of the colon and is eliminated through the anus.

Changes of Aging in the Digestive System. Changes of aging that occur in the digestive system can cause problems with nutrition. There is a decrease in saliva, and in the number of taste buds. These changes, combined with a reduced sense of smell, can affect the appetite. Swallowing is affected by a weakening of the gag reflex, which increases the chance of choking. The absorption of vitamins and minerals is reduced. The whole digestive process is less efficient as peristalsis slows and gastric juices decrease.

Common Problems of the Digestive System. Many problems of the digestive system are affected by nutrition. Some of these conditions present mild symptoms (heartburn, for example) that can be easily controlled. Others, like diabetes, can have serious complications that may last for a lifetime.

Heartburn and indigestion are the most common complaints. Almost everyone has experienced one or both of these problems at some time in their life. Heartburn or indigestion can be caused by eating too fast, eating too much, or eating certain foods. Emotional stress, disease, and medications may contribute to these problems. Indigestion may progress to nausea or vomiting. Treatment may include offering liquids, soups, and other easily digested foods. Medications are also available to treat these conditions.

Constipation is caused by a combination of factors, but diet plays a major role. An adequate fluid intake is necessary to keep the feces soft and moist. High-fiber (high-residue) foods create bulk and stimulate peristalsis. Prune juice and fresh fruits are helpful. Constipation can be treated with laxatives, suppositories, and enemas, but the best method is prevention. A well-balanced diet helps to prevent constipation.

Diabetes, heart disease, hypertension, anemia, osteoporosis, and gallbladder disease are also affected by nutrition. Diabetes is discussed in detail in Chapter 12. One of your duties is to assist the resident to follow the diet that has been ordered. You must observe and report the food intake accurately and be aware of complications that might develop.

Nutrition and the Elderly Resident

Most older people require fewer calories, because a decrease in metabolism and activity reduces the body's need for fuel. However, the amount of protein, minerals, and vitamins needed does not change. The diet that is usually recommended for the elderly includes foods that are high in the necessary nutrients and low in fat. Foods that have a high fiber content are also helpful.

Factors That Affect Nutrition. Some elderly residents have difficulty meeting their nutritional needs. Some factors that affect nutrition in the elderly are

- Physical changes of aging
- Difficulty chewing and dental problems
- Impaired mobility
- Disease or illness
- Decreased appetite

A decrease in appetite is a common problem in the elderly. Physical changes of aging can cause difficulty. Appetite is affected by more than the body's need for food. The smell of an apple pie in the oven makes the mouth water, and suddenly hunger strikes. The elderly person, however, with a decreased sense of smell and less saliva in the mouth, is not affected. You may hear the resident say that "food doesn't taste like it used to," and that is probably true. A decrease in taste buds has changed the ability to taste accurately.

The resident may be confused, or have emotional problems that cause a decrease in appetite. The confused resident may not recognize the signs of hunger, or may be afraid to eat. Medications affect appetite. Some drugs reduce hunger or leave an unpleasant taste in the mouth.

Sometimes the resident doesn't eat well because the food is different, or meal time is not the same as at home. The resident comes to the facility with eating habits that have developed over a lifetime, and may find it difficult to adjust to a new routine. There are foods that are liked and foods that are not liked. The resident may want to eat only special ethnic foods.

Factors that influence eating habits include culture, religion, finances, and personal preference. Food preferences may depend on where a person was born and raised. Ethnic foods are a part of every culture. Many people eat the same kinds of food that they grew up eating. As people age, the desire for favorite foods may grow stronger. It is a real challenge for the staff in the long-term care facility to meet the resident's individual needs and preferences.

Nutritional Care Plan. A nutritional assessment is completed on the resident at admission and is revised as necessary. The doctor orders the type of diet the resident will have. The dietitian is responsible for setting up a nutritional plan of care for each resident. The care planning team attempts

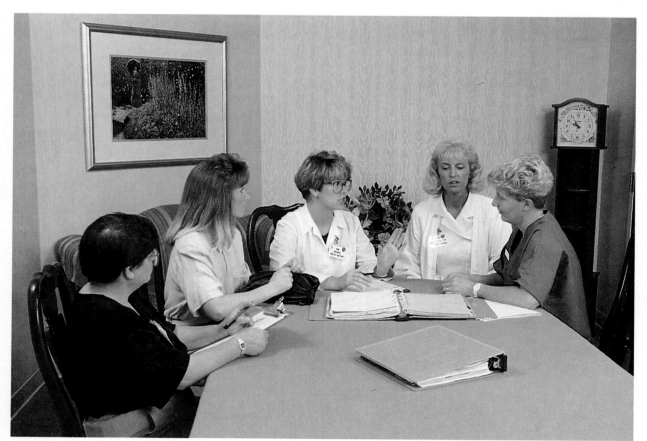

Fig. 21-6 Planing the nutritional care plan.

to create a plan that is as close as possible to the resident's usual eating habits. The goal of the nutritional care plan is to help the resident meet nutritional needs.

Residents' Rights as Related to Nutrition. The residents' bill of rights addresses nutrition and food. The facility and the caregivers must ensure that these rights are honored. They include the right to

- Be served food according to ethnic, cultural or religious beliefs
- Be served food according to personal preferences
- Be served attractive, tasty food at correct temperature, in a pleasant environment, in a pleasant manner
- Participate in traditional holiday meals

Assisting the Resident to Eat

As a nursing assistant, you will have the opportunity to provide physical assistance and emotional support to help the resident meet nutritional needs. You may be the one who hears about food likes and dislikes. Be sure to make the nurse aware of those preferences. Observe behavior and emotional state because eating habits may change when a person is upset. Encourage the resident to share feelings and listen respectfully.

Identify problems quickly, and offer help as necessary. Encourage physical activity to improve appetite and digestion.

Observe and record intake accurately. Measure and record height and weight as ordered. The resident's diet is based on those measurements. Offer and encourage between-meal nourishments or snacks as ordered.

Adaptive Equipment. There is adaptive equipment available to assist the resident in eating. The occupational therapist will recommend and obtain adaptive equipment that is specific to the resident's needs. This equipment may be useful to the resident who has weakness, paralysis, or impaired coordination. The chart in Fig. 21-7 lists some adaptive equipment that is commonly used.

Preparing the Resident for Meals. Take the resident to the bathroom or offer the bedpan before the meal is served. Assist with handwashing and oral care. A clean, fresh mouth makes eating more pleasant. Make sure clothes are clean and neat. Hair should be combed and the male resident should be shaved. Do you like to look nice when you go to dinner? The resident may feel the same way. Encourage and assist the resident to go to the dining room if possible. Most residents will eat better there, because the dining room is a more normal setting. Dining is

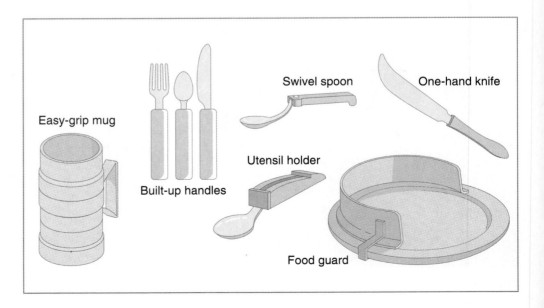

Fig. 21-7
Adaptive dining equipment.

Easy-grip mug

Built-up handles

Swivel spoon

One-hand knife

Utensil holder

Food guard

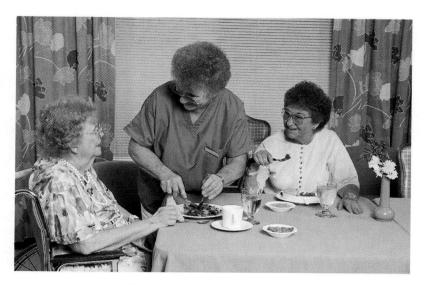

Fig. 21-8
Cutting up the resident's meat makes it easier for her to feed herself.

a social activity, and the dining room provides opportunities for socialization.

Assisting the Resident in the Dining Room. Help the resident to be seated and positioned in correct body alignment. Introduce residents seated at the table, if they do not already know each other. Bring the food tray to the table. Check to be sure the tray has the correct name on it and that it contains the proper diet. Remove the food from the tray and arrange it in front of the resident. Be sure there is a napkin, silverware, beverage, and other necessities. Provide special equipment if required by the resident.

Assist as needed by buttering the bread, cutting up the meat, and opening cartons. Offer salt, pepper, and other condiments that are allowed on the diet. Encourage the resident to be as independent as possible.

Stay near the table and observe for problems such as swallowing or chewing.

Observe the amount of food that is eaten. Report to the nurse if the resident has not eaten well, or has eaten only certain foods. If there is a food on the plate that the resident doesn't like, offer to get something else. Do not rush—allow time for eating and socializing. Assist the resident to leave the dining room when the meal is finished and offer oral hygiene.

Assisting Residents to Eat in Their Rooms. Assist the resident with toileting and personal hygiene. It may be important to be well groomed, even when eating alone. The resident should sit up in a chair, if possible. If bedrest is necessary, sitting up as straight as possible improves digestion and helps to prevent choking.

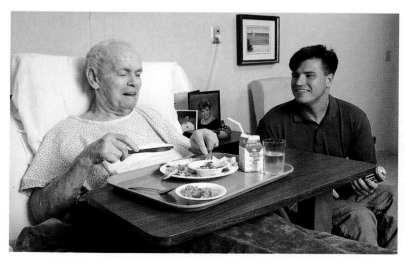

Fig. 21-9
The resident should sit up as straight as possible while eating in bed.

Clean the overbed table, place the tray on it, and remove the food covers. The resident may want to use a clothing protector. Assist as necessary, while encouraging independence and self-care. Be a pleasant companion and allow as much time as necessary. When you leave the room, place the call signal in reach, and check back frequently. Observe and report the amount of food eaten.

Assisting the Vision-Impaired Resident with Meals. Use of the clock method helps the blind or vision-impaired resident maintain independence. This means that placement of food is compared to the face of a clock. The following example shows how you can describe the food on the resident's plate. "Three slices of roast beef are at 9:00, two slices of bread are at 11:00, a baked potato is at 2:00, green peas are at 3:00, and carrots are at 5:00." You have described the food that is on the plate and its location. Remember, the vision-impaired resident cannot see what is on the plate and has no idea what to expect.

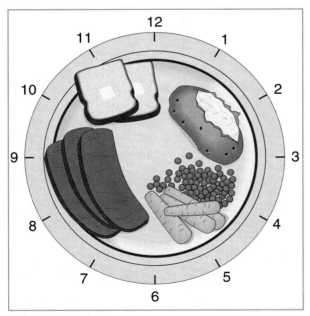

Fig. 21-10 Use the clock method to describe food placement to the blind resident.

Provide special equipment that might help the resident to eat independently. Do not assume that the vision-impaired person will want a lot of help. Regular dining utensils might be preferred, even though a plate guard or scoop plate might make it easier to eat.

Feeding the Resident Who Cannot Eat Independently. Some residents may have physical or emotional problems that interfere with their ability to feed themselves. For example, a paralyzed resident might be unable to handle utensils. A resident who has Alzheimer's disease may be too confused for self-feeding. In these situations, the resident will need to be fed. It is important to observe for any sign that the resident is improving. The resident who shows the ability or desire for self-feeding may need to be in a restorative dining program.

The helpless resident may be fed in the dining room, in the room, or in the bed. Make sure the resident is positioned correctly, sitting up as straight as possible. If a geri-chair is used, bring the recliner forward to an upright position. Do not attempt to feed the resident while the head is tilted back. Remember, when you tilt the head back, and bring up the chin, you open the airway. When the head is tilted downward, and the chin is tucked in toward the chest, the airway is closed. The resident may **aspirate** (choke), if you try to offer food while the airway is open because food will enter the airway instead of the esophagus.

Sit down beside the resident you are feeding, so that you are at eye level. This permits eye contact, and the resident will not have to look up at you. It is more comfortable to be on the same level with another person. Think how you feel when someone is standing over you, looking down. When you are sitting down, the resident does not feel rushed.

Some measures to use when feeding the helpless resident include the following:

- Provide a clothing protector.
- Tell the resident what is on the tray.
- Season the food as the resident desires.
- Serve the food as desired.
- Name each food as it is offered.
- Be sure that liquids are not too hot.
- Tell the resident when you are offering hot liquids or food.

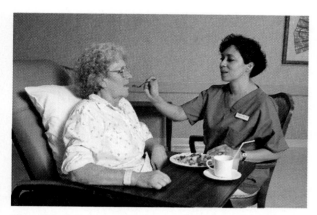

Fig. 21-11 When feeding a resident, sit down so that you are at eye level with the resident.

- Encourage the resident to help (hold the bread or cracker).
- Alternate foods and offer fluids frequently.
- Fill the spoon no more than half full.
- Feed with the tip of the spoon.
- Feed on the unaffected side if the resident is paralyzed.
- Use a different straw for each liquid.

Communicate with the resident, even if there is no response. Do not rush—allow time for chewing and make sure that swallowing is completed. Gently stroke the resident's throat if swallowing does not occur. Wipe the resident's mouth as needed. Make sure the resident is clean, neat, and comfortable after completing the meal. Record the amount eaten, and report to the nurse if the resident did not eat well.

Restorative Dining

Any assistance that is given the resident in dining should be given in a restorative manner. Encourage the resident to eat as independently, as possible. Eating in the dining room, with other people is important. Provide adaptive equipment as needed, and help maintain proper positioning. Offer praise and encouragement frequently. These techniques help the resident to maintain independence and self-esteem.

Restorative Dining Program. The residents may be divided into groups, according to their dining needs. Residents who are alert, and need no assistance, usually eat in the main dining room. They should be seated in a way that promotes socialization. Tables for four or six are better than long tables.

Residents who need assistance or supervision may also be seated in the main dining room. These residents may have physical or emotional problems that interfere with their ability to feed themselves. Seating the residents across from one another is helpful. Looking across the table at someone else who is eating may remind the residents of why they are in the dining room.

They may need to be reminded frequently to resume eating. Often, a simple statement such as, "Would you like a drink of milk, now," is all that is necessary. A staff member should be available for every eight to ten residents in this group. Nurses, speech therapists, social workers, and other personnel often assist in the dining room.

Retraining may be needed by some residents. Residents who have had strokes, for example, may need to learn how to feed themselves again. This group will need one staff member for three or four residents. Each resident is carefully assessed for problems, strengths, weaknesses, and motivation. Both short-term and long-term goals are set. Measures are suggested to help meet those goals and evaluations are made on a regular basis. Doesn't that sound like the requirements for a care plan? It is, in fact, a plan of care for meeting nutritional needs.

Creating the right environment is an important part of the restorative dining program. The area should be well-lit, without glare. The temperature should be at a comfortable setting. Tablecloths and centerpieces add a nice touch. Seating should be comfortable, and the residents should have plenty of room. The area must not appear cluttered, and distractions should be avoided. Soft music is soothing, as long as it does not interfere with communication. Residents who are relearning a skill need a quiet, peaceful atmosphere, free from distractions.

The area should be separated from the main dining room, if possible. If there is not a separate room for restorative dining, screens can be used to create a special area. This provides a cozy atmosphere and allows the staff to concentrate on those who need help.

To be successful, the retraining program should be consistent. This means that the resident should participate in the program three meals a day, seven days a week. The resident should be seated in the same area, at the same time of day. The same staff members should work with each resident as much as possible. This prevents the resident from having to adjust to a new environment or a change in technique.

GUIDELINES TO ASSIST THE RESIDENT TO EAT INDEPENDENTLY

- Provide adaptive equipment as needed.
- Place only one dish at a time in front of the resident who is easily distracted or lacks confidence.
- Place food within the resident's reach.
- Use the "clock method" to place food in front of the vision-impaired resident.
- Give directions one step at a time. For example, "Pick up your spoon. Put the spoon in your mashed potatoes. Bring the spoon to your mouth. Now swallow. That's great!"
- You may need to place your hand over the resident's hand to guide it.
- Allow time for the resident to chew and swallow.
- Repeat instructions patiently, as often as necessary.
- Use praise frequently.
- Encourage the resident to try; don't point out mistakes.

Do not be disappointed if the resident doesn't do well every day. Everybody has an "off" day from time to time. Do you ever have days when nothing goes right, and you seem to have forgotten everything you learned? The residents are no different. You can help by praising them on their good days and encouraging them on their bad days.

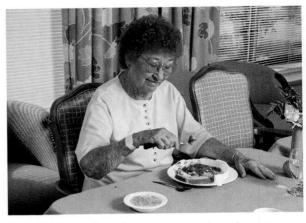

Fig. 21-12 The right environment, the right equipment, and the right attitude will help the resident maintain independence.

It is important to accurately record the amounts and types of food that the resident has eaten. Make note of food or fluids that the resident prefers and report any change in the resident's eating pattern to the nurse. Do not assume that the resident is just having a "bad day." There could also be a physical or emotional change taking place. The plan of care is continually evaluated and changed as necessary.

Working with residents who need to be retrained is rewarding. As you watch the helpless, discouraged resident regain the ability to eat without assistance, you can feel proud of the part you played in recovery. No matter how hard it seems or how long it takes, it is well worth the effort. Your pride in the residents' progress will help them to regain their pride. This, in turn, increases self-esteem and independence. Your belief in the success of this program can make it happen.

Supplemental Nutrition

Oral Supplements. Residents who do not eat well may be offered supplemental feedings. This type of feeding is also provided for the resident who has an increased need for calories. For example, some cancer patients need to follow a diet that is nutritionally high in calories.

To meet their needs, nutritious foods are provided for between-meal snacks. Milk shakes, ice cream, cheese, and peanut butter are examples of these snacks. It is important that you serve the snacks to the residents, and that you encourage them to eat. Many times, however, the resident who doesn't eat well at meals, will also refuse nourishment that is offered between meals. In that situation, the doctor may order a liquid nutritional supplement.

Liquid supplements provide the necessary nutrients and calories in a small amount of fluid. Many products are available that are equal to a well-balanced meal. They are nutritious enough to be used as a complete diet, or they may be added to a standard diet. Liquid supplements come in a variety of flavors. They may be mixed with ice cream, bananas, or other fruit, into a nutri-tious milkshake. Some are tasty enough to drink directly from the container.

Tube Feedings. The resident who is unable to take food or fluids by mouth, or is unable to swallow, may be fed through a tube. The two types of tubes most commonly used in a long-term care facility are nasogastric tubes and gastrostomy tubes.

A **nasogastric (NG)** tube is a tube that is placed through the nose into the stomach (see Fig. 21-13). ("Naso" is the medical term for nose and "gastric" means stomach.) It may also be called a Levine tube or abbreviated as NG tube.

An NG tube may also be used to suction and remove fluids from the body. Do not give the resident, who has an NG tube, any-thing to eat or drink, without checking with the nurse. Residents with feeding tubes are

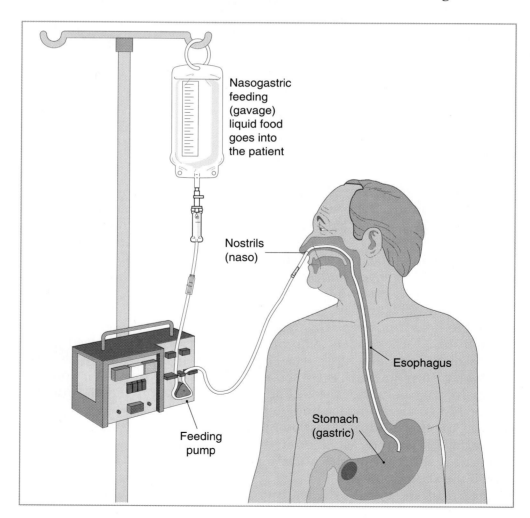

Nasogastric feeding (gavage) liquid food goes into the patient

Nostrils (naso)

Esophagus

Feeding pump

Stomach (gastric)

Fig. 21-13
A nasogastric tube.

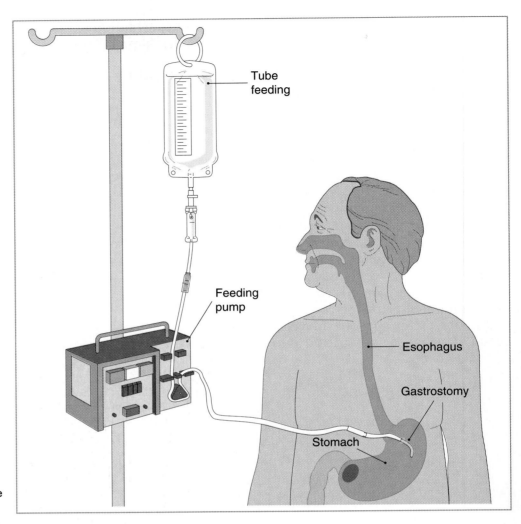

Tube feeding

Feeding pump

Esophagus

Gastrostomy

Stomach

Fig. 21-14
A gastrostomy tube is placed directly into the stomach for feeding.

often NPO. **NPO** is the abbreviation for nothing by mouth. **PO** is the abbreviation used when a person can have something by mouth.

A **gastrostomy tube** is a tube that is placed directly into the stomach for feeding. A small surgical opening is made through the abdominal wall into the stomach, and the tube is sutured to hold it in place. This type of tube is often used for a resident who may need tube feedings for a long time. The abbreviation for a gastrostomy tube is G-tube.

Usually the NG tube or the G-tube will be attached to an electronic feeding pump that controls the flow of fluid. Most pumps have an alarm that sounds when something is wrong. You must notify the nurse immediately if the alarm sounds.

The resident who has a feeding tube should be observed frequently. If the pump is not working properly, the resident may receive the wrong amount of food. The fluid may enter too quickly. This can cause nausea, vomiting, and aspiration. The NG tube may have moved out of the stomach and into the lungs. Aspiration pneumonia may result if tube feeding enters the lungs.

The NG tube is uncomfortable and irritating to the nose and throat. The G-tube may become dislodged from the stomach, or the skin may become irritated at the site of insertion. Infection can occur with either tube, if aseptic practices are not carefully followed.

The resident with a feeding tube should not lie flat. The head of the bed should be elevated. Some procedures will need to be changed slightly for the resident with a feeding tube. For example, if the resident has a feeding tube, an occupied bed cannot

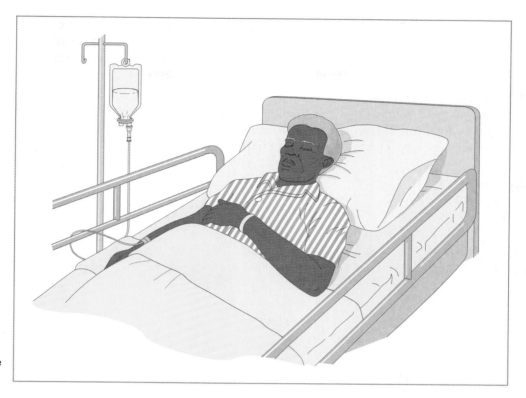

Fig. 21-15
Liquid nutrients can be given through a needle inserted into the vein.

be flattened to change the linen. Your major responsibility concerning the resident with a feeding tube is to make regular observations and promptly report any problems.

Parenteral Nutrition. The resident may need to receive parenteral nutrition (not in or through the digestive system). One form of parenteral nutrition is intravenous. **Intravenous (IV)** means into the vein. In this type of feeding, liquid nutrients are given through a needle that is inserted into a blood vessel (see Fig. 21-15). Care of the resident receiving parenteral nutrition is discussed in the chapter on fluid intake.

Conclusion

Remember these important points:

1. Dining meets physical, emotional, social, and spiritual needs.

2. Food is used to create energy for all body functions.

3. The diet is always ordered by the doctor.

4. The resident has the right to be served food according to individual needs and food preferences.

5. Encourage the resident to eat in the dining room, if possible.

6. Do not rush the resident; allow time for eating and socialization.

7. The location of food should be described for the blind resident by using the clock method.

8. Provide adaptive equipment and help the resident maintain proper positioning while eating.

9. Your attitude toward a restorative dining program contributes to its success or failure.

10. Check with the nurse before giving a resident with an NG tube anything to eat or drink.

Discussion Questions

1. How does dining help meet your emotional, social, and spiritual needs?

2. How is your appetite affected when you are upset?

3. How do the changes of aging affect nutrition in the elderly person?

4. A resident has right-sided weakness. How would you assist her in dining? What adaptive equipment would be helpful?

5. *Why is a quiet, peaceful environment helpful in restorative dining?*

Application Exercises

1. Each student will plan a well-balanced menu for one day. The menus will be shared and evaluated by the class. The instructor will point out how many differences there can be in a well-balanced diet.

2. The class will have a covered-dish luncheon. Each student will bring an ethnic food that represents his or her culture. The students will also discuss the cultural significance of special foods.

Fluid Balance

OBJECTIVES

Upon completing this chapter, you will be able to do the following:

1. Explain the importance of fluids.

2. Explain the meaning of fluid balance.

3. List four measures to prevent dehydration.

4. Identify reasons why the elderly do not drink enough fluids.

5. List two alternative measures of hydration.

6. List six guidelines for caring for a resident with an IV.

7. List four guidelines for emptying a urinary drainage bag.

8. List four guidelines for accurate intake and output.

9. Calculate fluid intake and output correctly using the metric system.

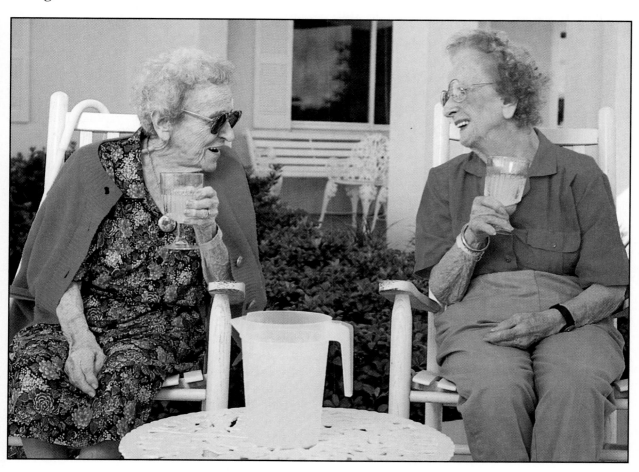

The Importance of Fluid

Water is essential to life. Wars have been fought and the course of history changed over water rights. In settling new lands, early pioneers built homes and towns near a water supply. They knew that if water was not readily available, they would not survive.

The human body needs water. A person might live for weeks without food but would die in a few days without water. It is more important than food, and is necessary for all body processes. If the amount of water in the body changes, cell activity is affected. When the amount of water in the body is very low, cells will die.

The body signals its need for water by the sensation of thirst. When you are thirsty, your throat feels dry and scratchy. You may have a cough, or a change in your voice. You react to these sensations by reaching for something to drink. Think about how satisfying a cool drink of water is when you are thirsty.

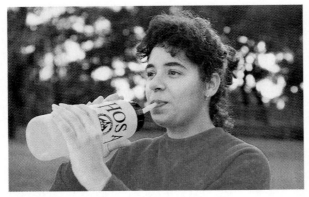

Fig. 22-1 A drink of water satisfies thirst.

The Functions of Water. The body uses water in many ways. It is needed inside the cells and between the cells. Water provides fluid for the body's transportation system. It is the major element of blood. The functions of water in the body include the following:

- Transports oxygen, nutrients, and other substances to the cells
- Carries waste products away from the cells
- Provides lubrication to body tissues
- Helps to control body temperature
- Helps to regulate the body's chemistry balance
- Helps to regulate fluid balance

Maintaining Fluid Balance

The human body is over 60 percent water. Food and fluid provide water for the body. The average fluid intake for an adult is between two and three quarts (2000–3000 cc) daily. Because the body is continually using water, fluid must be replaced daily. It is important that a person maintain fluid balance. This means that the amount of fluid taken in must equal the amount of fluid that is lost (eliminated). A person who receives adequate **hydration** (supply of fluids) will usually be in fluid balance. There may be an increased need for fluids during hot weather, or if the resident is ill.

Water is important to maintain the chemical balance of the body. Chemicals, such as sodium and potassium, are necessary for cell function. A change in the fluid balance causes a change in the chemical balance. If the chemicals in the body are not balanced, physical or mental problems may result.

Fluid balance is affected by the changes of aging. The skin loses some of its fluid and becomes drier. A decrease in activity of the sweat glands interferes with normal perspiration. As circulation slows, fragile blood vessels transport fluid less efficiently. A decrease in kidney function slows filtration and elimination of wastes.

Edema and Dehydration

Medical problems occur when the body is not in fluid balance. Either too much fluid or not enough fluid can have serious effects on the body. Measures must be taken to restore the balance as soon as possible.

Edema. When there is too much fluid, it tends to pool in parts of the body. The swelling of a body part with fluid is called **edema**. The swelling is usually noticed first in the hands and feet. Edema may be caused by poor circulation, fluid retention, or medications. It may be a complication of heart or kidney disease. Symptoms of edema include swelling, weight gain, increased blood pressure, and wet, noisy respirations.

An extremity that is swollen should be elevated whenever possible. When the resident is sitting in a chair, place a foot stool under the feet. A swollen hand can be elevated on a pillow. Restorative skin care will be necessary.

The resident with edema may be on a sodium-restricted diet. It will help to remember the saying that "water follows salt." When a person takes in too much sodium (salt), the body tends to retain water. It is very important that you encourage the resident to follow the diet that is ordered.

Restrict Fluids. The doctor may order "restrict fluids" for the resident with edema. A specific amount of fluid will be ordered daily, with the total amount divided between shifts. Fluids may be offered in small amounts. The amount of fluid taken in and eliminated will be carefully recorded. The resident and visitors, as well as staff members, must be aware that the resident is on restricted fluid intake. The resident on "restrict fluids" will need frequent oral care.

Medications (diuretics) may be ordered to reduce edema. They increase the residents need to urinate. Answer the call light promptly as urination may be an urgent

need. The medication may also increase the frequency of urination.

Dehydration. The condition of having less than the normal amount of fluid in the body is called **dehydration**. Dehydration occurs when the resident loses too much body fluid or does not take in enough fluid. A person with low body weight can dehydrate very quickly. Infants and the elderly are especially at risk.

The signs and symptoms of dehydration include

- Thirst
- Very dry skin that is much less elastic
- Pale or ashen skin color
- Sunken eyes
- Dry mouth and tongue
- Dry mucous membranes
- Weight loss
- Decreased urinary output
- Concentrated urine
- Constipation
- Rapid heart and respiratory rate
- Fever
- Irritable, confused, or depressed
- Weakness, twitching, or convulsions

The symptoms can be mild or severe, depending on the degree of dehydration. A 10 percent loss of body fluid can cause serious problems, while a 20–22 percent loss results in death. It is important to observe early signs of dehydration, before they become more serious.

Fluid is normally lost through urine, respirations, perspiration, and feces. Abnormal losses of fluid can be caused by vomiting, diarrhea, bleeding, or excessive perspiration. Dehydration may occur as a complication of an illness or as a side effect of medication.

The most common cause of dehydration in the elderly is an inadequate intake of fluid. Reasons why the elderly resident may not drink enough include

- Weakness and decreased mobility (difficulty reaching, opening, or pouring fluid)
- Difficulty swallowing
- Confusion (fails to recognize thirst, forgets to drink, is unable to work the water fountain, or fears being poisoned)

- Lack of assistance (fluids offered infrequently or failure to assist)
- Fear of urinary incontinence (inability to control urine)
- Dislikes fluid offered (many people do not like water)

The nursing assistant plays a major role in preventing dehydration. It is important to observe for signs and symptoms of dehydration. Be aware of the amount of fluids the resident is taking. Careful observation of fluid intake may prevent dehydration. Other measures to prevent dehydration are

- Offer fluids frequently and place them within the resident's reach
- Open containers and assist as needed
- Provide adaptive equipment if necessary
- Remind and encourage the resident to drink
- Find out what fluids the resident likes and check the care plan for suggestions

Share information that will assist the staff in meeting the resident's needs. For example, if you have learned that the resident will nearly always drink a particular kind of juice, that information needs to be on the care plan.

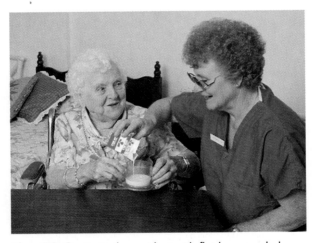

Fig. 22-2 Assist the resident with fluids as needed.

Encourage Fluids. If a resident is not taking adequate fluid, the nurse will call the doctor for specific orders. The doctor may order "encourage fluids." This means that fluids will be offered frequently, and the resident will be encouraged to drink. The nurse will tell you how much fluid the resident should drink on your shift. Fluids will need to be measured and recorded for the resident. It is necessary to keep accurate records in order to know exactly how much fluid the resident has taken. If you cannot get the resident to drink enough, tell the nurse right away. Do not wait until the end of the shift to report this information to the nurse.

Alternative Methods of Hydration

Sometimes, despite all your efforts, the resident will not drink enough fluids. In that case, the doctor may order fluids by a different route. Some alternative methods for giving fluid are by nasogastric tube (NG tube), gastric tube (G-tube), or intravenous (IV). NG tubes and G-tubes are explained in Chapter 21. A review of that section may be helpful.

Intravenous. Intravenous (IV) means into the vein. The resident can receive water, nutrients, and medications through the IV. A needle is inserted into the vein to give fluids by this method. A sterile dressing covers the insertion site. Tubing extends from the needle to a bag or bottle of fluids, which hangs from an IV pole (see Fig. 22-3A). The pole may be attached to the bed, or a portable IV stand may be used. There may be a pump attached to control the flow rate of the fluid.

A nursing assistant may not start, stop, or adjust the rate of an IV. You are not allowed to change the sterile dressing. These tasks are the responsibility of licensed nurses. Observe the resident frequently and report any problems to the nurse immediately.

GUIDELINES FOR CARING FOR THE RESIDENT WITH AN IV

- Call the nurse if the pump alarm sounds.
- Report swelling, redness, bleeding, or leaking at the insertion site. Wear gloves if you will be in contact with blood.
- Report breathing problems or an elevated temperature.

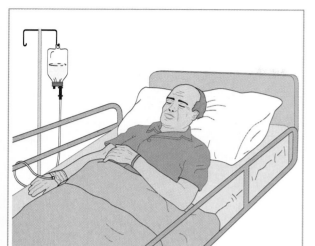

A A resident may receive fluids by IV.

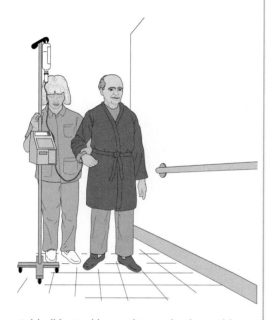

B A portable IV stand is used to assist the resident to ambulate.

Fig. 22-3 The resident with an IV.

- Report complaints of pain or burning at the site of insertion.
- Report to the nurse if the flow rate changes or stops.
- Call the nurse if the tubing disconnects. Do not attempt to reconnect it.
- Make sure the tubing is not kinked, tangled, or under the resident's body.
- Allow slack in the tubing to prevent pull on the needle.

- Give proper restraint care if the IV arm is restrained or splinted.
- Take blood pressures on the arm that does not have an IV.
- Assist the resident to turn and reposition, avoiding tension on the tubing.
- Keep the bag or bottle above the level of the insertion site.
- Use a portable IV stand to assist the resident in ambulation (see Fig. 22-3B).

Your major concern is to keep the resident with an IV as comfortable as possible, without disturbing the IV. The guidelines for changing the clothes of the resident with an IV, are described in Chapter 19. Always ask the nurse to check the IV, after you have completed the resident's care.

Measuring Fluid Intake and Output

Intake and Output. Intake and output (**I&O**) includes all fluids that are taken into the body and all fluids that are eliminated. The doctor orders I&O to observe fluid balance. It is very important to measure and record all fluids accurately, because this information is used in planning the resident's care and treatment. A **graduate**, a container that is used to measure fluid, will be needed (see Fig. 22-4). The graduate may be a measuring cup, bottle, or pitcher.

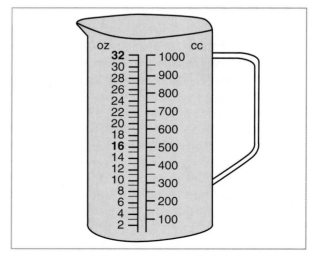

Fig. 22-4 A graduate is used to measure fluids.

INTAKE AND OUTPUT SHEET

Identification # ___125689400-2___   Resident's Name ___Mary Smith Jones___

Date ___12-1-98___   Room # ___4011A___

Time 11–7	INTAKE			OUTPUT			
				URINE		GASTRIC	
	BY MOUTH	TUBE	PARENTERAL	VOIDED	CATHETER	EMESIS	SUCTION
7:30a	120cc			250cc			
9:45	240cc						
10:30	60cc						
11:00				350cc			
11:20						200cc	
12:Noon	N.P.O.						
TOTAL	420cc	——	——	600cc	——	200cc	——
Time 7–3	NPO						
2:50p				450cc			
3:00			1000cc	200cc			300cc
TOTAL	——	——	1000cc	650cc	——	——	300cc
Time 3–11	NPO						
5:00p				200cc			
11:00			1000cc	480cc			250cc
TOTAL	——	——	1000cc	680cc	——	——	250cc
2 HOUR TOTAL	320cc	——	2000cc	1930cc	——	——	550cc
24 Hour Grand Total•Intake 2320cc				24 Hour Grand Total•Output 2480cc			

Fig. 22-5 Intake and output sheet.

Recording Fluid Intake and Output. An I&O recording form is placed in the room of a resident whose fluid intake and output is being measured. The amount of intake or output is listed in the proper column, beside the correct time. The type of fluid is also recorded in some facilities. At the end of each shift, the amount of fluid intake and output is totaled. The amount of fluid taken in and eliminated on all shifts is totaled every 24 hours. An example of an I&O recording form is shown in Fig. 22-5. Explain the need for recording I&O to the resident and visitors, and encourage their cooperation.

Measuring Fluid Intake. Fluid intake includes water and all liquid foods that are taken into the body. Tube feedings and IV solutions are counted as fluid intake. Juice, milk, soup, coffee, and tea are examples of liquid foods. Solid foods that will melt at room temperature are also counted as fluid. Ice chips, popsicles, ice cream, sherbet, pudding, and custard are examples of this type of food. Be sure that the solid foods you count can become liquid. For example, a dish of ice cream, left on the table for two hours would melt, but what would happen to a bowl of oatmeal? The cereal would not melt; in fact, it would become more solid. So, in measuring the fluids in a bowl of oatmeal, you would count only the milk that was added.

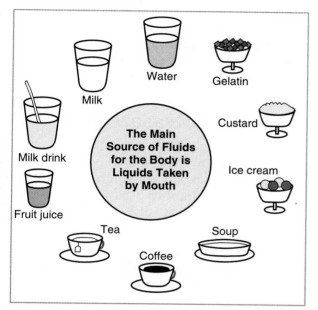

Fig. 22-6 Examples of fluid intake.

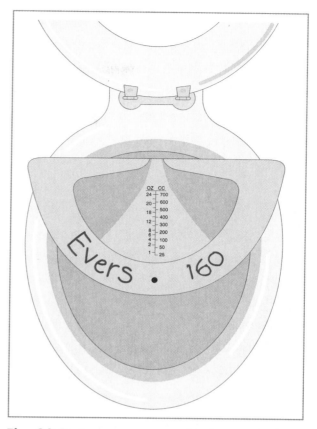

Fig. 22-7 A specimen pan may be placed under the toilet seat to collect the urine for measuring.

Record fluid as soon as the resident is finished eating or drinking. Mark the I&O sheet before the tray is removed at mealtime. If you do not write the amount down immediately, you may forget it or remember it wrong. The nursing assistant is responsible for recording oral fluid intake (all fluids taken by mouth). Usually, the nurse records the amount of tube feeding and IV fluids.

Measuring Urinary Output. Urinary output is measured after each voiding. A specimen pan can be placed under the seat of the toilet or bedside commode to collect and measure the urine (see Fig 22-7). The resident who is not able to get out of bed may use a bedpan or a urinal. Ask the resident not to put toilet tissue in the bedpan, urinal, or specimen pan. Instruct the resident to signal when through urinating, so that you may measure and discard the urine.

I&O is usually ordered for a resident with a Foley catheter. A catheter is a tube that is inserted into the bladder to drain urine. A **Foley catheter** is a urinary catheter that is left in place. It is attached to a urinary

drainage bag, which must be emptied to measure urine output. Use universal precautions and wear disposable gloves to empty the urine directly into a graduate (see Fig. 22-8). Do not allow the drainage bag to touch the floor or the inside of the graduate. When the bag is empty, replace the clamp into the holder and record the output immediately. Do not use the measurements on the side of the drainage bag, as they may be inaccurate.

The urinary drainage bag is emptied at the end of every shift and recorded on the I&O form. If the bag fills before the end of your shift, empty it and record the amount. Let your charge nurse know if this happens. The amount of urine from all shifts is totaled every 24 hours.

When I&O is ordered, you will measure and record emesis (vomitus), as well as urine. You must report bleeding, drainage, diarrhea, and excessive perspiration. The nurse will help you estimate these fluids.

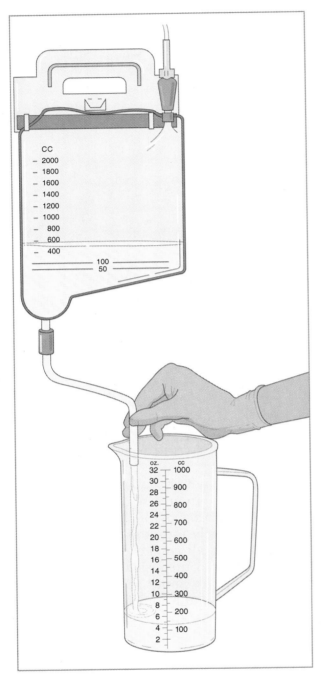

Fig. 22-8 Empty the urine directly into a graduate.

Accurate Intake and Output. There may be problems with keeping accurate I&O. The resident may drink something and forget to tell you. Visitors may not keep a record of fluids that they have given to the resident. If any of these things occur, report to the nurse.

GUIDELINES FOR ACCURATE I&O

- Inform the resident and visitors of the need to measure fluids.
- Place the I&O sheet in the proper place.
- Record intake promptly.
- Measure fluids accurately.
- Figure the amounts correctly.
- Report problems to the nurse immediately.

Systems of Measurement

Metric System. The metric system is an international system of weights and measures that is commonly used in health care. The terms used most often are cubic centimeter (cc) and milliliter (ml). These two units are equal (1 cc = 1 ml).

Customary System. The United States uses the customary system of measuring. This is the system you are probably more familiar with. It include ounces, pints, and quarts.

Household System. The household system of measuring includes teaspoons, tablespoons, and cups. You use this system at home in cooking, but you also use it in health care.

Code of Measurement. The systems include many other measurements, some of which you will learn in other chapters. This chapter will deal with those that are used in measuring fluids. Since you will frequently need to convert ounces to cubic centimeters, it is important to remember that 30 cc = 1 oz. The chart in Fig. 22-9 shows equivalent (approximately equal) measurements to be learned.

EQUIVALENT MEASUREMENTS

1 cc = 1 ml
30 cc = 1 oz
240 cc = 8 oz or 1 cup
1000 cc = 1 qt or 4 cups

Fig. 22-9 It is helpful to know equivalent measurements.

To total I&O, it will be necessary to know how much fluid various containers hold. For example, how much fluid does a coffee cup or a soup bowl hold? This information can usually be found on the I&O sheet and may be posted in the nourishment room or the utility room. It is your responsibility to know the code of measurements in your facility. They are not necessarily the same in all facilities. An example of a measurement chart can be seen in Fig. 22-10.

CODE OF MEASUREMENTS
coffee pot - 240 cc
coffee cup - 120 cc
milk carton - 240 cc
sm. juice glass - 120 cc
paper cup - 150 cc
soup bowl - 160 cc
water glass - 240 cc
ice cream - 120 cc
jello - 120 cc

Fig. 22-10 Sample code of measurements from a long-term care facility.

Using Math Skills. A graduate may be marked in cubic centimeters (cc), milliliters (ml), ounces (oz), or a combination. Look at Fig. 22-4 again. The graduate is marked in cubic centimeters and ounces. That works well in measuring output, but to measure intake, you will need to use your math skills. The math used in figuring I&O is very simple, when you work the problems one step at a time. Let's look at some examples. You will need to refer to Figs. 22-9 and 22-10.

Example 1: If you know how many cubic centimeters the container holds, all you need to do is add the amounts the resident drank.

Problem: The resident drank 150 cc of coffee, 120 cc of milk, and 90 cc of juice. What is the total amount of intake?

150 cc coffee
120 cc milk
90 cc juice
360 cc

The correct answer is 360 cc.

Example 2: You might use multiplication to figure the amount of intake.

Problem: The resident drank three cans of a feeding supplement. Each can contains 240 cc. What is the total intake?

240 cc
× 3
720 cc

The correct answer is 720 cc.

Example 3: Sometimes you will know how many ounces is in a container, and you will need to figure the total in cubic centimeters. In this situation, you will multiply the number of ounces by 30. (Remember, there are 30 cc in 1 ounce.)

Problem: The resident drank one 3-ounce glass of juice. What is the intake in cubic centimeters?

30 cc
× 3
90 cc

The correct answer is 90 cc.

Example 4: You might use a combination of methods.

Problem: The resident drank two 8-ounce cans of feeding supplement. What is the total intake in cubic centimeters?

Step 1. Figure the amount of cubic centimeters in one can. Multiply 8 ounces (each can) by 30 cc (the amount in each ounce).

30 cc
× 8
240 cc

Each can contains 240 cc.

Step 2. Figure the amount of cubic centimeters in two cans. Multiply the answer in step 1 by 2.

240 cc
× 2
480 cc

The correct answer is 480 cc.

Example 5: Probably the most difficult math will involve fractions. A fraction is a part of something. The fractions you will usually work with are quarters, halves, and thirds (see Fig. 22-11).

Problem: The resident drank three-fourths of a glass of water that contained 240 cc. How much water did he drink? Carefully follow these two steps to figure fractions.

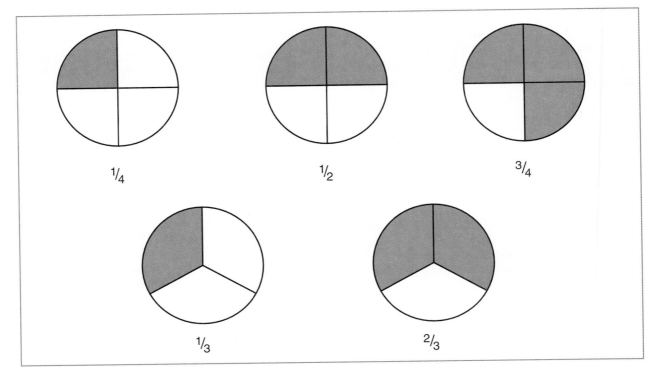

Fig. 22-11 A fraction is a part of something. The dark sections represent the fractions.

Step 1. Divide the bottom number of the fraction into the total amount in the glass.

3/4 of 240 cc
4 into 240 = 60 cc

Step 2. Multiply the answer to step 1 by the top number of the fraction.

60 × 3 = 180 cc

The correct answer is 180 cc.

Example 6: Most of the time you will use a combination of methods, when figuring the total intake for the day. The following example shows the intake for one meal, using the code of measurements in Fig. 22-10. Use the math techniques given earlier.

Problem: At breakfast, Mrs. Ryan ate one bowl of oatmeal, one-half carton of milk, two pieces of toast, one-half of a banana, one-third glass of orange juice, and two cups of coffee. What is her fluid intake for this meal?

Step 1. List the fluids: (a) 1/2 carton milk, (b) 2/3 glass juice, (c) 2 cups coffee. (The oatmeal, toast, and banana are not fluids.

Step 2. Figure the number of cubic centimeters in each item.

(a) 1/2 carton milk; 1 carton = 240 cc
1/2 of 240 = 120 cc

(b) 2/3 glass juice; 1 juice glass = 120 cc
2/3 of 120 = 80 cc

(c) 2 cups coffee; 1 china cup = 150 cc
2 × 150 = 300 cc

Step 3. Add the answers to a, b, and c.

120 cc
80 cc
300 cc
500 cc

The correct answer is 500 cc. This is the total amount of fluid that Mrs. Ryan took in at breakfast.

You can substitute milliliters for cubic centimeters in any of these problems. Remember, cubic centimeters and milliliters are equal (l cc = l ml).

Conclusion

Remember these important points:

1. Water is essential for life and is necessary for all body processes.

2. Edema or dehydration can occur when there is a fluid imbalance in the body.

3. The most common cause of dehydration in the elderly resident is not drinking enough fluid.

4. A resident who is not drinking enough may receive fluids through an NG tube, a G-tube, or an IV.

5. A nursing assistant may not start, stop, or adjust the flow rate of an IV.

6. Follow universal precautions and wear gloves, if there is a chance that you might be in contact with body fluids.

7. Use a graduate to measure fluids accurately.

8. Intake and output must be recorded accurately.

9. Empty urine from a urinary drainage bag directly into a graduate for measuring.

10. Encourage the resident and visitors to help with I&O.

Discussion Questions

1. What nursing measures could you use in caring for a resident who has edema?

2. Why are elderly residents at risk of developing dehydration?

3. You are assigned to care for a resident who needs more fluids. You are having difficulty getting her to drink. What will you do?

4. The resident is drinking a milkshake, brought from home. How will you figure the intake when he finishes?

Application Exercise

1. The instructor will put varying amounts of fluid in common facility containers. The containers will be placed on three food trays. Each student will be provided with a copy of an I&O form. These will be used by the students to calculate and record the amount of fluids on each food tray. The instructor will collect the forms and evaluate the students' efforts.

Elimination

OBJECTIVES

Upon completing this chapter, you will be able to do the following:

1. Explain the importance of privacy and positioning when assisting with elimination.

2. Identify two infection-control measures to be followed when assisting with elimination.

3. Describe the structure and function of the urinary system.

4. List three common urinary problems.

5. List two nursing measures to stimulate urination.

6. Describe the physical and emotional affects of incontinence on the resident, family, and staff.

7. List four guidelines for emptying a urinary drainage bag.

8. Identify the four basic steps of the restorative bladder program.

9. List three methods of preventing constipation.

10. Identify the general steps of a restorative bowel program.

11. List four guidelines each for giving a cleansing enema and a commercially prepared enema.

12. List six guidelines for providing ostomy care.

13. Perform the procedures described in this chapter.

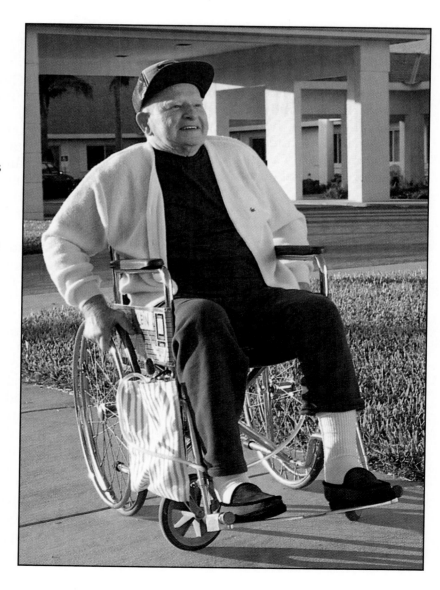

VOCABULARY

The following words or terms will help you to understand this chapter:

Feces	Foley catheter	Constipation
Incontinence	Intake and output (I&O)	Fecal impaction
Bedside commode	Graduate	Diarrhea
Fracture pan	Peristalsis	Enema
Urinal	Defecation	Ostomy
Void	Colon	Stoma
Urinary meatus	Flatus	Colostomy

As the body performs its many functions, waste material is produced. The body must eliminate those wastes to remain healthy. The two major systems involved in elimination are the urinary system and the digestive system. Some waste products are also eliminated through the skin and the lungs. The urinary system eliminates liquid waste, in the form of urine. The digestive system eliminates **feces** (solid waste). Feces may also be called stool, bowel movement, or BM. Normally, an adult has the ability to control elimination. The inability to control urine or feces is called **incontinence**.

Assisting the Resident with Elimination

Privacy, positioning, and infection control are important restorative measures during resident elimination. These measures assist the resident to optimum urinary and bowel function.

Privacy. The resident's privacy must always be maintained during elimination. Many people have difficulty urinating or having a bowel movement, if another person is present. Privacy can be protected by closing the door or pulling the curtain. When the resident's room or bathroom door is closed, knock and wait for a response before entering.

Positioning. Whenever possible, the resident should be sitting upright, to have a bowel movement. The normal position for a woman when urinating is sitting. The male normally stands to urinate. Correct body position allows the organs to be in natural alignment and provides for more efficient elimination. Residents should be assisted to a position that is as nearly normal as possible.

Infection Control. There will be times when you will wear disposable gloves while assisting a resident with elimination. Remember, one of the rules of universal precautions is to wear gloves when in contact with body fluid. Always wash your hands before and after using gloves. Dispose of gloves according to facility policy. They should not be discarded in an open wastebasket.

Bedpans and urinals should be covered as you take them to the bathroom for emptying. If there is no cover provided, use paper towels. Wear gloves to thoroughly wash, rinse, and dry the bedpan or urinal before putting it away. If bedpans and urinals must be taken out of the room to be emptied and cleaned, follow the procedure of the facility.

Perineal care may be necessary after elimination. Residents who are able to do their own peri-care should be encouraged to do so. Instruct the resident to use toilet tissue correctly, and assist with handwashing after elimination. When it is necessary to perform peri-care for the resident, wear gloves, follow aseptic technique, and clean away from the urinary opening.

Using the Bathroom. The resident should be encouraged to go to the bathroom for

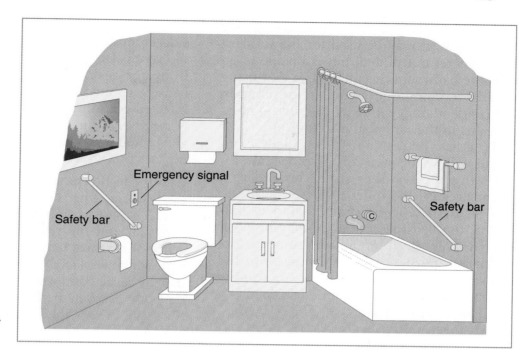

Fig. 23-1
Safety bars and an emergency signal make the environment safer.

elimination, whenever possible. This provides a more normal environment. Safety bars are provided to assist the resident on and off the toilet (see Fig. 23-1). Remind the resident to use the safety bars, not the sink or towel bar, for support. There is an emergency call signal in every bathroom that allows the resident to call for help, without getting up or leaving the bathroom (see Fig. 23-1). This notifies staff members immediately that there is an emergency. Be sure that the resident knows the location of the emergency signal.

The toilet may be fitted with a raised seat (see Fig. 23-2). This brings the seat to a height that is easier for the resident to use. The raised seat helps promote the independence of a resident who might otherwise need help in using the toilet.

Some residents will need assistance in getting to the bathroom. Residents who are weak or ill may need help getting out of bed or with ambulation. A cane or other prosthetic device might be necessary to promote independence. This information will be included in the resident's plan of care. Those who are confused may need to be reminded. The bathroom environment is restorative because it helps the confused resident recognize the need for elimination. Help resi-

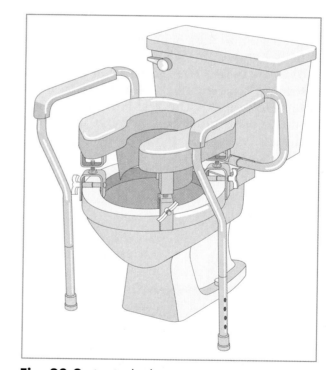

Fig. 23-2 A raised toilet seat.

dents wash their hands after using the bathroom.

Using a Bedside Commode. A bedside **commode** is a portable chair with a toilet seat that fits over a container or regular toilet (see Fig. 23-3). Sitting on a bedside commode positions the resident correctly for elimination. It may be used for the resident who can get out of bed, but is unable to go into the bathroom. If you believe that using a bedside commode would help maintain the resident's independence, be sure to mention this in the care plan meeting.

To assist the resident to a bedside commode, follow the steps of the procedure for assisting the resident from the bed to a chair. Because the toilet may feel unsafe to the resident who is weak or poorly balanced, the bedside commode may be positioned over the toilet. This promotes the resident's independence. Holding onto the arms of the bedside commode, or leaning against the back of the commode, provides a sense of security. Hands should be washed after using the bedside commode.

If the bedside commode has wheels, lock them, when it is positioned correctly. Some residents should not be left alone on the bedside commode. A bedside commode is usually lightweight, which makes it easier to move, but also easier to upset. Never restrain a resident to the toilet or the bedside commode. If the resident is weak or confused, you must be nearby at all times. Although you must remain close, give the resident as much privacy as possible.

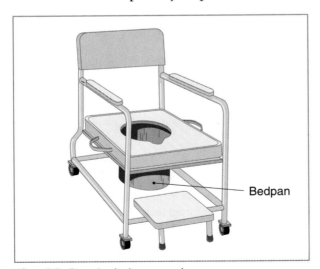

Fig. 23-3 A bedside commode.

The bedside commode must be cleaned every time it is used. This helps to eliminate odor and prevent the spread of infection.

Many facilities provide a cover for the bedside commode, to make it less obvious in the room. Do not take a bedside commode from one resident's room to another. The bedside commode must be cleaned and disinfected according to facility policy, when it is removed from the resident's room. Wear gloves and follow universal precautions during this procedure.

Using the Bedpan. A bedpan is a pan that the resident, who is in bed, uses for elimination. The most commonly used are the fracture pan and the regular bedpan (see Fig. 23-4). A **fracture pan** is a bedpan with a flat end, which is placed under the resident. It is usually more comfortable and has less effect on body alignment. Provide privacy when the resident uses the bedpan. Close the door and pull the curtain. Do not expose any more of the resident's body than necessary. You must wear gloves while assisting with the bedpan.

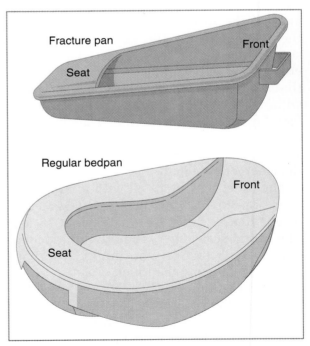

Fig. 23-4 A regular bedpan and a fracture pan.

One way to assist with a bedpan is to ask the resident to raise the hips, while you slide the bedpan under the buttocks (see Fig. 23-5A). Bending the knees and pushing up with the feet will also help the resident

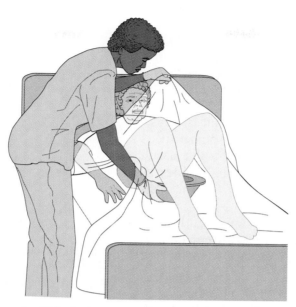

A Slide the bedpan under the resident's buttocks.

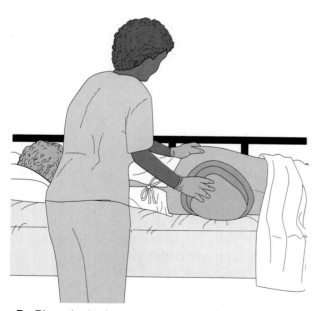

B Place the bedpan against the resident's buttocks and turn her back onto the bedpan.

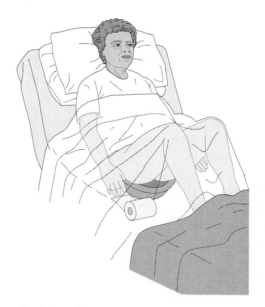

C Adjust the head of the bed so that the resident is in a sitting position.

Fig. 23-5 Assisting the resident onto the bedpan.

to assume the correct position. This procedure allows the resident to use and maintain muscle strength.

If this is not possible, assist the resident to turn onto the side, while you place the bedpan against the buttocks. Then turn the resident back onto the bedpan (see Fig. 23-5B). When the bedpan is correctly placed, adjust the head of the bed, so that the resident is in as normal a sitting position as possible (see Fig. 23-5C). Place toilet tissue and the call signal within the resident's reach. Raise the side rails, and tell the resident to signal when through.

Remove your gloves, wash your hands, and leave the room, if the resident can be left alone on the bedpan. Answer the call signal promptly. Check back frequently to see if the resident needs assistance. Do not leave the resident on the pan for a prolonged period. The pressure of the bedpan can cause discomfort and skin breakdown.

When the resident is finished, assist in raising the hips, or turn the resident onto the side, and remove the bedpan. Wear gloves and follow aseptic practices. Hold the pan to prevent spilling, when turning the resident. Place a bedpan cover over the pan as soon as you remove it. Be sure the resident has thoroughly cleaned the perineal area, and assist as necessary.

Take the bedpan to the resident's bathroom. Check urine or feces for unusual odor or appearance. Measure the urine, if the resident is on intake and output. Empty the bedpan into the toilet. Clean the pan and put it away. Remove the gloves, wash your hands, and assist the resident with handwashing. Return the bed to a comfortable position, and open the privacy curtain and the door. Report your observations to the nurse, and record the necessary information.

Using the Urinal. A **urinal** is a container that the male resident uses when urinating. It usually has a handle and is marked with measurements (see Fig 23-6). The resident may stand to use the urinal or he may use it while in bed. Many male residents like to keep the urinal within reach when they are

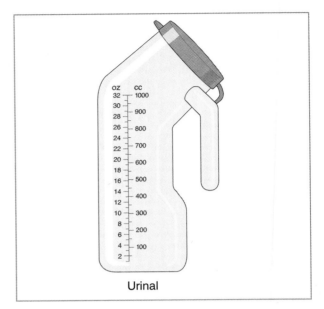

Fig. 23-6 A urinal.

in bed. This allows them to remain independent. Empty and clean the urinal promptly after it has been used to prevent odor and maintain asepsis.

Some residents may need your assistance with the urinal. Close the door and pull the curtain. If the resident is unable to position the urinal properly, you will need to put on gloves and help him. Raise the head of the bed to a sitting position, if possible. Place toilet tissue and the call signal within reach. Adjust the covers for privacy, and step outside the curtain or leave the room. If you leave the room, remove your gloves and wash your hands.

Answer the call signal promptly. Put on gloves, cover the urinal, and take it to the resident's bathroom. Measure the urine if intake and output are to be recorded. Empty and clean the urinal and return it to its proper place. Remove the gloves, wash your hands, and assist the resident to wash his or hers. Make sure the resident is comfortable and the call signal is within reach.

Urinary Elimination

The major organs of the urinary system are the kidneys, ureters, bladder, and urethra (see Fig. 23-7). The kidneys filter waste

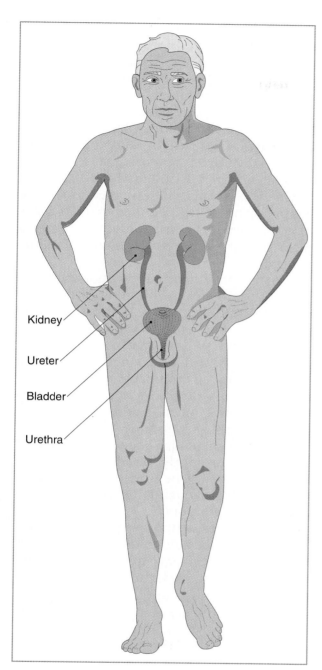

Fig. 23-7 The urinary system.

Kidney

Ureter

Bladder

Urethra

body. The outer opening of the urethra is called the **urinary meatus**.

Most people are able to control urinary elimination. When they feel the urge to urinate, they can wait until they get to a bathroom. However, if the urge is ignored, or delayed too long, the bladder will empty and release the urine.

Urine is normally pale yellow (straw colored) and clear. It has a very distinct odor. A change in urine clarity (clearness), color, or odor occurs in many disease conditions. Notify the nurse if you observe any of the following in urinary drainage:

- Blood or mucus
- Stones, gravel, or sediment
- Dark color or concentration
- Unusual odor

Report resident complaints of pain, burning, or itching in the perineal area. These symptoms may indicate a urinary tract infection. Careful observation helps to prevent infection and other urinary problems.

Common Urinary Problems

Some of the urinary problems that occur in residents are a result of aging. Muscles weaken and control of urinary elimination decreases. The urge to urinate may occur more frequently, and the resident may pass only a small amount of urine each time. The need to urinate often is called urinary frequency. The resident may not be able to hold the urine after feeling the urge to void. The sudden, strong urge to urinate is called urinary urgency. Although these problems can occur in any elderly person, they are more common in women.

Many elderly men have difficulty in starting to urinate. This problem may be caused by the prostate gland, which tends to enlarge and cause constriction of the urethra. Male residents will be able to urinate easier if they are in a standing position. Using measures to stimulate urination may be helpful. These measures may be included in the resident's care plan.

material from the blood to produce urine. The urine flows from the kidneys, through the ureters, to the bladder, where it is stored until it is eliminated. The average adult bladder can hold about 1000 cc of urine. When it contains about 350 cc, the brain sends a signal that causes the urge to void (urinate). Urine flows from the bladder, through the urethra, to the outside of the

Nursing Measures to Stimulate Urination.

Sometimes a resident may have difficulty urinating. Water can be an effective tool to use in solving this problem. Have you ever noticed that you usually feel the urge to urinate while you are running water in the tub? Measures used to stimulate urination include turning on the faucet, placing the resident's fingers in warm water, or pouring warm water over the genitals. Offering a drink of water may also help.

Elderly residents may need to urinate several times during the night. This is called nocturia. Nocturia can interfere with rest and sleep and may result in incontinence. Staff members who work the night shift should check frequently to see if a resident needs to go to the bathroom.

The Effects of Urinary Incontinence.

Although elderly residents may be incontinent, it is not a normal change of aging. The changes of aging do, however, contribute to urinary incontinence, because they make it more difficult to control elimination. Other causes of incontinence include

- Disease
- Confusion
- Medications
- Failure to toilet frequently

While incontinence affects everyone who is involved, the impact on the resident can be devastating. It can have physical, emotional, and social effects. Incontinence is a major cause of skin breakdown because urine provides a warm, moist environment for pathogens, which may attack the skin or lead to a urinary tract infection. It is difficult to maintain healthy skin when a person is frequently wet with urine.

Emotional effects of incontinence include feelings of embarrassment, shame, anger, and frustration. The loss of urinary control can damage self-esteem. Depression is not uncommon. The resident may withdraw and avoid social activities, for fear of "having an accident."

Family relationships may suffer. Incontinence makes it more difficult to take the resident out of the facility for family visits.

In many cases, incontinence is the reason for long-term care placement. The family may become unable to cope with the physical and emotional demands. As a result, they may feel frustration, guilt, or failure.

Urinary incontinence also affects health care workers. Caring for an incontinent resident is time consuming and the resident may be incontinent several times a day. It is difficult for the nursing assistant to remain organized. No matter how well you have planned your time, or how much you have to do, an incontinent resident becomes a priority. Preventing incontinence benefits everyone.

Urinary incontinence presents a challenge to infection control. Follow universal precautions and wear gloves when handling soiled linen. Immediate attention should be given to urine spills. Constant effort is necessary to prevent odors and maintain a clean, pleasant environment.

Many times incontinence can be prevented. Offering toileting at regular intervals helps to establish a routine. Explain to the resident and encourage cooperation. Answer call signals promptly, because the elderly resident may not be able to wait. Check your residents frequently to see if they need to go to the bathroom.

Confused residents present a challenge. They may not be able to tell you when they need to urinate or have a bowel movement. If they are ambulatory, they may not be able to locate the bathroom. Remember, it is easier to toilet the resident than to change linen and clothing. Observe carefully for signs that the resident might need to go to the bathroom. These signs include

- Restlessness
- Fidgeting
- Pulling at clothes or undressing
- Holding or pointing at the genitals
- Crying

If incontinence is a temporary result of an illness or medication, the problem may be relieved by treating the illness or changing the medication. Long-term urinary incontinence is usually managed by restorative bladder retraining. That program is explained later in this chapter. Measures to use in treating incontinence are included in the resident's plan of care.

The resident who is incontinent must be changed immediately. If the bed is wet, the linen will need to be removed. Place a bath blanket under the resident, while you are bathing. Wear gloves and use aseptic technique to clean the wet area of the skin with soap and water. Rinse and dry well. Wiping the urine with a dry towel, without washing it well, leaves microorganisms and chemicals on the skin.

Urinary Tract Infection. A urinary tract infection (UTI) results when pathogens enter the urinary system. UTI is more common in women, because the opening of the urinary system is close to the opening of the rectum. The female bladder is also nearer to the outside of the body.

A urinary tract infection may occur because of improper cleansing of the perineal area. Always cleanse from the urinary meatus to the anus, when performing perineal care. If this procedure is not done correctly, pathogens from the rectal area may be brought forward to the urinary tract.

Most urinary tract infections can be prevented by practicing aseptic technique at all times, and by changing the incontinent resident immediately.

Urinary Catheters

A urinary catheter is a tube that is inserted through the urethra, into the bladder to drain urine. A catheter may be inserted temporarily and then removed after the bladder is drained. Another type of catheter is left in place to drain urine continuously. A urinary catheter that is left in place is called a **Foley catheter** or an indwelling catheter. The nurse inflates a balloon on one end of the catheter with sterile water (see Fig. 23-8). The balloon is inside the bladder and keeps the catheter in place. The other end of the catheter is attached to a drainage bag.

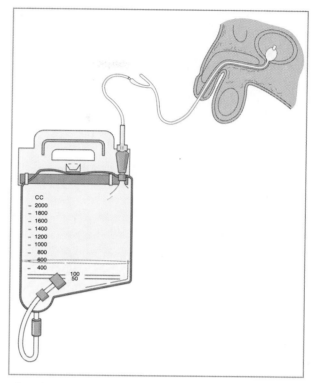

Fig. 23-8 A balloon is inflated to hold the urinary catheter in place.

Nursing Care. Urinary catheterization is a procedure that is performed by a nurse or doctor and requires a doctor's order. Nursing assistants do not insert catheters. Special precautions are necessary when caring for a resident with a Foley catheter. The drainage bag must always be kept below the level of the bladder. Urine drains from the bladder to the drainage bag, by gravity. If the bag is higher than the bladder, contaminated urine from the bag may return to the bladder and cause an infection.

It is important to keep the catheter and drainage tubing free of kinks or pressure. A kink in the tubing will obstruct the flow of urine. Be careful, when assisting a resident to move, that you do not kink the tubing or pull on the catheter. Remember, it is held in place by a small balloon. Too much tension will cause discomfort or pull out the catheter.

Urinary drainage systems should be left closed and connected as much as possible to prevent infection. Any time the catheter is disconnected from the drainage tubing, contamination may occur. Report any leaks in the drainage system. If urine can get out, germs can enter through the same opening.

The drainage bag should be attached to the bed frame when the resident is in bed (see Fig. 23-9). Never attach the bag to the side rail or any other moving part of the bed. Do not allow the bag or tubing to touch the floor.

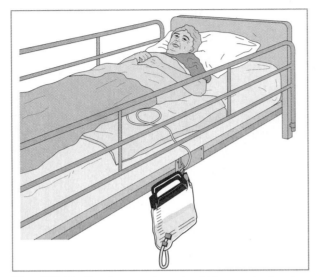

Fig. 23-9 The drainage bag should be attached to the bedframe.

If the resident is in a wheelchair, the drainage bag is attached to the chair, below the level of the bladder. Many facilities have covers available for the bag. Having a Foley catheter should not interfere with mobility. The drainage bag does not have to be disconnected for ambulation.

Urinary Leg Bags. Some residents may feel more comfortable with a leg bag. This is a small drainage bag that is worn on the upper leg. It may be held in place by a Velcro® band (see Fig. 23-10). If the resident is to wear a leg bag, it will be indicated in the care plan.

The risk of infection is increased when a leg bag is used. It holds a smaller amount of urine and must be emptied more often. Each time it is emptied, the urinary tract is exposed to infection. Care must be taken to prevent contamination of the catheter and urinary drainage tubing. Follow facility policy and procedure in changing to and from the use of a leg bag.

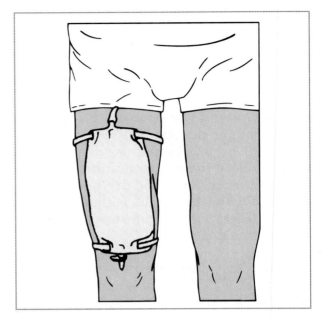

Fig. 23-10 A urinary drainage leg bag.

Providing Catheter Care. A tube placed into the body creates an entry for germs. Using aseptic technique helps to prevent infection. The resident with a Foley needs special cleansing of the perineal area. This procedure is called catheter care. The catheter care procedure begins with pericare. Before you touch the catheter, the perineal area needs to be as clean as possible.

A catheter care kit may be used to perform catheter care. These kits may contain antiseptic, swabs, cotton balls, and disposable gloves. The most common method is washing with soap and water. Follow the policy of your facility. Although catheter care procedures vary, the principles remain the same. The principles of catheter care include the following:

- Wear gloves and follow universal precautions.
- Wash away from the urinary meatus.
- Use a different part of the washcloth or a separate wipe, for each stroke.

Equipment and Supplies. The equipment and supplies needed to perform catheter care include a protective pad, towel, washcloths, soap, bath basin, gloves, catheter care kit (optional), and solution (optional).

PROCEDURE

Providing Catheter Care

Before any procedure you must always follow the five basic steps: wash your hands, collect the equipment, identify the resident, explain the procedure, and protect privacy.

Follow universal precautions and wear gloves when appropriate.

1. Raise the bed to a correct working height and lock the brakes.
2. Raise the side rail on the opposite side, and lower the rail on the side nearest you.
3. Assist the resident to a supine position with the legs separated and the knees bent, if possible.
4. Place a protective pad or towel under the resident's buttocks, and drape as you would for perineal care.
5. Put on disposable gloves.
6. Perform perineal care, following the procedure found in the personal care chapter.
7. Check carefully for dried secretions.
8. Using a clean washcloth, wash the catheter for three or four inches, beginning at the urinary meatus and washing away from it (see Fig. 23-11).
9. Rinse and dry the tubing thoroughly.
10. Make sure there are no kinks in the tubing.
11. Raise the side rail.
12. Empty, rinse, and dry the basin.
13. Remove the gloves and wash your hands.
14. Return equipment and supplies to the proper location.
15. Remove the bath blanket, after covering the resident with the top linen.
16. Lower the bed and position the side rails as required.
17. Be sure the resident is comfortable and place the call signal within reach.
18. Wash your hands.

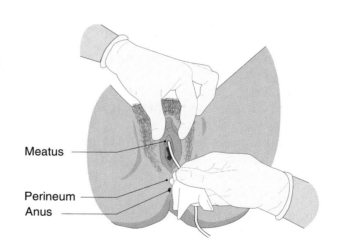

Meatus

Perineum

Anus

Fig. 23-11 Wash the catheter for three or four inches, beginning at the urinary meatus.

External Catheter. The doctor may order an external catheter for the incontinent male resident. An external catheter (Texas catheter) is a soft rubber sheath that is applied over the penis (see Fig. 23-12). A tube leading from the sheath, connects to a urinary drainage bag. The external catheter may have an adhesive tape attached to it. There is less chance of infection with this device, and it is more comfortable.

However, the external catheter can present problems. It can irritate the skin or interfere with circulation if not applied correctly. An inch of space must be left between the end of the catheter and the tip of the penis. When tape is used it is applied spirally, and must not completely encircle the penis (see Fig. 23-12). Care must be taken not to interfere with circulation or urinary output. There are many different types of external catheters that are kept in place by various methods. Follow the procedural steps used in your facility.

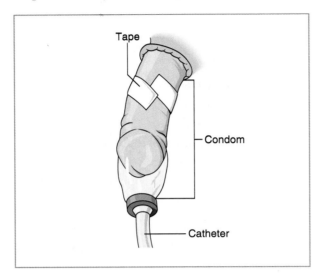

Fig. 23-12 An external urinary catheter must be applied and taped correctly.

GUIDELINES FOR ASSISTING THE RESIDENT WITH AN EXTERNAL CATHETER

- Follow universal precautions and wear disposable gloves.
- Provide perineal care.
- Roll the catheter onto the penis, leaving an inch of space at the end.
- Apply tape spirally and do not completely encircle the penis with tape.
- Attach the catheter to drainage tubing and bag.

The external catheter should be changed daily, and as often as needed. To change the catheter, remove the tape and roll the sheath off the penis. Observe for skin irritation.

Emptying the Urinary Drainage Bag. The urinary drainage bag is emptied at the end of every shift, and the amount of urine measured is recorded on the intake and output record. **Intake and output (I&O)** includes all fluids that are taken into the body and all fluids that are eliminated. Empty the urine bag into a **graduate** (a container used to measure fluids). Do not use the measurements on the side of the drainage bag as they may not be accurate.

GUIDELINES FOR EMPTYING A URINARY DRAINAGE BAG

- Follow universal precautions and wear disposable gloves.
- Empty the drainage bag into a graduate (see Fig. 23-13).
- Do not allow the drain to touch the inside of the graduate.
- Do not allow the drainage bag to touch the floor.
- Replace the closed clamp in the holder.
- Record output immediately.

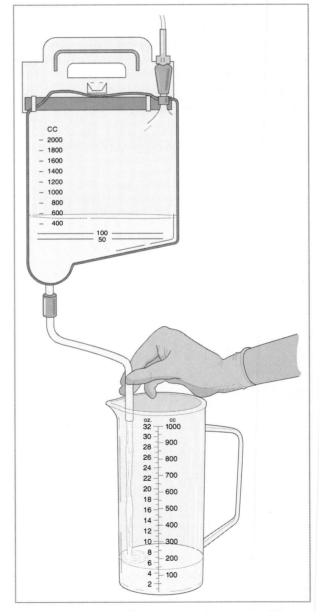

Fig. 23-13 Empty the urine directly into a graduate.

Check the amount of urine in the drainage bag frequently. Although this does not give you an accurate measurement, it allows you to observe if urinary output has decreased or increased. If it fills before the end of the shift, empty and measure the urine. Record this information and notify the nurse. When you make rounds to check on your residents at the beginning of your shift, carefully observe those with catheters. Make sure that the bag has been emptied and the tubing is free of kinks. Refer to the section in Chapter 22 entitled "Maintaining Fluid Balance" for a thorough description of the procedure for intake and output.

Restorative Bladder Retraining

Restorative bladder retraining is a program that is used to prevent incontinence and to restore urinary elimination to as near normal as possible. It involves establishing a routine of emptying the bladder at regular intervals. An individual plan of retraining is developed for each resident in the program. Successful retraining requires the cooperation of staff members and the resident. Be sure that the resident understands what the staff will be doing and what is expected. Close observation by the staff will be necessary during the retraining period.

Restorative bladder retraining is basically a four-step program. These steps are:

1. Determining normal voiding habits
2. Establishing a regular routine
3. Evaluating results
4. Adjusting the routine as necessary

Determining Normal Voiding Habits. The first step is to determine the resident's normal pattern of voiding. The need to empty the bladder varies from person to person. Some people can go all day without urinating, while others must use the bathroom every two or three hours. It is important that the plan meets the resident's personal needs. Think about your own habits. Do you need to go to the bathroom every

three or four hours? If so, what would happen if you were asked to wait until the end of your shift?

The resident's normal urinary pattern is determined by careful observation and recording. Usually, the resident's voiding will be checked every two hours for one week. If the resident is frequently incontinent at the two-hour checks, one-hour checks will be necessary. A special form is provided to record information that is collected (see Fig. 23-14). Recording is done every two hours, indicating whether the resident has voided, is dry, or is incontinent. Correct abbreviations to be used in recording are listed on the form. The only way to determine the urinary pattern correctly is by accurate recording. The staff must be consistent on every shift during the observation period.

Establishing a Regular Routine. The second step of a bladder retraining program is to establish a routine. This is based on the resident's normal pattern of voiding that was determined in step 1. For example, if a resident voids approximately every two hours, toileting would be offered every two hours. Fluids are increased and the resident is encouraged to try to urinate each time. Although the resident is encouraged to go to the bathroom for urination, bladder retraining can be accomplished using a bedpan or bedside commode, if necessary. Once the routine is established, it becomes a part of the resident's plan of care.

Evaluation. The retraining program is usually continued for six to eight weeks. Evaluation of the results is an ongoing process. Some people respond more quickly than others. If the plan has not succeeded at the end of two months, retraining may be discontinued temporarily.

Adjusting the Routine. Changes in the routine are made as often as necessary. For example, an extra voiding may be necessary after lunch, or when the resident first wakes up in the morning. If incontinence continues to occur prior to scheduled toileting, shorter intervals may be established to prevent it. If the goal of the bladder training is for the resident to be able to hold urine for a longer time, the routine may be changed to every three hours.

Factors that affect the success of restorative bladder retraining include:

- Toilet residents as soon as they ask.
- Use methods to stimulate urination as needed.
- Build trust, so the resident can depend on you.
- Be consistent—24 hours a day, 7 days a week.
- Maintain a positive attitude—your belief in retraining will help the resident to believe in it.
- Establish and maintain accurate recording procedures.

Proper recording is necessary if the program is to succeed. It shows whether or not the retraining is effective. It also indicates changes that are needed in the resident's plan of retraining. The nursing assistant plays an important role in restorative bladder retraining. You make observations that help to determine the normal voiding pattern. Your duties include answering call signals and assisting the resident with toileting. It is often your attitude that influences the resident's attitude. When you are assigned a resident who is on bladder retraining, their schedule must be a priority as you organize your work. Regardless of the resident's response to retraining, you must be aware of his or her need for urinary elimination. You will help to prevent incontinence by toileting the resident according to the established schedule.

Special Situations. The resident with an indwelling catheter (Foley) may also be on a restorative bladder program. In this case, the goal is to remove the catheter and prevent incontinence. The catheter may be clamped for a period of time, so that urine will not drain. The clamp would be opened at specific times to allow the bladder to empty. The nursing assistant may be asked to clamp or unclamp the catheter. Report

RESIDENT VOIDING CHART

Week of:_____ Resident's Name:_____ Room No:_____

Code: [I] in red—Incontinent   [V] in black—Voided   [NV] in black—Dry, Unable to Void

Day of Week and Date	7 AM	8 AM	9 AM	10 AM	11 AM	12 N	1 PM	2 PM	3 PM	4 PM	5 PM	6 PM	7 PM	8 PM	9 PM	10 PM	11 PM	12 M	1 AM	2 AM	3 AM	4 AM	5 AM	6 AM
	7 AM	8 AM	9 AM	10 AM	11 AM	12 N	1 PM	2 PM	3 PM	4 PM	5 PM	6 PM	7 PM	8 PM	9 PM	10 PM	11 PM	12 M	1 AM	2 AM	3 AM	4 AM	5 AM	6 AM

Fig. 23-14 A sample bladder retraining record.

any complaints of pain or discomfort to the nurse. Remember, while the catheter is clamped, urine cannot drain from the bladder. Clamping and unclamping the catheter as scheduled will prevent injury to the bladder, which could occur from overfilling. Wear gloves and follow universal precautions when performing this procedure.

Bowel Elimination

The digestive system breaks down the food that is eaten into a form that the body can use. It also provides for the elimination of wastes by peristalsis. **Peristalsis** is the muscular contractions that push food through the digestive system. Most of the food is digested in the small intestine, where nutrients are absorbed through the villi, into the bloodstream. The nutrients are delivered, by the bloodstream, to all the cells. Waste material, fluid, and undigested food continue through the digestive system for elimination. This material is called feces, bowel movement, or BM. The act of eliminating solid wastes is called **defecation**.

When waste material reaches the **colon** (large intestine), it is mostly liquid. The purpose of the colon is to remove water from the feces for the body's use. Feces is stored in the rectum until nerve receptors

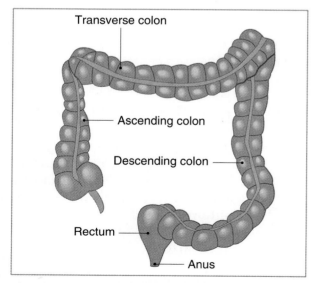

Fig. 23-15 The colon (large intestine).

- Transverse colon
- Ascending colon
- Descending colon
- Rectum
- Anus

signal the urge for defecation. Feces is eliminated from the body through the anus (the outer opening of the rectum). Normally, defecation takes place once every day or two. Feces should be soft formed and brown colored. Let the nurse know if the stool is too soft or too hard or has an unusual color. Always report the presence of blood in the stool or during defecation. Bowel elimination is affected by diet, fluid intake, exercise, and medication.

Diet and Bowel Elimination. Drinking adequate fluids and eating a well-balanced diet help to promote proper bowel elimination. Water and other fluids are necessary to keep the stool soft formed and the body well hydrated. Some foods, like beans or cabbage, produce **flatus** (gas or air expelled from the digestive system).

Common Problems of Bowel Elimination

Constipation. The most common problem of bowel elimination is constipation. **Constipation** is the passage of hard, dry stool. Hard, dry stool collects in the rectum, because it cannot pass easily through the anus. A person who is constipated has to strain to have a bowel movement, which may cause pain or bleeding from the rectum.

Constipation can be caused by any of the following:

- Poor fluid intake
- Lack of exercise
- Eating the wrong foods
- Ignoring the urge to defecate
- Medication
- Disease

Many elderly people suffer from constipation. It can be caused by any of the situations listed above or may be related to some of the changes of aging. Peristalsis slows, allowing the colon to absorb more water from the stool. The result is hard, dry feces.

Constipation may be treated with laxatives, suppositories, or enemas. However, the best plan is to prevent constipation.

Restorative methods to prevent constipation include the following:

- Increase fluid intake.
- Increase activity and exercise.
- Offer foods that stimulate peristalsis, such as whole-grain cereals.
- Answer call signals promptly, and assist the resident as needed.
- Observe and record bowel movements, noting color, amount, and consistency (hard or soft).
- Remind the resident to toilet as needed.

The methods used to prevent constipation will be included on the resident's care plan. Let the nurse know if you have any suggestions that might be added to the plan.

Constipation that is not relieved can result in an impaction. A **fecal impaction** is a large amount of hard, dry stool. It is often too large to be expelled from the rectum. The resident with a fecal impaction may complain of pain or nausea. The abdomen may appear swollen and hard. Smears of stool may be noticed on clothing or linen. Dark liquid feces may leak from the anus. Don't assume that the resident has diarrhea, as it may be liquid stool going around the large mass of solid stool. An impaction may affect urinary elimination because of pressure exerted on the bladder by the mass of stool. Always report these signs and symptoms to the nurse. Impaction is a serious complication that may completely block the bowel and prevent elimination of wastes. Enemas may be given for a fecal impaction, or it may have to be manually removed by the nurse.

Diarrhea. **Diarrhea** is loose, watery stool. It occurs when peristalsis pushes food too rapidly through the intestines. This results in insufficient time for the colon to absorb water, leaving the feces very watery. Diarrhea can be caused by food, medication, infection, or other diseases. Diarrhea can be very serious for the frail, elderly resident. The rapid loss of water from the body can result in dehydration. Diarrhea requires immediate medical attention to find the cause and treat the condition.

The resident with diarrhea will need to defecate frequently and urgently. Bowel incontinence may occur. Answer call lights promptly, and provide toileting when needed. Thorough cleansing of the rectal and perineal area is important to prevent skin damage. Empty bedpans immediately to reduce odor and prevent the spread of infection. Wear gloves whenever there is a possibility of contact with feces, and use aseptic technique at all times. Report each occurrence of diarrhea to the nurse. Note the time, amount, and frequency of the diarrhea.

Fecal Incontinence. Fecal incontinence is the inability to control bowel movements. It can be caused by poor muscle tone, a change in peristalsis, or nervous system damage. Confusion is frequently the cause of incontinence in the elderly resident. Confused residents may not be able to understand and respond correctly to the urge to defecate. They may not be aware that the need to empty the rectum has been signaled.

Fecal incontinence can cause skin breakdown and urinary tract infection. Feelings of embarrassment, guilt, and depression may result. The resident who cannot control bowel movements often feels as if life were out of control.

An illness, such as infectious diarrhea, may cause temporary incontinence. Usually, the incontinence stops when the illness is brought under control. Long-term fecal incontinence is best treated by restorative bowel retraining.

Restorative Bowel Retraining

The goal of restorative bowel retraining is to prevent fecal incontinence, constipation, and other bowel problems. The retraining program usually includes increased activity, adequate fluid intake, and a high-fiber diet. Residents are encouraged to go to the bathroom for defecation, if possible. They should sit as upright as possible, to assist in complete emptying of the rectum.

Although each bowel retraining program is individualized, the general steps are as follows:

- Evaluate bowel function.
- Normalize stool consistency.
- Determine the regular pattern of elimination.
- Establish a schedule.
- Stimulate the bowel to empty on schedule.

Evaluate Bowel Function. Bowel function is evaluated to determine the cause of incontinence. This information is used to plan the steps to be taken in retraining.

Normalize Stool Consistency. Successful retraining will not be possible until the consistency of the stool is normal. Feces should be soft formed. Constipation or diarrhea will interfere with retraining.

BOWEL HABIT ASSESSMENT SHEET

Resident's Name_____ Room Number:_____

CHECK OFF OR FILL IN THE APPROPRIATE RESPONSE

1. Frequency of defecation:

    _____Daily   _____Varies
    _____Every other day   _____Unknown
    _____Every third day   _____Other_____

2. Usual time of defecation:

    Give hour, if known _____AM   _____PM
    _____Several times a day
    _____Varies
    _____Unknown
    _____Other_____

3. Usual place of defecation:

    _____Toilet   _____Bedpan
    _____Commode   _____Incontinent

4. Consistency of stool:

    _____Hard   _____Soft   _____Liquid

5. Size of stool:

    _____Large   _____Medium   _____Small

6. Fluid intake:

    _____Good   _____Fair   _____Poor

7. Eating habits:

    _____Good   _____Fair   _____Poor

8. Amount of exercise:

    _____Ambulate   _____Range of motion
    _____Sits in chair   _____None
    _____Other

Fig. 23-16 A sample bowel retraining record.

Determine the Pattern of Bowel Elimination. Some people have a bowel movement every morning or every evening. Others may defecate every other day. The resident may use coffee, tea, hot water, or prune juice to regulate bowel movements.

Establish a Schedule. It is important to build on the routine that is already established. For example, if the resident usually defecates in the morning, after drinking a hot cup of coffee, that should be a part of the retraining program. If a resident has an irregular pattern of elimination, a regular routine will be planned. This may involve establishing a schedule of defecation every morning, after breakfast.

Stimulate the Bowel to Empty on Schedule. The bowel may be stimulated by using a combination of stool softeners, laxatives, suppositories, or enemas. Although the nurse is responsible for carrying out the treatment, you may be asked to assist.

Bowel retraining may take several weeks to accomplish. It is difficult to evaluate the results, because bowel elimination may take place only once every day or two. The nursing assistant can help to make restorative bowel retraining successful. Develop a positive attitude, and let the resident know that you believe it will work. Remember, your expectation of success will help the resident to feel more confident.

Offer fluids frequently, and encourage the resident to eat foods that create bulk. Provide prune juice, orange juice, coffee, and tea as desired, if allowed on the resident's diet. Encourage ambulation and activity. Suggest that the resident attend exercise programs, whenever possible. Provide range-of-motion exercises for residents who have limited mobility.

Assist the resident with toileting at regular intervals and encourage the resident to go to the bathroom, whenever possible. Be alert for signs that indicate a need for defecation. The resident may complain of fullness or abdominal cramps. Nonverbal clues include perspiration, goose pimples, holding the abdomen, frowning and straining movements, crying, or restlessness. Offer toileting immediately, if any of these signs are present.

Sometimes the bowels cannot be retrained. However, careful planning can prevent fecal incontinence, most of the time. This type of plan is called bowel management. Toileting is offered at regular intervals, according to the resident's normal pattern. Assist the resident to follow this schedule.

As in any restorative program, reporting and documenting are vital. Your facility may use a special form for recording (see Fig. 23-16 on page 355). Always record amount, frequency, and consistency of the stool. The information you provide is used in evaluating and changing the plan of care.

Enemas

An **enema** is the introduction of fluid into the rectum and colon. Enemas are used to remove feces and cleanse the lower bowel. Some X-ray tests require the bowel to be cleansed. The doctor may order an enema to relieve constipation or an impaction. The two basic types of enemas are cleansing enemas and commercially prepared enemas.

Cleansing Enemas. A cleansing enema must be prepared before it is given. The doctor orders the type of solution to use. The solution may be plain tap water (1,000 cc), soap suds (1,000 cc water and 5 cc liquid soap), or saline (1,000 cc water and 2 teaspoons salt). The water temperature for the enema solution should be 105°F or 40.5°C.

Most facilities have disposable enema kits. The kit usually contains an enema bag, tubing with a clamp and a bed protector. Some kits may contain a package of liquid soap or salt. If the tubing is not already lubricated, a lubricant will be necessary. A bedpan and toilet paper will be needed.

PROCEDURE

Giving a Cleansing Enema

Before any procedure you must always follow the five basic steps: wash your hands, collect the equipment, identify the resident, explain the procedure, and protect privacy.

Follow universal precautions and wear gloves when appropriate.

1. Close the door and pull the privacy curtain.
2. Raise the bed to a comfortable working height and lock the wheels.
3. Raise the side rail on the opposite side, and lower the rail on the side nearest you.
4. Assist the resident into the left-sided Sims' position (see Fig. 23-17A), and cover with a bath blanket.
5. Place an IV pole beside the bed, and raise the side rail.
6. Clamp the tubing on the enema tube, and prepare the solution that is ordered to 105°F or 40.5°C.
7. Allow a small amount of solution to run through the tubing. Clamp the tubing.
8. Hang the enema bag on the IV pole with the tubing at the bottom. Make sure that the enema bag is no more than 18 inches above the bed or 12 inches above the anus (see Fig. 23-17B).
9. Wash your hands and put on disposable gloves.
10. Lower the side rail, and uncover the resident enough to expose the anus.
11. Place the disposable bed protector under the resident's buttocks. Place the bedpan close to the resident's body.
12. Lubricate four inches of the tip of the enema tubing.
13. Ask the resident to breathe deeply during the procedure, to help relieve cramps.
14. With one hand, lift the upper buttock to expose the anus. With the other hand, insert the tip of the tubing into the rectum (see Fig. 23-17C).
15. Rotate the tubing two to four inches into the rectum. Stop if you feel resistance, or the resi-

dent complains of pain. If this happens, clamp the tubing and call the nurse.
16. Allow the solution to flow slowly into the rectum. If the resident complains of cramping, clamp the tubing and stop for a minute or so. Encourage the resident to take as much of the solution as possible.
17. When the solution is almost gone, clamp the tubing, and remove the tip from the rectum. Place the tip of the tubing into the empty enema bag. Do not let it contaminate you or the linens.
18. Ask the resident to hold the solution as long as possible.
19. Assist the resident onto the bedpan or bedside commode, or into the bathroom.
20. Place toilet paper and the call signal within reach. Ask the resident not to flush the toilet when finished.
21. Discard the disposable equipment, and clean up the area.
22. Remove your gloves and wash your hands.
23. If the resident can be left alone, leave the room for a few minutes. Remind the resident to use the call signal. Check back frequently.
24. When the resident is through, put on gloves and assist the resident to clean the perineal area and remove the bed protector. Assist the resident from the pan.
25. Empty the bedpan and observe the enema results for amount, color, and consistency. Clean the bedpan and put it away. Check the contents of the toilet, if the resident was in the bathroom.
26. Remove your gloves and wash your hands.
27. Assist the resident with handwashing.
28. Remove the bath blanket and make the resident comfortable. Open the privacy curtains. Place the call signal within reach.
29. Return equipment to its proper place.
30. Wash your hands.
31. Record your observations and report to the nurse.

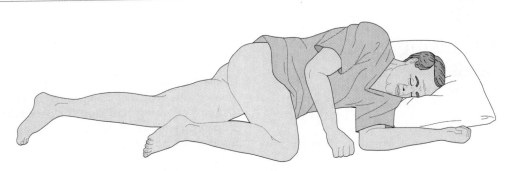

A Assist the resident onto the left side.

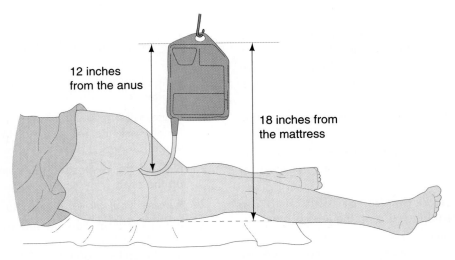

12 inches
from the anus

18 inches from
the mattress

B The enema bag should be no more than 18 inches from the bed
or 12 inches from the anus.

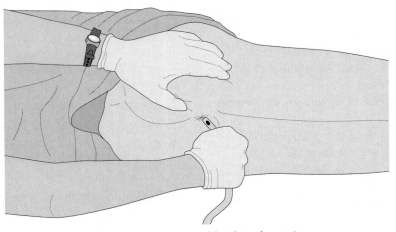

C Insert the tip of the tubing into the rectum.

Fig. 23-17 Giving a cleansing enema.

GENERAL GUIDELINES FOR GIVING A CLEANSING ENEMA

- Collect all equipment. Once you begin the procedure, you will not be able to leave the resident.
- Follow universal precautions and wear disposable gloves.
- Hold the tubing in place while giving the enema.
- Usually 750–1,000 cc is given.
- If the resident complains of cramps, close the clamp and wait a few minutes before resuming the enema. Remind the resident to breathe deeply through the mouth.
- Report to the nurse if the resident is unable to hold the solution or does not release all the solution that has been given.

Many long-term care facilities do not allow nursing assistants to give cleansing enemas. It is your responsibility to know the policy where you work. The procedure for giving a cleansing enema is located on pages 357–358.

Equipment and Supplies. The equipment and supplies needed for a cleansing enema include an enema bag or can, solution bed protector, gloves, lubricant, toilet tissue, and a bedpan.

Commercially Prepared Enemas. The commercially prepared enema comes prepackaged and ready to use. The most common type is a disposable, plastic bottle filled with solution (Fig. 23-18A). The tip of the bottle is lubricated and inserted into the rectum. The bottle is squeezed and rolled from the bottom, until all the solution has been given. The directions for giving the enema are usually found on the con-

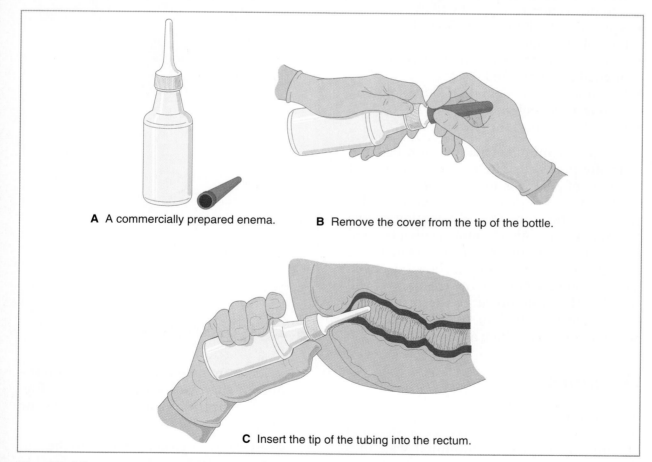

A A commercially prepared enema.

B Remove the cover from the tip of the bottle.

C Insert the tip of the tubing into the rectum.

Fig. 23-18 Using a commercially prepared enema.

tainer. Some facilities do not allow nursing assistants to give commercially prepared enemas. It is your responsibility to know the policy of the facility where you work.

Giving a commercially prepared enema is similar to the procedure for giving a cleansing enema. The steps for maintaining privacy, protecting bed linens, positioning, and asepsis are the same.

GUIDELINES FOR GIVING A COMMERCIALLY PREPARED ENEMA

- Collect your equipment before you begin.
- Follow universal precautions and wear disposable gloves.
- Position the resident on the left side.
- Remove the protective cover from the tip of the squeeze bottle (see Fig. 23-18B).
- Gently insert the lubricated tip two inches into the rectum (see Fig. 23-18C).
- Squeeze and roll the bottle from the bottom until all the solution is used.
- Place the squeeze bottle, tip first, into its original container, and discard.
- Encourage the resident to hold the solution as long as possible.
- Record and report the enema results.

The oil retention enema may also be commercially prepared. The primary purpose of this type of enema is to soften and lubricate stool. This makes defecation easier and helps relieve constipation. The oil retention enema is given like any other commercially prepared enema. The solution should be retained long enough for the oil to soften the stool. Even though you may not give the enema, you will care for the resident after the procedure. Encourage the resident to lie quietly and hold the solution as long as possible.

Ostomies

An **ostomy** is a surgical opening into the body. Some ostomies involve a surgical opening through the abdominal wall into the intestines or urinary tract. The mouth or opening of the ostomy is called a **stoma**. An ostomy is necessary when disease or injury

prevents normal elimination. An ostomy may be permanent or temporary and an appliance may be worn to collect the waste material. This may include a bag that fits over the stoma and supplies to keep the bag in place. There are many types of ostomy appliances (see Fig. 23-19). The type used depends on the size and location of the stoma, as well as personal preference. This information is a part of the resident's plan of care. Some ostomies do not require an appliance. A gauze or large Band-Aid® may be placed over the stoma.

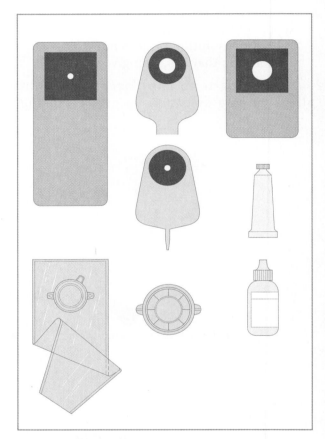

Fig. 23-19 Ostomy appliances.

The location of an ostomy depends on the location of the disease or injury (see Fig. 23-20). Examples of ostomies include the following:

- colostomy—a surgical opening into the colon
- ileostomy—a surgical opening into the ileum

- jejunostomy—a surgical opening into the jejunum
- ureterostomy—a surgical opening into a ureter

Note that the first part of the word indicates the location and the last part of the word indicates the procedure.

Psychosocial Considerations. The resident with an ostomy may have feelings of anxiety, embarrassment, and anger. Having an artificial opening in the body affects self-image. The change in body image can lead to depression and social withdrawal. These reactions will affect independence and self-esteem. This is especially true when the ostomy surgery was fairly recent. As time passes, most people adjust to the ostomy, both physically and emotionally. They usually learn to care for their own ostomy and continue to live normal lives.

As a nursing assistant, you can help the resident adjust to the ostomy. Be familiar with the problems listed in the care plan. Encourage the resident to express feelings, and listen attentively. Refer questions that you cannot answer to the nurse. Allow the resident to do as much of the ostomy care as possible. This helps build confidence and promote independence.

Colostomy. A **colostomy** is a surgical opening into the colon. A section of the colon is brought to the surface of the abdomen for defecation. Feces and flatus are eliminated from the body, through the stoma.

The consistency of feces from the colostomy depends on its location in the colon. Water is removed from the feces as it moves through the colon. If the colostomy is near the beginning of the colon, the feces will be watery. The nearer the colostomy is to the rectum, the more normal the feces will appear (see Fig. 23-21).

The colostomy appliance may develop an odor. Proper hygiene and asepsis help to eliminate unpleasant odors. Wear gloves and follow universal precautions when caring for the ostomy. The bag should be emptied every time soiling occurs. It should be cleaned or replaced immediately. Certain foods are gas forming. Because the escape of gas cannot be controlled, embarrassment may occur. The dietitian will work with the resident if that becomes a problem. Special deodorants may be available to place in the bag.

Be aware of your feelings while providing care for the resident with an otomy. Avoid facial expressions that indicate distaste for the procedure. The resident will be aware of your reactions. If you care for the ostomy in a comfortable manner, you will help the resident to feel more relaxed.

Colostomy Irrigation. Sometimes, a colostomy will need to be irrigated. This procedure is much like that of giving an enema. An irrigation might be given to treat constipation, cleanse the bowel, or regulate elimination. Ostomy irrigations are usually done by licensed nurses.

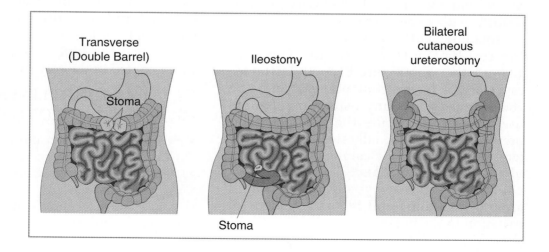

Fig. 23-20
Types of ostomies.

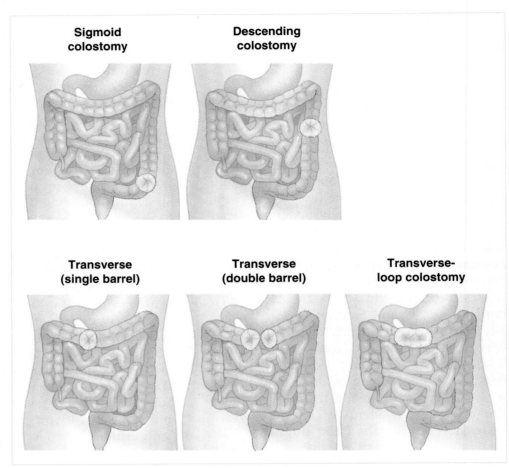

Sigmoid colostomy

Descending colostomy

Transverse (single barrel)

Transverse (double barrel)

Transverse-loop colostomy

Fig. 23-21
Examples of colostomy stoma locations.

Providing Colostomy Care. Colostomy care should be provided every time the resident has a bowel movement. The care might involve emptying and cleaning the bag, or it might include changing the entire appliance. Check with the nurse or the care plan to determine what care is necessary for each resident with a colostomy.

Providing skin care is very important for the resident with an ostomy. The skin around the stoma may become irritated, especially if bowel contents leak onto the abdominal skin. Many ostomy appliances use adhesive to secure the appliance and prevent leaking. The adhesive can also irritate the skin. Proper cleaning and emptying of the ostomy appliance help to prevent complications. Always observe the skin around the stoma and report any signs of irritation to the nurse.

The procedure for providing colostomy care depends upon the type of appliance that is used. A belt may be worn, with an attached bag that fits over the stoma. Sometimes, an adhesive wafer (see Fig. 23-22) is applied to the skin around the stoma. The bag is attached to the wafer. Some bags are emptied and discarded after each bowel movement. Others are emptied and cleaned each time. The type of appliance required will be noted in the care plan.

GENERAL GUIDELINES FOR PROVIDING COLOSTOMY CARE

- Follow universal precautions and wear gloves.
- Carefully and gently remove appliances that are applied to the skin.
- Empty and clean a reusable bag after each bowel movement.

- Observe the skin around the stoma for redness and irritation.
- Use lubricant, skin protector, or skin cream around the stoma, as ordered.
- Attach appliances securely to prevent leaking.
- Clean the reusable bag with soap and water.
- Fasten the clamp securely when you are finished.
- Observe the contents of the bag. Record and report as necessary.
- Wipe around the stoma with toilet tissue to remove feces. Use soap and water to clean around the stoma, unless otherwise ordered.
- Use the following steps to apply an adhesive wafer around the stoma (see Fig. 23-22).

    Step 1. Cut the hole in the center of the wafer 1/8 inch larger than the stoma (see Fig. 23-22A).

Step 2. Apply adhesive stoma paste around the stoma, as ordered.

Step 3. Peel the backing from the wafer (see Fig. 23-22B).

Step 4. Place wafer, adhesive side down, over the stoma.

Step 5. Attach a clean bag to the wafer (see Fig. 23-22C).

Bowel and bladder elimination are private and personal body functions. Privacy, infection control, and careful observation are very important restorative measures in urinary and bowel care. Sensitivity to the resident's emotional needs must be combined with thorough and consistent physical care to maintain healthy elimination for the elderly resident.

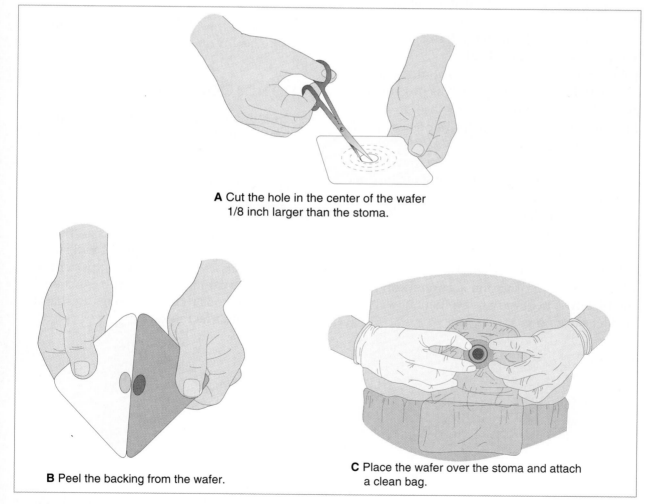

A Cut the hole in the center of the wafer 1/8 inch larger than the stoma.

B Peel the backing from the wafer.

C Place the wafer over the stoma and attach a clean bag.

Fig. 23-22 Applying an adhesive wafer around a colostomy stoma.

Conclusion

Remember these important points:

1. The resident should go to the bathroom for elimination, whenever possible.

2. Do not leave a weak or confused resident alone on the toilet or bedside commode.

3. Never restrain a resident to the toilet or bedside commode.

4. Empty and clean the bedpan and the urinal promptly after every use.

5. Incontinence affects the resident physically and emotionally.

6. The resident who is incontinent must be changed immediately.

7. Follow universal precautions and wear gloves when appropriate.

8. Always clean from the urinary meatus to the rectum.

9. Always keep the urinary drainage bag below the level of the bladder.

10. Urinary drainage systems should be left closed and connected as much as possible to prevent contamination.

11. Careful observation helps to prevent infection and other urinary problems.

12. Restorative bladder retraining involves establishing a routine of emptying the bladder at regular intervals.

13. Bowel and bladder retraining must be consistent, 24 hours a day, 7 days a week.

14. Constipation can often be prevented by increasing fluids and exercise.

15. Recording information accurately and completely is necessary to evaluate bowel and bladder retraining.

16. Encourage the resident who has had an enema to hold the solution as long as possible.

17. The resident may feel embarrassed or depressed about having an ostomy.

18. Ostomy care should be provided every time the resident has a bowel movement.

Discussion Questions

1. Why is it necessary to follow universal precautions when assisting the resident with elimination?

2. How does incontinence affect the resident? How would you feel if you were incontinent?

3. What should you do if the resident's Foley catheter isn't draining?

4. What does the nursing assistant's attitude have to do with the success of bowel or bladder retraining?

5. Why might it be difficult for a resident to adjust to having an ostomy?

Application Exercise

1. The students will role play, setting up a restorative bladder retraining program. The class will divide into two groups. One group will be nursing assistants, and the other group will act as residents. The instructor will assign a "resident" to each "nursing assistant." The "nursing assistant" will explain how the retraining works and will try to convince the "resident" that it will succeed. The class will share their experiences, including problems the "nursing assistants" had and methods that were used. "Residents" will share their feelings.

Specific Types of Care and Procedures

OBJECTIVES

Upon completing this chapter, you will be able to do the following:

1. List six guidelines for care of the resident receiving oxygen.

2. Identify four guidelines for cast care.

3. Describe three types of scales and their use.

4. Explain how to measure the resident's height.

5. Identify four general guidelines for collecting specimens.

6. List three guidelines for performing a sugar and acetone test.

7. List two purposes of a vaginal irrigation.

8. List four guidelines for applying elastic support hose.

9. Identify six general guidelines for heat and cold applications.

10. Perform the procedures described in this chapter, as allowed.

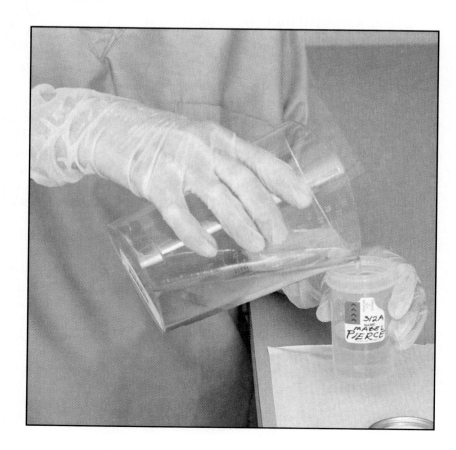

VOCABULARY

The following words or terms will help you to understand this chapter:

Oxygen	Fracture	Sputum	Expectorate
Dyspnea	Specimen	Stool	S&A test

This chapter contains procedures that are not done as part of routine care. In some facilities, they may be performed by licensed nurses. It is your responsibility to know your facility's policy in regard to these procedures.

Care of the Resident Receiving Oxygen

One of the main purposes of respirations is to obtain **oxygen** (a gas) from the air. Sometimes illness affects the balance of oxygen obtained and used by the body. The doctor may order additional oxygen for a resident who needs it. The method, rate, and length of oxygen administration are indicated in the doctor's order.

Nursing assistants may not begin, discontinue, or adjust the flow rate of oxygen. However, nursing assistants meet other special needs of residents receiving oxygen. Your observation and awareness of the resident and the environment, where oxygen is being administered, is important. In many facilities, nursing assistants are responsible for the care of oxygen equipment. Follow the policy of the facility where you work.

Oxygen may be administered from piped-in wall outlets, tanks, and concentrators. Many long-term care facilities depend upon oxygen tanks or concentrators to supply oxygen. Oxygen concentrators may look like small pieces of furniture. Inside the framework is equipment that pulls oxygen from the air and provides it to the resident in a concentrated form (see Fig. 24-1).

Because oxygen is very drying, it may be passed through moisture before reaching the resident. The device that provides moisture is a humidifier, in which oxygen bubbles

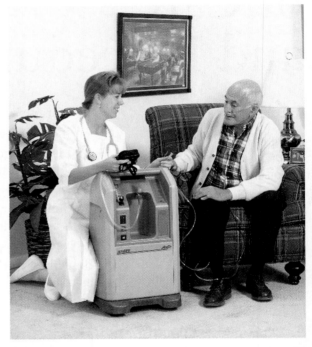

Fig. 24-1 An oxygen concentrator.

through water. The water level in the humidifier must be kept at proper levels (see Fig. 24-2).

Oxygen from tanks or wall outlets is regulated by a flow gauge. Although it may not be your responsibility to adjust the flow, your observation, awareness, and reporting of changes in the flow gauge are important to the resident's well-being. If a tank is used, be observant of the pressure gauge. This gauge indicates the amount of oxygen that remains in the tank, so that staff members will know when a new supply tank is needed. Follow the policy of your facility.

Many methods of oxygen administration are available. These include the mask, cannula (prongs), nasal catheter, and tent (see Fig. 24-2). The type of device to be used is ordered by the doctor. In an emergency, masks are usually used with a small portable

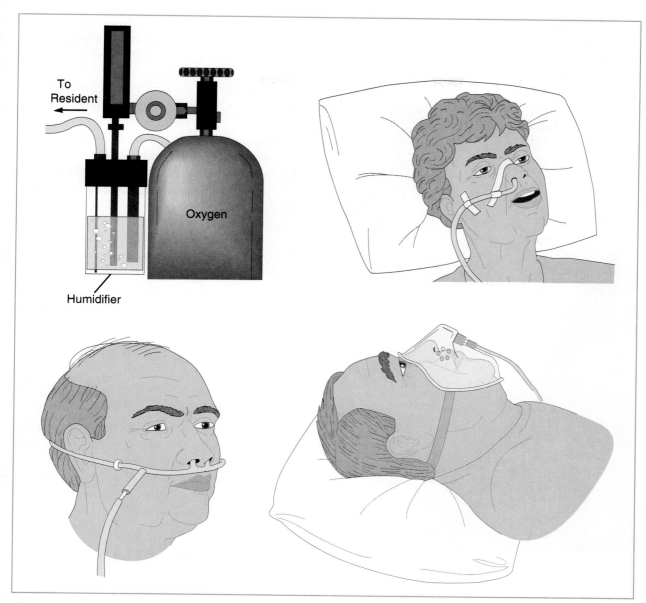

Fig. 24-2 Oxygen equipment.

canister of oxygen. This equipment is kept in a convenient location on each nursing unit. A humidifier is not usually necessary for short-term emergency use.

Because oxygen supports combustion, smoking materials are removed from the room. "No Smoking" signs are placed at the bedside and on the door of the resident's room. Check with the charge nurse before using any electrical equipment in the room. Wool blankets and fabrics that create static should be avoided. The resident and visitors must be advised of the safety precautions.

Universal precautions must be followed any time you are in contact with mucus, sputum, or other body fluids. Do not handle contaminated tissues without gloves. Provide the resident with a convenient container or bag for disposing of tissues. Always wash your hands after removing gloves, and assist the resident with handwashing.

The resident who requires oxygen administration has increased needs. **Dyspnea** (difficult or labored breathing) is tiring and uncomfortable. The resident may perspire heavily and may become too warm or too cool. Finding a comfortable position that eases breathing can be difficult. Dizziness may occur and interfere with safety. Check the care plan daily for changes or additions.

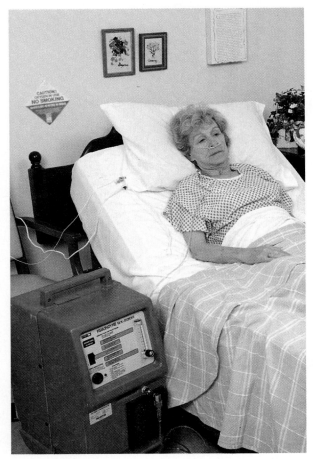

Fig. 24-3 It can be a challenge to meet the needs of the resident receiving oxygen.

Experiencing dyspnea is frightening. Even though the administration of oxygen is helpful, it can increase fear and cause discomfort. Maintaining the resident's independence, function, and comfort requires time, effort, and empathy.

GUIDELINES FOR ASSISTING THE RESIDENT WHO IS RECEIVING OXYGEN

- Recognize the resident's fear and suffering. Provide emotional support and reassurance as needed.
- Check on the resident frequently and spend as much time as possible.

- Recognize the resident's limitations of physical and emotional energy and strength.
- Activity may require frequent periods of rest.
- Frequent mouth care and lubrication are necessary. Oxygen dries the nose and mouth.
- Observe and relieve pressure on the skin or discomfort caused by oxygen devices.
- Frequent bathing, skin care, and clothing changes may be necessary due to perspiration.
- Adjust the room temperature and clothing as needed for the resident's comfort.
- An upright position often makes breathing easier (see Fig. 24-4).
- Allow the resident to sit on the side of the bed before standing to prevent dizziness.
- Observe for dizziness and weakness, and stay with resident as necessary.
- Observe and report changes in gauges and water level.
- Observe and report changes in the resident's condition.

Helping the resident who is receiving oxygen to maintain independence, while providing the assistance that is needed, can be challenging. You must remain very observant, aware, and sensitive to the resident's physical and emotional needs.

Care of the Resident with a Fracture

A **fracture** is a broken bone. Residents who have a fractured bone may be treated with a cast, splint, or traction. These treatments are used to immobilize (prevent movement of) the bone to promote proper healing. Restorative care is especially challenging, because residents who are immobilized are more dependent on others to meet their needs. Encourage the resident to be as active as possible.

The probability of skin problems increases when the resident has a fracture. Nutrition, elimination, and exercise may cause additional concern. It may be difficult to provide comfort. Always check with the

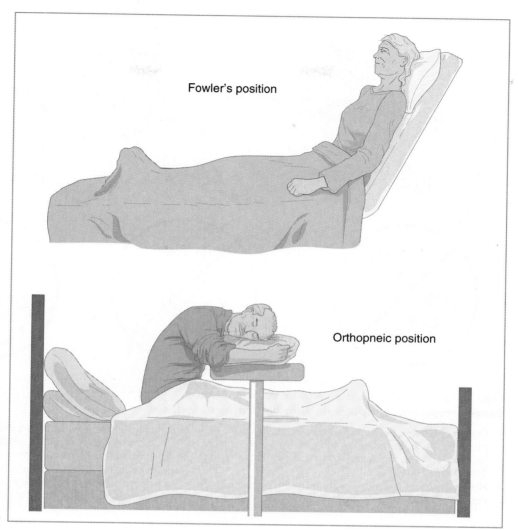

Fig. 24-4
An upright position makes breathing easier.

charge nurse and obtain specific directions before caring for a resident who has been immobilized. Check the care plan daily.

Residents who have hip fractures must not rotate the affected leg outward. The knee must be kept below the hip, and the resident is not allowed to bend more than 90° from the waist. A special pillow or cushion is used between the resident's legs to support the leg in an abducted position (away from the midline of the body). Always check with the charge nurse regarding movement and positioning of the resident with a hip fracture (see Fig. 24-5).

Casts, Splints, and Traction. All casts, splints, and traction require special care for positioning. Skin must be observed carefully for pressure that may result from the appliance or from immobilization. Nursing assis-

tants are not allowed to adjust traction equipment. Observation of equipment, body alignment, and skin problems is the responsibility of the nursing assistant. A new cast requires additional observation and care.

GUIDELINES FOR CAST CARE

- Elevate and support a casted extremity with pillows.
- Observe fingers and toes for color, swelling, or temperature changes that may indicate impaired circulation.
- If the resident complains of numbness, pain, or tingling, report this immediately to your charge nurse.
- Observe stains or color changes in the cast material. This may indicate bleeding or drainage inside the cast. Report these changes to the nurse.

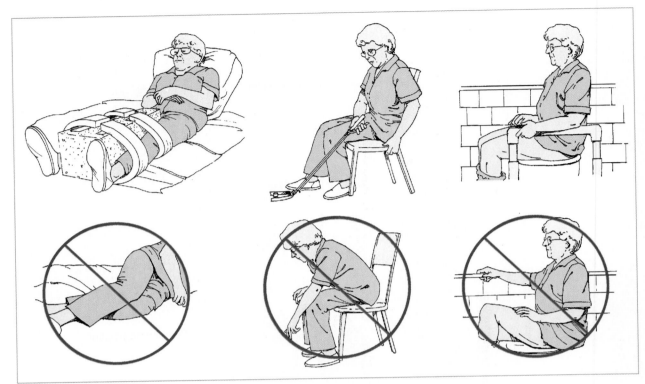

Fig. 24-5   Correct position for a resident with a hip fracture.
Some precautions for patients with hip fractures include:

- Use an abduction device to keep the fracture in the proper position. Do not allow the patient to lie on his or her side with legs together. Do not rotate or turn the operated leg outward.

- Have the patient use a device for reaching objects on the floor or shelves. Do not allow the patient to bend forward from the waist more than 90 degrees—to pull up blankets or socks, for example, or to tie shoes. Provide adaptive devices for these purposes.

- Have the patient sit in a high chair. Do not allow the patient to cross his or her legs or raise the knee on the affected side higher than the hip.

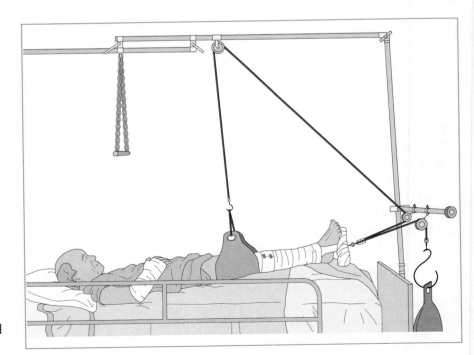

Fig. 24-6
Residents with casts, splints, and traction require special care.

- Wear gloves and follow universal precautions any time there is a possibility of contact with blood or drainage.
- Foul odor must be reported to the charge nurse.
- Taping or padding rough edges of the cast may be necessary. Report any problems to the charge nurse.
- Keep the cast dry.

Close observation may prevent complications and promote a smoother return to normal function.

Measuring the Resident's Weight

Residents are usually weighed on admission to a facility and regularly thereafter. Monthly weights are frequently the established routine. Sometimes the physician will order weight to be measured more often. Accuracy of measurement is important because weight changes may indicate progress or decline in the resident's condition. Nutritional status is also evaluated by weight measurement. Treatments and dietary changes may be ordered as a result of weight measurements.

GUIDELINES FOR ACCURATE WEIGHT MEASUREMENT

- The resident should be weighed at approximately the same time of day, wearing the same type of clothing.
- The resident should urinate before being weighed.
- Heavy clothing and shoes should be removed before weight is measured.
- Moving the scale as little as possible helps maintain accuracy.

Types of Scales. Residents are usually weighed on the standing balance scale or a bathroom scale. Other styles of scales are available that can be used for residents who are unable to stand. These include the bed scale, mechanical lift scale, chair scale, and wheelchair platform scales (see Fig. 24-7).

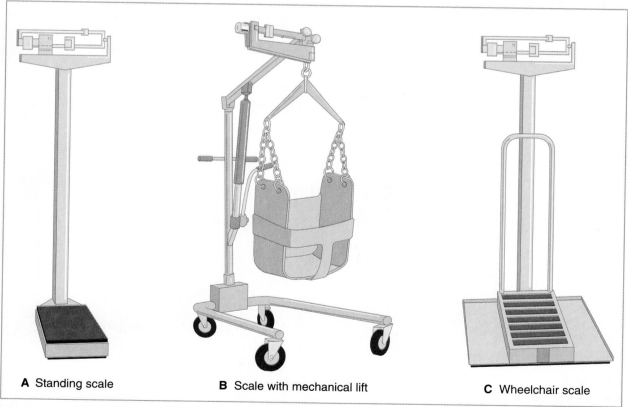

A Standing scale   **B** Scale with mechanical lift   **C** Wheelchair scale

Fig. 24-7 Types of scales.

The bed scale is a padded platform on wheels that can be adjusted to bed height. The resident is turned to the side of the bed, and the platform is placed on the bed behind the resident, who is then turned to a supine position on the scale. Usually, the scale is then raised above the bed for the weight to be taken. Facility policy should be followed to ensure infection control. This might include the use of clean linen between the resident and the platform. A disinfectant may be used between weight measurements.

The mechanical lift scale may be used to weigh residents who must be lifted to be transferred. After balancing the scale, follow the procedure for using a mechanical lift in Chapter 17. Place a clean sheet between the resident and the sling for infection control. When the resident's body is no longer touching the bed surface, adjust the weights to balance them, and note the weight measurement. Return the resident to bed following correct procedure. You may wish to review the procedure for using a mechanical lift in Chapter 17.

The chair scale allows a weak resident to sit while being weighed. This scale consists of an armed chair which is balanced on the weight mechanism. A footrest is attached to support the resident's feet.

The wheelchair platform scale allows the resident to be weighed without transferring from the wheelchair. The resident is wheeled onto the scale for weight measurement. The empty wheelchair must be weighed and its weight subtracted from the total weight of the resident and the chair. In some facilities the wheelchairs that are used with this type of scale have been weighed and a record is kept, so that the chair does not have to be weighed each time.

The standing balance scale requires a scale and clean paper towels. Clean paper towels are placed on the platform for each resident to stand on. This prevents the transmission of microorganisms between residents who are being weighed without shoes. Assist the resident to step on and off the scale. Do not leave the resident unattended while standing on the scale.

Before the resident steps on the scale, set both weights at zero (see Fig. 24-8). If the balance bar pointer is not in the middle of the designated area, the balance adjustment must be set. Some scales have a level bar with a bubble that must be floating in the center when balance is obtained.

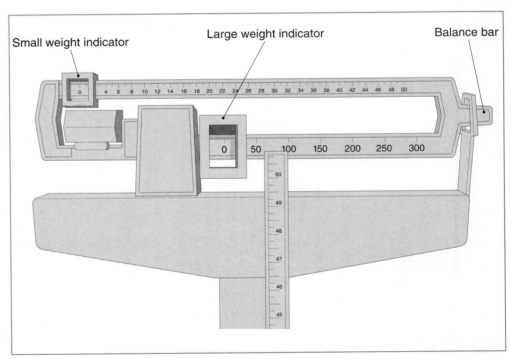

Fig. 24-8
The scale must be balanced before weighing the resident.

PROCEDURE

Using a Standing Balance Scale

Before any procedure you must always follow the five basic steps: wash your hands, collect the equipment, identify the resident, explain the procedure, and protect privacy.

1. Assist the resident to the scale.
2. Balance the scale, so that the balance bar is level.
3. Place clean paper towels on the platform.
4. Assist the resident to step out of shoes onto the center of the scale platform.
5. Adjust the weights until the scale is balanced.
6. Note the resident's weight.
7. Assist the resident off the scale, and into shoes.
8. Assure the resident's comfort and safety.
9. Dispose of paper towels and wash your hands.
10. Record the weight and report to the nurse.

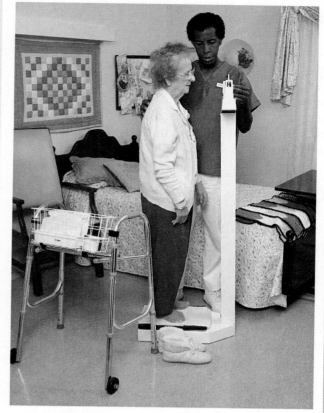

Fig. 24-9 Weighing the resident on the balance scale.

Measuring the Resident's Height

The height of the resident is usually measured on admission. If the resident is able to stand, you may use the height measurement rod that is attached to the standing balance scale. Raise the rod to a level above the resident's head, before assisting the resident onto the scale (see Fig. 24-9). After the weight is measured, ask the resident to stand very straight. Lower the height measurement device until it rests flat on the resident's head. Note the height and record it after the resident is comfortable and safe.

The rod measures the height in inches and fractions of inches. It is calibrated (marked) in 1/4-inch segments. You may be required to record the height in feet and inches. To convert a total number of inches to feet and inches, you must divide 12 into the total number of inches measured. (There are 12 inches in a foot.) The answer will be the number of feet, and the remainder will be the number of inches in the resident's height (see Fig. 24-10).

$$\begin{array}{r} 5 \text{ feet} \\ 12\overline{)62\ 1/2 \text{ inches}} \\ \underline{60} \\ 2\ 1/2 \text{ inches} \end{array}$$

ANSWER: 62 1/2 inches = 5 feet, 2 1/2 inches

Fig. 24-10 Converting inches to feet and inches.

Measuring Height for the Resident Who Cannot Stand. A resident's height may be measured in bed with a tape measure if standing is not possible. Flatten the bed and place the resident in a supine (back-lying) position. Place a mark on the sheet at the top of the head and another at the bottom of the feet. The distance between the marks is the resident's height.

If the resident has contractures and cannot lie in a straight position, a tape measure may be used to measure the height. Begin at the top of the head and continue to the base of the heel, following the curves of the spine and legs. All height measurements may be converted to feet and inches as explained previously.

Collecting Specimens

A **specimen** is a sample of material from the resident's body. Nursing assistants collect specimens of urine, feces, and **sputum** (mucus from the lungs). The purpose of collecting specimens is to identify and treat disease. Although collection procedures vary, certain guidelines apply to collecting any specimen.

GENERAL GUIDELINES FOR COLLECTING SPECIMENS

- Wear gloves and follow aseptic practices (see Fig. 24-11A).
- Identify and label the specimen accurately (see Fig. 24-11B).
- Use the correct specimen container.
- Follow the correct procedure for collecting each type of specimen.
- Take the labeled specimen to the designated area as soon as you have collected it.
- Record and report to the nurse.

In the hospital, most specimens are taken directly to the laboratory. However, in the long-term care facility, the specimens are usually taken to the nurse's station. Notify the charge nurse as soon as you collect the specimen, and take it to the designated area. Follow facility policy for packaging, storing, and labeling specimens.

ASEPTIC PRACTICES

- Use universal precautions.
- Wash your hands.
- Don't touch the inside of the container.
- Place the lid upside down on a clean surface.
- Clean and dry the bedpan or urinal before collecting the specimen.

A Follow aseptic practices when collecting specimens.

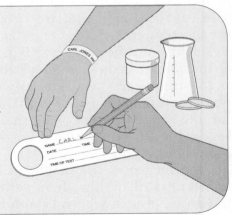

BE ACCURATE...

- Check identification bracelet.
- Print clearly so the label can be easily read.
- Put label on specimen container.
- Check identification bracelet.
- Copy the resident's name from the bracelet.

Fig. 24-11
Infection control and accuracy are important when collecting specimens.

B Accuracy is necessary in collecting specimens.

Collecting a Urine Specimen. Urine specimens are studied to determine kidney function, infection, and other disease conditions. Urine may also be tested to determine treatment. The urine specimens that are most commonly collected in the long-term care facility include routine urine specimens, clean-catch urine specimens, fresh-fractional urine specimens, and 24-hour urine specimens.

Wash and dry the urinal or bedpan before collecting any urine specimen. Ask the resident not to have a bowel movement or place toilet tissue in the pan. These measures help to prevent contamination of the specimen.

A *routine urine specimen* is collected whenever the doctor orders it. In hospitals, and some long-term care facilities, it is a part of the admission procedure. Be aware of the policy where you work. This procedure is located on page 376.

The equipment needed to collect a routine urine specimen includes a bedpan, urinal, graduate, urine specimen container, label, and disposable gloves.

A *clean-catch urine specimen* is collected when the specimen must be free from contamination. It is also called a midstream urine specimen. A clean-catch urine specimen is collected between the time the resident starts to urinate and the time he stops. To do this, the resident must interrupt the flow of urine.

Perineal care is performed before collecting a clean-catch urine specimen. This helps to prevent contamination. You may already be familiar with this type of specimen collection. It is commonly used in doctor's offices.

Interrupting urination may be difficult or impossible for the elderly resident. Report to the charge nurse if you are unable to collect the specimen correctly.

GUIDELINES FOR COLLECTING A CLEAN-CATCH URINE SPECIMEN

- Wear gloves and follow the guidelines for collecting urine specimens.
- Perform perineal care before collecting the specimen.
- Ask the resident to begin voiding, and then stop.

- Position the container and ask the resident to begin voiding again.
- Ask the resident to stop voiding, and remove the container when it is three-fourths full.
- Allow the resident to finish voiding.
- Record and report.

A *fresh-fractional urine specimen* requires the resident to void twice. It is also called a double-voided specimen. The purpose of a fresh-fractional urine specimen is to obtain "fresh" urine. The results are more accurate when the urine that is tested has been freshly produced by the kidneys and has not been stored in the bladder for a prolonged period of time. The word "fractional" refers to the small amount of urine that is voided on the second urine. One of the uses of the fresh-fractional urine specimen is to test for diabetes.

If you are to collect a fresh-fractional urine specimen, ask the resident to void at the specified time. Return in 30 minutes and ask the resident to void again. Explain that you need only a small amount of urine. Some people who empty their bladders are unable to void again in 30 minutes. Let the nurse know if you were unable to obtain a second specimen. Follow the guidelines for collecting urine specimens when collecting a fresh-fractional urine specimen.

A *24-hour urine specimen* requires collecting all the urine that is voided during a 24-hour period. The collection begins after the first voiding. The urine from the first voiding is discarded because it has been in the bladder for some time. For example, if the resident voids at 7 A.M., the urine is discarded, and the test begins. All urine is saved for the next 24 hours. At 7 A.M., the next morning, ask the resident to void before the test ends. Do not discard the last voiding, as it is part of the test.

A large container will be provided for collecting the urine. The urine that is collected must be kept chilled to prevent the growth of microorganisms. The container may be kept in a bucket of ice. Nursing assistants are responsible for keeping the bucket filled with ice (see Fig. 24-13).

PROCEDURE

Collecting a Routine Urine Specimen

Before any procedure you must always follow the five basic steps: wash your hands, collect the equipment, identify the resident, explain the procedure, and protect privacy.

Follow universal precautions and wear gloves when appropriate.

1. Select and label the specimen container.
2. Put on disposable gloves and follow aseptic practices.
3. Ask the resident to urinate into a clean bedpan or urinal. Assist as necessary.
4. Pour the urine from the bedpan or urinal into a clean graduate.
5. Measure the urine if the resident is on I&O.
6. Pour the urine from the graduate into the specimen container. Fill the container three-fourths full, if possible (see Fig. 24-12).
7. Place the lid on the container, being careful not to touch the inside.
8. Clean and replace the equipment.
9. Remove the gloves and wash your hands.
10. Assist the resident with handwashing.
11. Assure the resident's comfort and safety.
12. Take the labeled container to the designated area.
13. Wash your hands.
14. Report and record that you have collected the specimen.

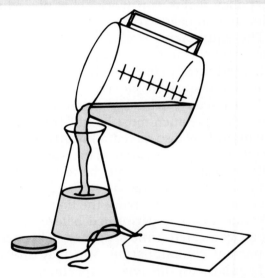

Fig. 24-12
Pour the urine from the graduate into the specimen container.

Explain to the resident and family members that a 24-hour urine test is in progress. Be sure that they are aware that all the urinary output must be saved. Staff members must also be aware of the test period. Incontinence, spilling, or accidental disposal of urine should be reported to the nurse immediately. The test will need to be discontinued and restarted for accurate results. Follow the general guidelines for collecting urine specimens when performing this procedure.

Collecting a Stool Specimen. Stool (feces, bowel movement, BM) is solid waste material from the digestive system. Stool specimens are collected to test for blood, fat, microorganisms, parasites (worms), or other abnormal conditions. When collecting a stool specimen, instruct the resident not to urinate or place toilet tissue in the bedpan. This will contaminate the specimen. Some tests require a warm stool specimen. In that case, the specimen must go to the laboratory promptly.

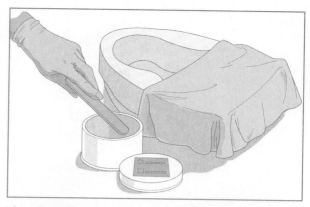

Fig. 24-14 Use a tongue blade to transfer a stool specimen from a bedpan to the specimen container.

Sometimes stool specimens are ordered to be collected three times. The specimen container is labeled with the appropriate number. Be sure to number the specimen correctly and let the nurse know that it has been collected.

Collecting a Sputum Specimen. Some disease processes cause the respiratory system to produce mucus. Mucus from the lungs or deep in the respiratory system is called sputum. Sputum is a thick, sticky substance. It differs from saliva.

Coughing and bringing up sputum can be difficult and painful for the resident. The resident is asked to cough and **expectorate** (spit) directly into the specimen container. Nursing assistants are not usually asked to collect sputum specimens.

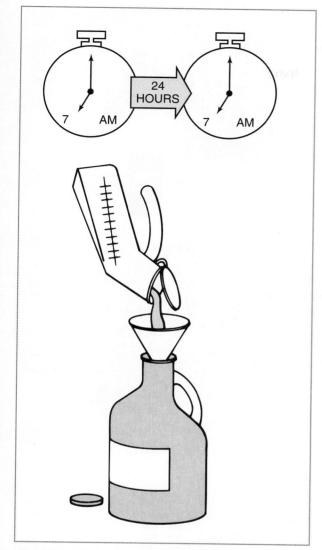

Fig. 24-13 Collecting a 24-hour urine specimen.

GUIDELINES FOR COLLECTING A STOOL SPECIMEN

- Wear gloves and follow aseptic practices.
- Follow the guidelines for collecting specimens.
- Use a tongue blade (tongue depressor) to transfer one or two tablespoons of stool from the bedpan to the specimen container (see Fig. 24-14).
- Place the lid on the container without contaminating it.
- Wrap the tongue blade in a paper towel and discard it in the biohazardous waste container.

GUIDELINES FOR COLLECTING A SPUTUM SPECIMEN

- Wear gloves and follow aseptic practices. Sputum is considered infectious.
- Sputum specimens are easier to collect in the early morning.
- The mouth should be rinsed with plain water before collecting the specimen. Do not use mouthwash.
- Instruct the resident to take three deep breaths and cough.
- The resident should expectorate directly into the container (see Fig. 24-15).
- Do not contaminate the container.
- Cover the container immediately.

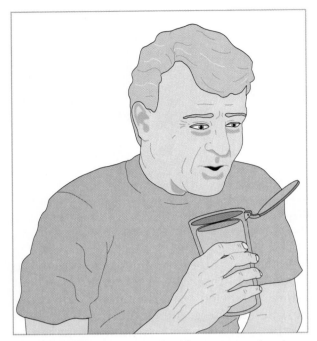

Fig. 24-15 The resident should expectorate directly into the sputum specimen container.

Diabetic Testing for Sugar and Acetone

Testing Urine. The urine of the resident with diabetes may be tested for the presence of sugar and acetone. Diabetes is a disease in which the body does not properly use insulin to change sugar to energy. This causes sugar to build up in the blood. If there is not enough sugar for energy, the body will use fat. The breakdown of fat produces acetone (ketones), which may also build up in the blood. Sugar and acetone may appear in the urine. Read the section on diabetes in Chapter 12 for a better understanding of this disease. The urine test for sugar and acetone is called an **S&A test.**

A fresh-fractional urine specimen is needed for the S&A. This procedure is described earlier in this chapter. It is important that the test be done on fresh urine to obtain results that are as accurate as possible. Although the second voided specimen is more accurate, you should also test the first specimen. This is in case the resident is unable to give another specimen when

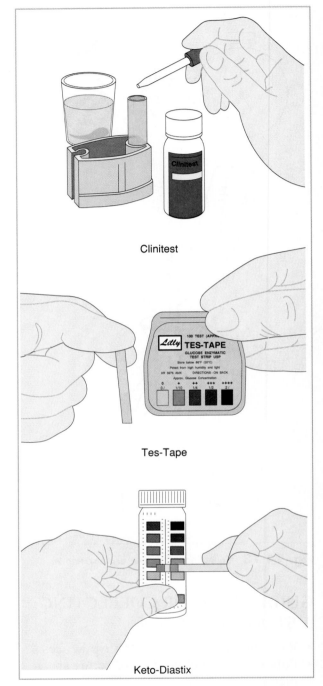

Clinitest

Tes-Tape

Keto-Diastix

Fig. 24-16 Types of diabetic urine tests.

needed. Be sure the nurse is aware of which urine test you are reporting.

There are many types of diabetic urine tests. Some test only for sugar in the urine, others test only for acetone, while some test for both sugar and acetone. For these tests, either a reagent tablet or a reagent strip is used. The word "reagent" refers to the chemical substance on the strip or tablet. The most common urine tests used are Clinitest®, Acetest®, Tes-Tape®, and Keto-Diastix®. Clinitest and Tes-Tape test for sugar in the urine. Acetest tests for acetone in the urine. Keto-Diastix tests for both sugar and acetone. The procedure is different for performing each of these tests. Directions for testing the urine, and reading the results, are on each container. Follow the directions carefully to ensure accuracy. Medication and other treatment are affected by the results of the sugar and acetone test.

The reagent on the tablets and strips is poisonous and is affected by light or air. Handle tablets and strips carefully and avoid touching the reagent. When taking a reagent tablet from a bottle, pour the tablet into the lid (see Fig. 24-17). Then pour the tablet from the lid into a test tube or place it on a clean paper towel. Container lids should be closed tightly and the containers stored away from direct light.

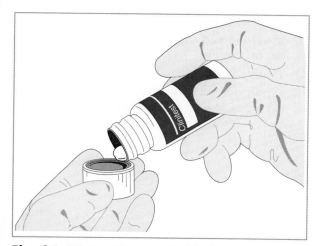

Fig. 24-17 Pour the reagent tablet from the bottle into the lid.

GENERAL GUIDELINES FOR PERFORMING A TEST FOR SUGAR AND ACETONE

- Wear gloves and follow aseptic practices.
- Collect a fresh-fractional urine specimen.
- Handle tablets and strips carefully.
- Follow the directions on the testing kit.
- Record and report results to the nurse immediately.

Today, most facilities test the blood for sugar and acetone. This may be done in place of or in addition to checking urine. Studies have shown that blood testing is more accurate than urine testing. In many facilities, urine testing is no longer done. Follow the policy and procedures of the facility where you work.

Vaginal Irrigations

The physician may order a vaginal irrigation (douche) to cleanse the vagina or relieve inflammation. A douche (vaginal irrigation) is given by allowing a solution to flow into the vagina, after which it returns by the force of gravity. Usually a douche is used to apply heat or cold, or to medicate the vaginal tissues. Frequent douches wash away the normal flora of the vagina. These normal flora are microorganisms that exist in the vaginal area and provide protection from other invading microorganisms.

Equipment needed to administer a vaginal douche includes a disposable vaginal irrigation kit, solution, bedpan, linen protector, and gloves. Universal precautions are required for the administration of a vaginal irrigation.

Elastic Support Hose and Bandages

Elastic support hose and bandages are often ordered for residents with heart disease and other circulatory problems. They improve circulation by exerting pressure on the veins, which promotes blood return to the heart. Support hose and bandages are used to prevent and treat blood clots. They may also be used to provide comfort and support. Elastic support hose are often ordered for the resident with limited mobility.

It is important for you to know how to apply elastic support hose and bandages properly. They can cause discomfort and injury if not correctly applied. Do not apply elastic support hose or bandages unless the nurse tells you to do so, or it is indicated in the resident's plan of care.

PROCEDURE

Administering a Vaginal Irrigation

Before performing any procedure you must complete the five basic steps: wash your hands, gather equipment, identify the resident, explain the procedure, and provide privacy.

Follow universal precautions and wear gloves when appropriate.

1. Ask the resident to urinate.
2. Raise the bed to a comfortable working height, lock the wheels, and lower the side rails on the side nearest you.
3. Cover the resident with a bath blanket and fold the top linen to the foot of the bed.
4. Place a protective pad under the resident's buttocks.
5. Put on gloves, and place the bedpan under the resident.
6. Provide peri-care (see the procedure for giving perineal care). Raise the side rail.
7. Clamp the tubing of the douche kit before pouring solution into the container.
8. Fill the douche container with warm solution (105°F or 40.5°C). Lower the side rail.
9. Expel air from the tubing by releasing the clamp and allowing the solution to flow through the nozzle and over the genitalia, without allowing the nozzle to touch the vulva.
10. While the solution flows, insert the nozzle 2–3 inches into the vagina, in an upward, then downward and backward motion (see Fig. 24-18).
11. Hold the solution container 12 inches above the vagina while the solution flows.
12. Gently rotate the nozzle.
13. Remove the nozzle after clamping the tubing, and place the nozzle inside the solution container.
14. Ask the resident to sit upright on the bedpan to allow the solution to drain from the vagina.
15. Assist the resident to dry the perineal area.
16. Empty the bedpan, and observe the solution. Rinse the pan, and return it to storage.
17. Remove the protective pad, and dispose of it.
18. Remove the gloves, and wash your hands.
19. Cover the resident with the top linen, and raise the side rail.
20. Lower the bed, and assure the resident's comfort and safety.
21. Wash your hands.
22. Report any unusual observations, and record the procedure on the resident's record.

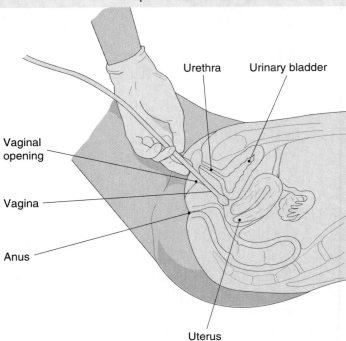

Fig. 24-18
Insert the douche nozzle 2–3 inches into the vagina, in an upward and then downward and backward motion.

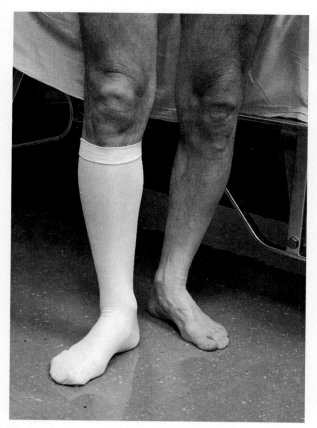
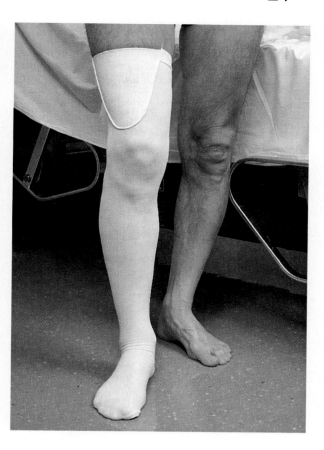

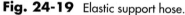
Fig. 24-19 Elastic support hose.

Elastic Support Hose. Elastic support hose are also called antiembolism stockings or T.E.D.® hose. They may be knee high or full length, and a variety of sizes are available (see Fig. 24-19).

GUIDELINES FOR APPLYING ELASTIC SUPPORT HOSE

- Be sure the hose are the correct size.
- Apply them before the resident gets out of bed.
- Hold the heel of the stocking, and gather the rest of the stocking in your hand.
- Support the resident's foot at the heel.
- Slip the front of the stocking over the toes, foot, and heel (see Fig. 24-20).
- Pull the stocking snugly and evenly up over the leg.
- Check frequently to see that the hose are not twisted or wrinkled.
- Remove the hose at least twice a day.
- Check for edema or discolored areas.

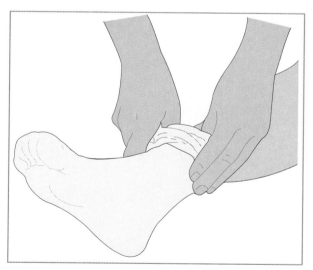

Fig. 24-20 Slip the front of the stocking over the toes, foot, and heel.

Elastic Bandages. Elastic bandages are often called ACE® bandages. They are strips of elasticized material of varying lengths and widths. Elastic bandages are sometimes used to reduce swelling from a musculoskeletal injury.

PROCEDURE

Applying Elastic Bandages

Before any procedure you must always follow the five basic steps: wash your hands, collect the equipment, identify the resident, explain the procedure, and protect privacy.

Follow universal precautions and wear gloves when appropriate.

1. Hold the bandage with the loose end at the bottom of the roll.
2. Make two circular turns, to anchor the bandage, around the smallest part of the extremity (see Fig. 24-21A).
3. Make overlapping spiral wraps in an upward direction. Each wrap should overlap about half the width of the bandage (see Fig. 24-21B).
4. Apply the bandage smoothly and firmly, being careful not to wrap it too tightly. Make sure that no skin is exposed.
5. Fasten the bandage with clips to hold it in place (see Fig. 24-21C).
6. Wash your hands.
7. Assure the resident's comfort and safety.
8. Record and report to the charge nurse.

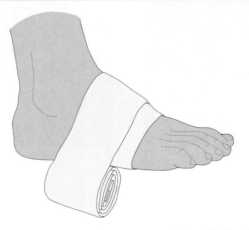

A Make two circular wraps to anchor the bandage.

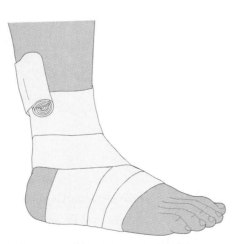

B With each spiral wrap, overlap about one-half of the width of the bandage.

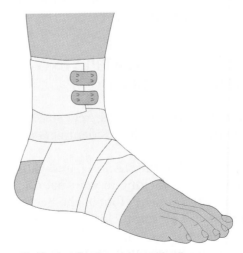

C Fasten the bandage with clips.

Fig. 24-21 Applying an elastic bandage.

The nurse will tell you what area should be bandaged. Begin applying the bandage at the smallest part of the extremity, leaving the fingers or toes exposed. Use as many bandages as you need to cover the area. Once you have applied elastic bandages, check frequently for edema, skin discoloration, or changes in skin temperature. Reapply bandages if they become loose or wrinkled.

The equipment needed for this procedure includes the proper size elastic bandage and clips to secure the bandage and hold it in place.

Hot and Cold Applications

Treatment with heat and cold is ordered by the physician to reduce swelling, relieve pain, stimulate circulation, and promote healing. Because heat and cold can cause injury, great care and constant attention are necessary in this type of application. Elderly residents may have decreased awareness or sensation of temperature changes and pain. Their skin is fragile and may be injured easily. They are at increased risk of burns. In many facilities, nursing assistants are not responsible for applying heat and cold, because of the risk involved. Be sure that you are familiar with the policies of your facility.

Heat and cold applications may be dry or moist. In a dry application, moisture is not in contact with the skin. Dry applications include ice bags, collars or packs, water bottles, heat lamps, and electric, fluid-filled warming pads (often called K-Pads®). These devices should be covered before application, to protect the skin. Because electric heating pads and heat lamps are extremely dangerous, many facilities do not allow their use.

Moist applications include soaks, compresses, wet packs, cooling sponge baths, and sitz baths. Moisture is in contact with the skin for these applications. Soaks, compresses, and wet compresses can be warm or cold. A wet cloth is wrung out and placed upon the skin for a wet compress. A device filled with ice or warm water may be applied to the moist compress to maintain the temperature. Soaks involve placing the resident (or a part of the resident's body) into warm water or solution.

A Cooling Sponge Bath. A cooling sponge bath may be ordered by the doctor to reduce a resident's fever. Evaporation of moisture from the skin has a cooling effect. Alcohol evaporates very quickly, and may cool more effectively than water. Alcohol or cool water is sponged onto the resident's skin and is left to evaporate. The application is repeated as needed. Do not apply alcohol near the face. Check with your charge nurse to determine what areas should be sponged, and follow facility policy.

The Sitz Bath. The term "sitz bath" almost defines itself. To take a sitz bath the resident must sit in warm water (105°F or 40.5°C) for 20 minutes. This procedure relieves pain, improves circulation, and cleanses wounds. It may also be used to stimulate urination.

A disposable plastic sitz bath is available. This model fits into the toilet seat. Some facilities use portable sitz chairs or may have a permanent built-in model. A regular bathtub may be used for a sitz bath by filling it with warm water to a level that covers the pelvis.

You must assure the resident's safety by assisting the resident into and out of the tub. If a regular bathtub is used, the resident may not be left alone. The resident may experience fatigue, weakness, or faintness. Stay with the resident and observe for these conditions. Assist the resident to and from the sitz bath.

GENERAL GUIDELINES FOR HEAT AND COLD APPLICATIONS

- Proper temperature of heat applications must be maintained between 100° and 115°F (37.8° and 46.5°C) by frequently checking the application.
- Temperature of solutions should be checked with a bath thermometer, according to facility policy.
- Stop treatment, cover the resident, and notify the charge nurse if shivering occurs.

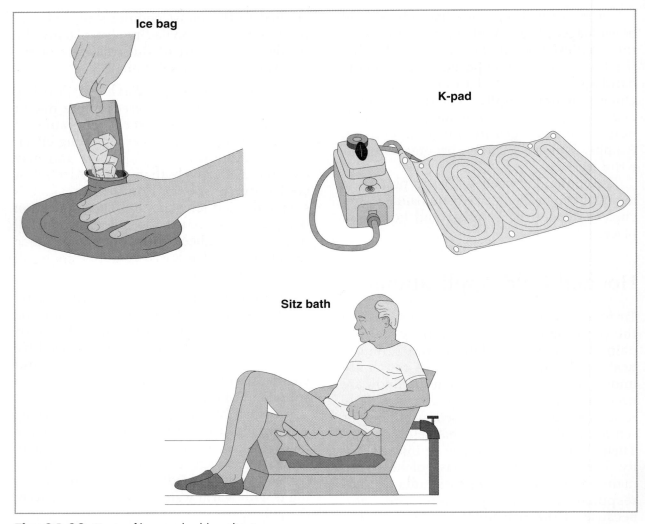

Ice bag

K-pad

Sitz bath

Fig. 24-22 Types of heat and cold applications.

- Add ice to cold applications as necessary to maintain constant temperature.
- Check for leaks in ice bags, collars, or packs and water bottles.
- Always be sure ice bags are dry before applying.
- Always cover ice bags, hot water bottles, or vinyl containers with cloth before applying to the skin.
- Be sure that caps, or firm parts of bags, are away from the skin.
- Remember, ice will burn.
- Check skin frequently, and report abnormalities or resident complaints to the charge nurse immediately.
- Remove the heat or cold application immediately, if you suspect burns. Report the situation immediately to your charge nurse.

- Be familiar with and follow the policies of your facility.

Conclusion

Remember these important points:

1. Positioning, skin care, and mouth care help provide comfort for the resident, who is receiving oxygen.

2. The resident who is having difficulty breathing may need extra reassurance and emotional support.

3. Check with the nurse regarding movement and positioning of the resident with a hip fracture.

4. Observe fingers or toes for circulation when the resident has a cast.

5. Make sure the scale is properly balanced before weighing the resident.

6. Diet, medications, and other treatments are based on height and weight measurements.

7. Wear gloves and follow aseptic practices when collecting a specimen.

8. The purpose of a fresh-fractional urine is to obtain urine that has not been in the bladder for long.

9. A 24-hour urine specimen must be kept chilled during the collection period.

10. When collecting a stool specimen, instruct the resident not to urinate or place toilet tissue in the pan.

11. A fresh-fractional urine specimen is needed for the sugar and acetone test.

12. Frequent douches wash away the protective normal flora of the vagina.

13. Elastic support hose and bandages improve circulation by exerting pressure on the veins.

14. Because heat and cold can cause injury, caution is necessary in this type of application.

Discussion Questions

1. What are some special needs of the resident requiring oxygen?

2. Why do residents who are immobilized need special care?

3. Why is it important to follow aseptic technique when collecting specimens?

4. What may happen if a woman douches frequently?

5. What are the dangers of using heat and cold applications for the elderly?

Application Exercise

1. The class will visit a long-term care facility. The instructor will assign the students (singly or in pairs) to a resident who is receiving one or more of the specific types of treatment discussed in this chapter. The students will visit for one to two hours with the residents and assist the C.N.A. as needed. The students will share their observations and experiences with the class. Observations should include

   a. Special needs of the resident

   b. The resident's feelings about the treatment

   c. Safety considerations

   d. Infection control concerns

   e. Special equipment needed

   f. Your own feelings

Coping with Death and Dying

OBJECTIVES

Upon completing this chapter, you will be able to do the following:

1. Explain how your attitude toward death affects your response to the dying resident.

2. Describe the stages of grief.

3. Explain how you can help meet the physical and psychosocial needs of the dying resident, the family, and other residents.

4. Identify three methods to cope with staff stress.

5. Describe hospice care.

6. Identify the signs of approaching death.

7. List six guidelines for providing postmortem care.

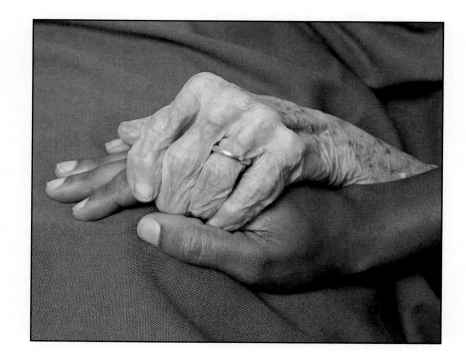

VOCABULARY

The following words or terms will help you to understand this chapter:

Terminal illness	Bargaining stage	Hospice
Denial stage	Depression stage	Cyanosis
Anger stage	Acceptance stage	Postmortem care

Death and dying is a subject that can be frightening and misunderstood. It involves a wide range of emotions such as fear, anger, guilt, empathy, and compassion. It is little wonder that many people avoid talking about death. All of us will face death someday and for the geriatric resident, that time may not be too distant. The more you learn about the dying process, the more you will be able to understand. Understanding can help you to release fear and gain acceptance. This, in turn, will allow you to become a more compassionate and effective caregiver. Keep that goal in mind as you study this chapter.

Terminal Illness

A **terminal illness** is an illness that is expected to end in death. There is little hope of recovery. Although many illnesses can be treated, controlled, or cured, there is usually no cure for a terminal illness.

Hope. The fact that recovery is not expected does not mean that there is no hope. Having hope is as necessary to the dying as it is to the living. Hope changes as the disease progresses. At first there may be hope that the doctor is wrong. Later, thoughts may change to hope for a peaceful death. As a nursing assistant, you can encourage feelings of hope by being a supportive listener and allowing the resident to express feelings.

Attitudes Toward Death and Dying

Attitudes are a combination of beliefs, feelings, and actions. Your attitude is influenced by culture, religion, experience, and age. People tend to act according to their beliefs and feelings.

Culture. You learned, very early in life, what your culture expected of you. You saw how your family and friends reacted to certain life events, such as birth, marriage, and death. If they feared death, you may share the same feelings. When you turn away from your cultural beliefs, you may feel guilty and uncertain.

Religion. Religion has a great influence on attitudes toward death. Most religions hold beliefs about what happens after death. If you believe that death leads to a place of peace and beauty, it is not so frightening. However, if death leads to eternal pain and suffering, fear is a normal reaction.

Personal Experience. If you have never experienced the death of a loved one, you do not know how you will react. Grieving is learned through experience. Your relationship with the dying person, your experience with grieving, and your expectations affect your attitude. You may find it easier to accept a death that is peaceful and expected than one that is sudden or violent.

Age. Age also affects your attitude toward death. Children do not fear death, until they learn it from others. Young children often believe that death is only temporary and expect the dead person to return someday. The elderly usually have less fear of death. In fact, some see death as a release from suffering and loneliness. There seems to be less fear of death at both the beginning and the end of life.

Most people are uncomfortable talking about death. They say "He passed away" or "We lost him." What they mean is, "He

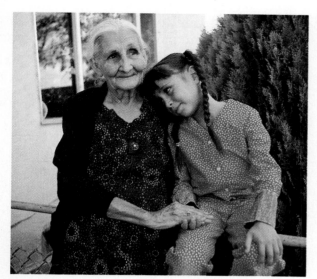

Fig. 25-1 There is often less fear of death in the very old and the very young.

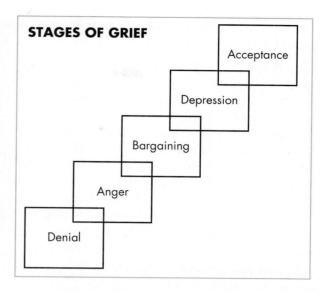

Fig. 25-2 The stages of grief.

died." This avoidance of the word "death" is caused by fear, and fear affects your attitude. Your attitude about death will affect the way you respond. If you feel frightened, you will feel uncomfortable caring for the dying resident. If you pretend that you are not afraid, the resident will usually sense your true feelings. Because your attitude about death and dying has such a great influence on the care that you give, it will help you to develop an attitude of acceptance about death.

The Stages of Grief

Elisabeth Kubler-Ross is a doctor who has devoted much of her life to working with terminally ill patients. She divided grief into stages. The "stages of grief" are sometimes called "stages of dying." The person who is dying feels intense grief. However, family members, friends, and caregivers also grieve. The five stages of grief, according to Kubler-Ross, are denial, anger, bargaining, depression, and acceptance.

Denial Stage. In the **denial stage**, the grieving person is refusing to believe what is happening. This first stage of grief is like a shock absorber, giving time to adjust. Denial delays the shock until a person has more emotional control. Sometimes people need denial because they are not ready for the

truth. This can be frustrating to others because the truth seems obvious. You cannot rush someone through denial. As much time as is needed should be allowed. A conflict can also arise when the resident is accepting while a family member is still in denial.

Anger Stage. During the second stage of grief, intense anger may be directed at anyone or anything. This is called the **anger stage**. The most common target of this anger is the person with whom the grieving person spends the most time. At home, that is usually a family member. In the long-term care facility, it might be you. Acting out in anger toward those who provide care may be the only way the grieving person can express hostility. The anger is not about you, it is about dying.

Bargaining Stage. The **bargaining stage**, the third stage of grief, is an attempt to gain more time by promising something in return. Have you ever heard a child say, "If you will let me stay up one hour longer, I'll be good all day tomorrow." That is an example of bargaining. Bargaining is often between the grieving person and God or a Higher Power. Sometimes bargaining is expressed in the form of prayer. If the grieving person wants to talk to you, encourage hope, and respect beliefs. Let the nurse know if the grieving resident indicates a need for spiritual assistance.

Depression Stage. The **depression stage** of grief is experienced with sadness and quiet. Denial and anger are gone in this fourth stage. There is a deep sadness, with thoughts of loss of health, loss of independence, and eventually loss of life. The grieving person may feel numb and unable to communicate. Your help may be refused as the grieving person withdraws. Do not feel hurt if this occurs. Your concern is comforting, so continue to offer your assistance, and spend time with the resident when you can.

Acceptance Stage. In the **acceptance stage**, the fifth and last stage of grief, the dying person is calm and peaceful. It is an easier time for everyone, as anger fades and depression lifts. You may hear the grieving resident say something like, "I'm ready to die now." This doesn't always mean that death is really desired. It simply means that the resident has accepted that there is limited time left to live. You can help by trying to understand and accept the situation. Being quiet yourself helps provide a calm environment. At this time, you might use some of your energy to assist family members, or other residents, with their grief. This helps to satisfy your own need to be needed.

People do not always experience all the stages of grief in the same order. Some who never accept death die in denial or anger. A person may repeat the stages. For example, the dying resident may work through grief to the stage of acceptance, as long as independence is possible. Later, when the dying person is unable to provide self-care, anger or depression might return. It is important that you are aware of the stages and know what to expect when they occur. Your understanding that these are normal reactions will help you and the grieving person.

Meeting the Needs of the Dying Resident

It is easy to focus on the approaching death and lose sight of the needs of the whole person. Providing care for the dying involves responding to the psychosocial needs, as well as the physical needs. The basic needs (physical, safety, love, self-esteem, and self-actualization) have the same effect on dying as they do on living. The basic needs are discussed in detail in Chapter 13. Measures for meeting the dying resident's needs are included in the care plan. Your reporting of observed needs contributes to the effectiveness of the plan of care.

Physical Needs. Keeping the resident comfortable should be your most important goal. Any complaint of pain must be reported immediately to the charge nurse. Watch for restlessness or facial expressions that may indicate pain. Many times, pain can be relieved by simple nursing measures, such as giving a backrub or helping the resident into a more comfortable position.

The terminally ill resident may have dyspnea (difficult breathing). This may be caused by disease or by anxiety and fear. It is frightening to have difficulty breathing. Anxiety and fear can be reduced by the presence of a calm, reassuring person. It is comforting to know that someone is nearby who can help. Encourage the resident to take slow, deep breaths. Do not leave the resident alone until the dyspnea is relieved.

The dying resident may lose interest in eating and drinking. Frequent, small amounts of soft feedings may be helpful. Mouth care must be done at least every two hours. The lips may need to be lubricated to prevent cracking. Difficulty swallowing, and a decreased cough reflex, make it more difficult for the resident to handle oral secretions. Oral tissues may dry out, as fluid intake decreases. Eventually, the dying resident may stop eating and drinking. This can be very upsetting to family members, who will need your support.

Slowed circulation, decreased activity, and poor nutrition increase the risk of skin breakdown. Frequent turning and positioning helps to prevent decubitus ulcers (bedsores). Position the resident for comfort, and in correct body alignment, when possible. Special equipment, such as air mattresses, foam pads, or heel protectors, can be helpful. It is important to keep the skin clean and dry and to massage with lotion each time the person is repositioned. Lotion and the touch of your hands are comforting.

The nursing assistant plays a very important role in providing physical comfort for the dying resident. Your observations and reporting help to assure prompt relief from pain. Your "hands-on" care of giving a back-rub or soothing a fevered brow may be the dying resident's last memory.

Safety Needs. It is important to provide a safe, secure environment. The dying resident may be frightened and insecure, because the future is uncertain and limited. Loss of control may cause the resident to feel helpless and powerless. Reassurance that you will do your best to maintain the resident's safety will be comforting. A review of the chapter on safety will be helpful.

Psychosocial Needs. Psychosocial needs may increase when the resident is dying. The staff must help meet the need for love, self-esteem, and self-actualization. Family and friends may not always be present. They may live far away, or the resident may have outlived close relatives. The long-term care facility becomes the resident's home, and the staff may become the resident's family.

You can help meet the dying resident's need for love by being caring, gentle and empathetic. There are no right or wrong words to comfort the resident. It is your presence that is comforting, not what you say. Touch and listening are important forms of communication. People who are dying often need to talk, but they do not always expect answers to their questions. Listen carefully, as speech may be difficult. Silence can truly be golden, so do not be afraid to be quiet. If you are not sure what to do, a hug or touch on the shoulder speaks louder than words.

It may be difficult for the dying resident to maintain self-esteem. Physical or mental changes such as incontinence or confusion may occur. Self-esteem is closely tied to independence. Allow the resident to make decisions, such as when to bathe, or what to

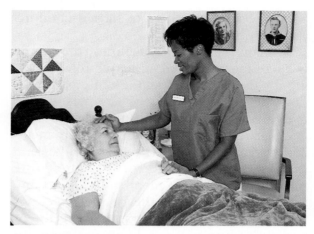

Fig. 25-3 The touch of your hand may be the dying resident's last memory.

eat. Maintaining some power and control increases self-esteem. Being treated with respect and dignity also helps to build feelings of value and worth.

It is important that the resident continues to set goals, even if the goals need to be changed frequently. An early goal might be to go to the dining room for dinner. As the resident gets weaker, that goal might change to sharing meals with a loved one at the bedside. Setting and striving for goals is a form of self-actualization. While you cannot set goals for the resident, you can encourage and assist as needed.

Spiritual Needs. Religion is usually a source of comfort to the dying resident and family members. Let the nurse know if the resident expresses a need for spiritual guidance. Assure privacy for spiritual visits and rituals. Because of the relationship that has developed with the dying resident, you may be the one the dying resident turns to for spiritual help. To understand the resident's needs, listen with care and respect.

The Dying Resident's Family

One of the greatest needs of the dying resident is to be with family members, who are also grieving. They need time to share memories and discuss the future. This provides an opportunity to make apologies and say goodbye. Visiting hours are usually extended to allow friends and family members to visit. Help them to have a comfortable, private visit.

In many health care facilities, the family is encouraged to take an active role in caring for the dying resident. Family participation can benefit everyone. The person who is dying is comforted to know that a loved one is caring for him or her. A family member may be aware of the resident's likes and dislikes. Being as helpful as possible increases the family member's self-esteem, and reduces some of the helpless feelings that death may bring. Straightening linens and adjusting pillows keep the resident more comfortable. Feeding or giving fluids relieve hunger and thirst. Participating in the dying resident's care helps to ease the feelings of guilt that may come later. The family member is comforted by being available and useful.

Family participation does not relieve the staff of responsibility for the care of the dying person. The dying resident should receive as much of your time as your other residents. However, you will feel better knowing that the resident is not alone.

The staff has a responsibility to the dying resident's family. Their problems may be included in the plan of care. Anything that you do for the family also helps the resident. You can help the family by assisting them to meet their basic needs. Orient them to the facility and be sure they know the location of bathrooms, water fountains, and vending machines. Tell family members about nearby restaurants. In some facilities, guest trays are available. A cup of hot coffee or tea may be welcome, especially during the long hours of the night. A pillow and warm blanket may also be appreciated.

You can help meet the family's psychosocial needs through communication and courtesy. Touch and listening are your most valuable tools. Remember that family members are also grieving and may need to express their feelings. Family members may

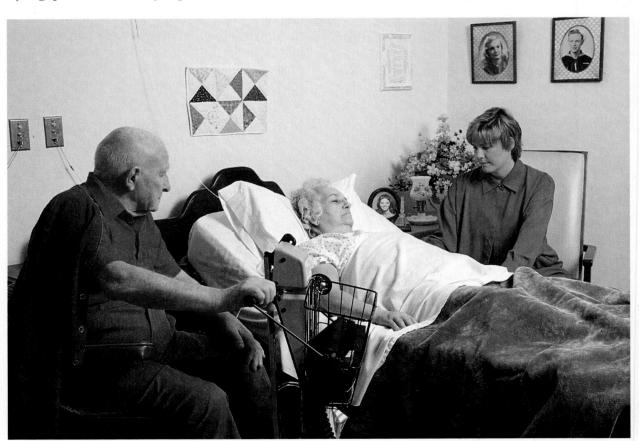

Fig. 25-4 The presence of family and friends comforts the dying resident.

have questions that you cannot answer. Usually, they are not looking for answers or advice—they may just want you to listen. Don't be afraid to say that you don't know. People do not expect answers to questions such as, "Why did this have to happen to my mother?"

The family member's behavior will be affected by the stage of grief that is being experienced. The dying resident and a family member may not be in the same stage at the same time. The resident may be in acceptance while the family member is still in denial. Open communication helps to solve this problem. Encourage them to share their feelings and provide opportunities for private conversations.

Family members can cause extra work for the staff as they deal with their own grief and try to keep the resident comfortable. There may be times when you wish they would go home and let you take care of the resident. If you find yourself feeling that way, remember how sad it is when a resident dies with no family member present.

The Other Residents

Residents of long-term care facilities often form close relationships. As they live together, they become a family. They share rooms, families, joys, and sorrows. Roommates frequently become close friends, who depend on each other for companionship. Is it any wonder that they are saddened by the death of one of their own?

When a resident is dying, other residents may be upset. They may act out their emotions in irritability and anger. Some may withdraw and become depressed. Anxiety and fear affect their feelings and reactions. "I may be next" is a thought that may enter the minds of many residents.

Some of the residents, especially the roommate of the dying resident, will be grieving. You can help by showing concern and understanding. Take time to listen when they want to talk, because talking helps them to work through their grief. Remarks such as, "I can see that you are very sad

about Mrs. Vargas. I'd feel the same way if I lost a good friend," assure the resident that those feelings are normal. Report any problems to the nurse so they can included in the grieving resident's plan of care.

Two or three weeks after a death, when the residents have gotten over the shock, they may need to talk. They may be beginning to adjust to life without the resident who died. You might notice behavior changes, such as pouting, crying, or frequent complaining. These may be clues that the resident needs to talk. Your attention and willingness to listen indicate that you care.

Coping with Staff Stress

When a resident dies in a long-term care facility, staff members may also grieve. Some residents have lived for years in the same facility. Because the staff knows and loves the residents, it is like a death in the family.

Working with dying residents can cause emotional conflict. Feelings of frustration, anger, and guilt are not uncommon. You may feel frustrated because you spend so much time with the resident, yet nothing you do seems to help. Frustration can quickly turn to anger. You may feel guilty because the resident called for you when you were busy, and someone else answered their call signal. These are all normal feelings, so don't be too hard on yourself. Do the best you can—that's all anyone can do.

You may have to cope with the anger of a resident or family member. When you feel that you have done your best, you can't understand why they are angry. They are not mad at you, so don't take it personally. Can you remember the last time you had a bad day at work? When you got home feeling tired and angry, what happened? Did your anger go away or was it still there? What did you do with it? Did you take it out on someone else?

Taking care of a dying resident is physically and emotionally stressful. You will need to take care of yourself by eating a balanced diet, exercising regularly, and getting plenty of rest. Develop the habit of leaving work problems at work and home problems at home. Suggestions for taking care of yourself can be found in Chapter 2.

Staff members need to help each other work through their own grief. A staff member who has been extremely close to a resident will be upset when that resident is dying. Sometimes health care workers are trying so hard to be brave and "put up a good front" that they fail to grieve. Your empathy and support will be needed. Be an active listener and encourage your coworker to talk about feelings.

Hospice

Centuries ago, in Europe, a hospice was a place of shelter for sick and weary travelers. Today, the old-fashioned idea of hospice has been updated to meet the special needs of the dying and their families. **Hospice** is a program that provides care for the terminally ill and their families. Pain control, comfort measures, and continuity of care are provided by a team of health care workers and volunteers. Their goal is to improve quality of life by assisting the dying person to be as comfortable as possible and by providing supportive services to the family.

Care may be provided in a hospice facility or at home. Some hospice patients may be in a long-term care facility. The family or doctor may have requested hospice care. There may be no one available to care for the person at home or the family may have been providing the care, but are unable to continue. It is very stressful to care for a loved one who is dying.

Hospice team members will visit the resident after admission to the facility. The hospice nurse will help the staff develop a plan that will provide continuity of care. The volunteer will make regular visits, and other hospice team members will be available as needed.

Signs That Death Is Near

All the systems of the body gradually slow down. The dying process varies from one person to another, and there is no set pattern. There are, however, some common signs that are often observed. Even when most of these signs are present, it is difficult to predict the time of death. Dying is as individualized as living.

Circulatory System. The signs of decreasing circulation may include **cyanosis**, a blue color of the lips, nails and skin, caused by a lack of oxygen. Cyanosis usually begins with the lips and around the mouth and nose. The feet and hands may also be cyanotic. The pulse may be weak, rapid, and irregular, while the blood pressure continues to drop. Although the skin feels cold, there may actually be a rise in body temperature, with fever and perspiration.

Respiratory System. Dyspnea (difficult breathing) may be present, with shallow, noisy respirations. This type of ineffective breathing is the reason for cyanosis. An increase in secretions, and a weak cough reflex, can result in a "death rattle." This occurs when the dying person cannot expectorate (spit) the secretions, and they tend to collect in the back of the throat. Cheyne-Stokes respirations may also occur. This is a repetitious pattern of breathing in which shallow breathing is followed by longer, deeper breathing and then apnea (no breathing). Generally, when Cheyne-Stokes begins, it continues until death occurs.

Digestive System. The dying resident may lose the desire to eat and drink. Swallowing becomes difficult, and digestion is affected. Peristalsis slows, and the abdomen may become distended (swollen). Nausea and vomiting may occur when the resident tries to take nourishment. Bowel incontinence and irregularity are common.

Urinary System. The resident who is dying may experience urinary incontinence. As fluid intake decreases and circulation slows, urine output also decreases. Kidney function is impaired and eventually fails. In the last hours or days, there may be no urine at all.

Muscular System. There is a decrease in body movement and in muscle tone. The muscles relax and become flaccid (limp).

When jaw muscles are affected, the jaw drops and the mouth remains partly opened.

Sensory System. A decrease in awareness takes place in most people, as death approaches. While the ability to feel pain is decreased, not everyone will be unconscious. The eyes may stare, and the pupils may be dilated. The last sense to go is hearing. You should always assume that the dying resident can hear, and continue talking, even though there may be no response.

Signs of Death. Death occurs when there is no pulse, no respirations, and no blood pressure.

Postmortem Care

Care of the body after death is called **postmortem care**. The purpose of postmortem care is to preserve the appearance of the body. The nurse will tell you when to begin this procedure. If you feel uneasy the first time you do postmortem care, talk about your feelings with the nurse.

Postmortem care includes positioning the body, straightening the room, and collecting the resident's personal belongings. The body should be placed in correct alignment, usually in the supine position. The body must be treated with respect, dignity, and privacy at all times. Show respect for the resident's belongings by packing them carefully.

If the family is present, they may want to view the body and say their goodbyes. Family members should be allowed to make this choice for themselves. Provide privacy, but be available for physical and emotional support if needed.

When the family leaves, you may resume postmortem care according to the policy of your facility. The procedure for postmortem care is not the same in all facilities. In some facilities a shroud will be used. A shroud is a cover for wrapping the dead body. It is your responsibility to know the procedure where you work.

GUIDELINES FOR PROVIDING POSTMORTEM CARE

- Wear gloves and follow universal precautions.
- Treat the body with respect and privacy.
- Remove tubes and catheters according to facility policy.
- Bathe as needed.
- Place protective pads under the body to absorb urine and feces.
- Comb or brush the hair.
- Place the body in a supine position, with the bed flat, if possible.
- Close the eyes gently.

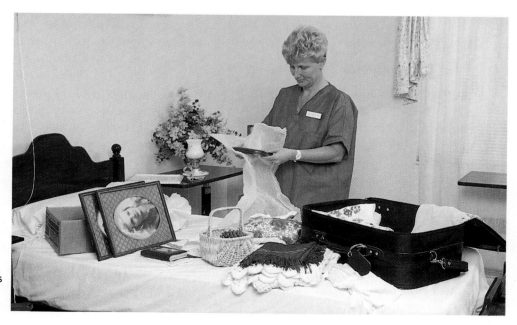

Fig. 25-5
Collecting the resident's belongings is part of postmortem care.

- Elevate the head on a pillow, and place the arms at the side.
- Replace the dentures, or put them in a labeled container.
- Cover the body with a clean sheet, leaving the head and shoulders exposed.
- Remove supplies from the room. Leave the room neat and orderly.
- Provide privacy for the family if they wish to view the body.
- Handle jewelry according to facility policy.
- Leave identification on the body. You may need to apply additional identification according to facility policy.
- Wrap the body in a shroud or sheet if facility policy calls for it.
- If belongings are not given to the family, they are cared for according to facility policy. A list of belongings may be required.
- Strip the unit after the body has been removed from the room.

As a nursing assistant your role in caring for the dying resident is very important. Because you provide so much of the hands-on care, the dying resident may turn to you in this time of need. Your comfort in working with the dying, as well as your knowledgeable and accepting attitude, can help the resident accept death more easily. Your presence at the bedside, as a caring compassionate friend will help the resident take that final step on the journey through life.

Conclusion

Remember these important points:

1. Your attitude toward death and dying affects your response to the dying resident.

2. People do not always experience all the stages of grief in the same order.

3. The most important physical need of the dying resident is comfort.

4. It is important to meet the dying person's psychosocial needs as well as the physical needs.

5. You can help the family by being a supportive listener.

6. Discuss your feelings with a coworker, and don't be ashamed to cry.

7. Hospice provides care for people who are terminally ill.

8. The signs of death are no pulse, no respirations, and no blood pressure.

9. Follow you facility's policy when performing postmortem care.

10. The body must be treated with respect, dignity, and privacy at all times.

11. Pack the resident's belongings in a way that shows respect and caring.

12. Provide privacy for the family if they wish to view the body.

Discussion Questions

1. *What can you do to meet the physical needs of the dying resident? How can you help him to be more comfortable?*

2. *How would you respond if a resident's wife told you she thought her husband was going to die soon? What if she started crying?*

3. *What observations could you make that might indicate that a resident needed to talk about the death of his roommate?*

4. *How could you help a friend or coworker who was grieving?*

5. *How does postmortem care differ in facilities in your area?*

Application Exercise

1. To develop self-awareness, spend a few minutes answering the following questions. You might want to write them down, so you can read them later and see if you still feel the same way.

   a. How do I feel about death? Has someone close to me died? How did I feel then, and how do I feel about it now?

   b. How do I feel when people talk about dying? Does it make me feel uncomfortable? What do I do or say that seems to be helpful?

   c. Do I ever think about dying? Do I think about it often? Does it make me feel afraid or depressed?

   d. If I were dying, what would I want to have done for me? Who would I want to be with me? How would I want people to act?

References

Musculoskeletal System

Skeleton

The skeleton is a living framework made by the joining of bones. It serves to provide support, body movement powered by muscular contractions, protection for the vital organs and other soft structures, blood cell production, and storage for essential minerals. There are 206 bones in the adult body, forming the two divisions of the skeletal system. The axial skeleton is comprised of skull, vertebrae, rib cage, and sternum. The upper and lower extremeties and the shoulder and pelvic girdles form the appendicular skeleton.

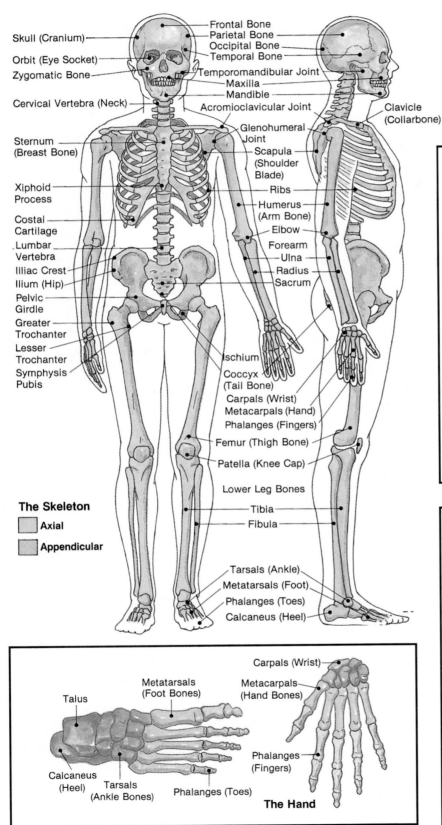

Skull (Cranium)
Orbit (Eye Socket)
Zygomatic Bone
Cervical Vertebra (Neck)
Sternum (Breast Bone)
Xiphoid Process
Costal Cartilage
Lumbar Vertebra
Illiac Crest
Ilium (Hip)
Pelvic Girdle
Greater Trochanter
Lesser Trochanter
Symphysis Pubis

Frontal Bone
Parietal Bone
Occipital Bone
Temporal Bone
Temporomandibular Joint
Maxilla
Mandible
Acromioclavicular Joint
Glenohumeral Joint
Scapula (Shoulder Blade)
Ribs
Humerus (Arm Bone)
Elbow
Forearm
Ulna
Radius
Sacrum

Clavicle (Collarbone)

Ischium
Coccyx (Tail Bone)
Carpals (Wrist)
Metacarpals (Hand)
Phalanges (Fingers)
Femur (Thigh Bone)
Patella (Knee Cap)
Lower Leg Bones
Tibia
Fibula

Tarsals (Ankle)
Metatarsals (Foot)
Phalanges (Toes)
Calcaneus (Heel)

The Skeleton
Axial
Appendicular

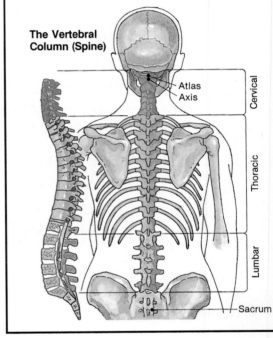

The Vertebral Column (Spine)

Atlas
Axis
Cervical
Thoracic
Lumbar
Sacrum

Talus
Metatarsals (Foot Bones)
Calcaneus (Heel)
Tarsals (Ankle Bones)
Phalanges (Toes)

Carpals (Wrist)
Metacarpals (Hand Bones)
Phalanges (Fingers)

The Hand

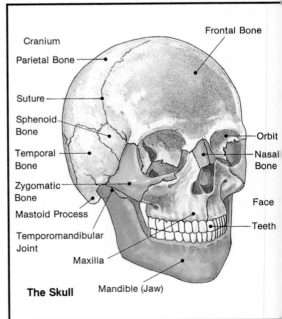

Cranium
Parietal Bone
Suture
Sphenoid Bone
Temporal Bone
Zygomatic Bone
Mastoid Process
Temporomandibular Joint
Maxilla
Mandible (Jaw)

Frontal Bone
Orbit
Nasal Bone
Face
Teeth

The Skull

The tissues of the muscular system comprise 40 to 50% of the body's weight. The skeletal muscles of the body are voluntary muscles, subject to conscious control. They exhibit the properties of excitability; that is, they will react to nerve stimulus. Once stimulated, skeleton muscles are quick to contract and can relax and very quickly be ready for another contraction. There are 501 separate skeletal muscles that provide contractions for movement, coordinated support for posture, and heat production. Muscles connect to bones by way of tendons.

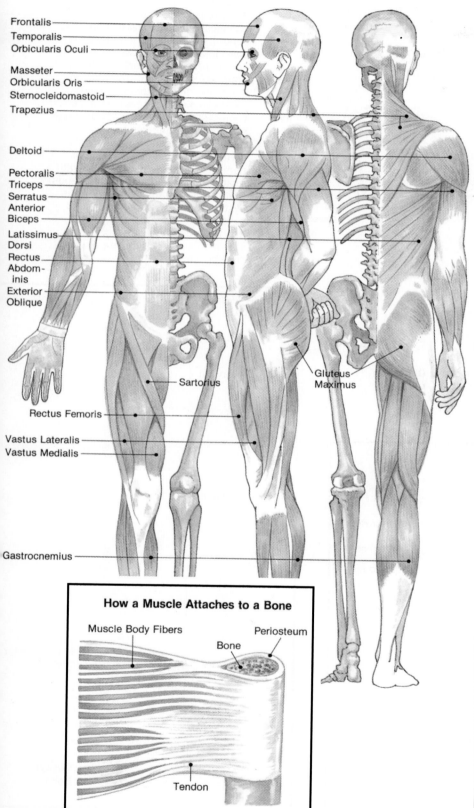

Frontalis
Temporalis
Orbicularis Oculi
Masseter
Orbicularis Oris
Sternocleidomastoid
Trapezius
Deltoid
Pectoralis
Triceps
Serratus Anterior
Biceps
Latissimus Dorsi
Rectus Abdominis
Exterior Oblique
Sartorius
Rectus Femoris
Vastus Lateralis
Vastus Medialis
Gastrocnemius
Gluteus Maximus

How a Muscle Attaches to a Bone

Muscle Body Fibers
Periosteum
Bone
Tendon

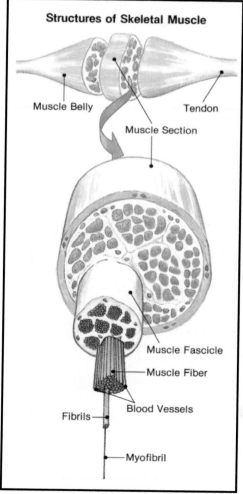

Structures of Skeletal Muscle

Muscle Belly
Tendon
Muscle Section
Muscle Fascicle
Muscle Fiber
Blood Vessels
Fibrils
Myofibril

399

Nervous System
Brain and Spine

The Brain

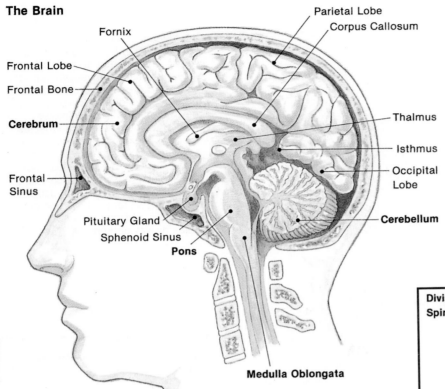

Fornix

Frontal Lobe

Frontal Bone

Cerebrum

Frontal Sinus

Pituitary Gland

Sphenoid Sinus

Pons

Parietal Lobe

Corpus Callosum

Thalmus

Isthmus

Occipital Lobe

Cerebellum

Medulla Oblongata

The nervous system includes the brain, spinal cord, and nerves. Structures within the system may be classified according to divisions: central, peripheral, and autonomic divisions of the nervous system. The central nervous system includes the brain and spinal cord. The sensory (incoming) and motor (outgoing) nerves make up the peripheral nervous system. The autonomic nervous system has structures that parallel the spinal cord and then share the same pathways as the peripheral nerves. This division is involved with motor impulses (outgoing commands) that travel from the central nervous system to the heart muscle, blood vessels, secreting cells of glands, and the smooth muscles of organs. The impulses will stimulate or inhibit certain activities.

The Spinal Cord

Sympathetic Trunk

Spinal Ganglion

Pia Mater

Dura Mater

Body of Vertebra

Intervertebral Disk

Spinal Cord

Posterior Root

Anterior Root

Arachnoid

Spinous Process of Vertebra

Spinal Nerves

Sympathetic Ganglion

Transverse Process of Vertebra

Divisions of the Spinal Cord

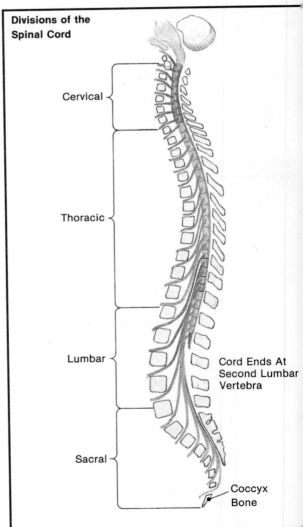

Cervical

Thoracic

Lumbar

Sacral

Cord Ends At Second Lumbar Vertebra

Coccyx Bone

Nervous System
Nerves

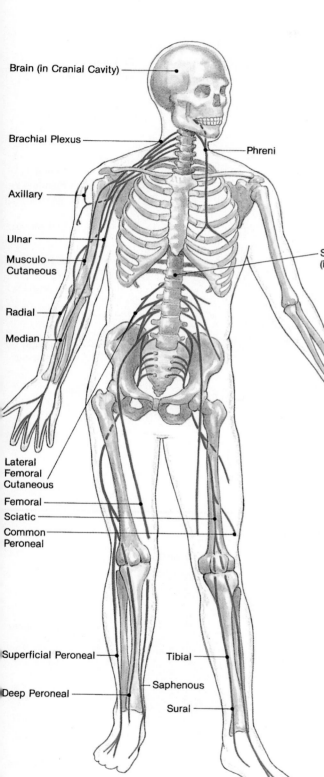

Brain (in Cranial Cavity)

Brachial Plexus

Phreni

Axillary

Ulnar

Musculo Cutaneous

Spinal Cord (in Spinal Cavity)

Radial

Median

Lateral Femoral Cutaneous

Femoral

Sciatic

Common Peroneal

Superficial Peroneal

Tibial

Deep Peroneal

Saphenous

Sural

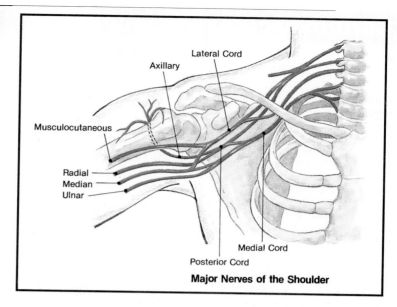

Lateral Cord

Axillary

Musculocutaneous

Radial
Median
Ulnar

Medial Cord

Posterior Cord

Major Nerves of the Shoulder

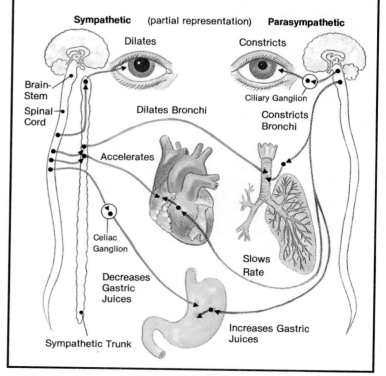

Autonomic Nervous System

The autonomic nervous system affects the heart, blood vessels, digestive tract, salivary and digestive glands, pancreas, liver, spleen, anal sphincter, kidneys, urinary bladder, urinary sphincter, adrenal glands, thyroid gland, gonads, genitalia, nasal lining, larynx, bronchi, lungs, iris and ciliary muscles of the eyes, tear glands, and hair muscles. Impulses can increase or slow heart rate, stimulate dilation or constriction of blood vessels, cause glands to secrete or decrease secretion, initiate or inhibit contractions in the bladder, stimulate or decrease a wave of muscle contraction along the digestive tract, and many other essential body activities.

Sympathetic   (partial representation)   Parasympathetic

Dilates

Constricts

Brain-Stem

Spinal Cord

Ciliary Ganglion

Dilates Bronchi

Constricts Bronchi

Accelerates

Celiac Ganglion

Slows Rate

Decreases Gastric Juices

Increases Gastric Juices

Sympathetic Trunk

The heart is a hollow, muscular organ that pumps 450 million pints of blood in the average lifetime. Its superior chambers, the atria, receive blood. Both atria fill and then contract at the same time. The inferior chambers are the ventricles. They pump blood out of the heart. Both ventricles fill and then contract at the same time. When the atria are relaxing, the ventricles are contracting.

The right side of the heart receives blood from the body and sends it to the lungs (pulmonic circulation). The heart's left side receives oxygenated blood from the lungs and sends it out to the body (systemic circulation).

The heartbeat originates at the sinoatrial node (pacemaker) and spreads across the atria to stimulate contraction. After a slight delay, the impulse is sent from the atrioventricular node, down the bundles of His, and out across the ventricles. This stimulates the ventricles to contract while the atria are relaxing.

The heart muscle (myocardium) receives its blood supply by way of the right and left coronary arteries. These vessels are the first branches of the aorta.

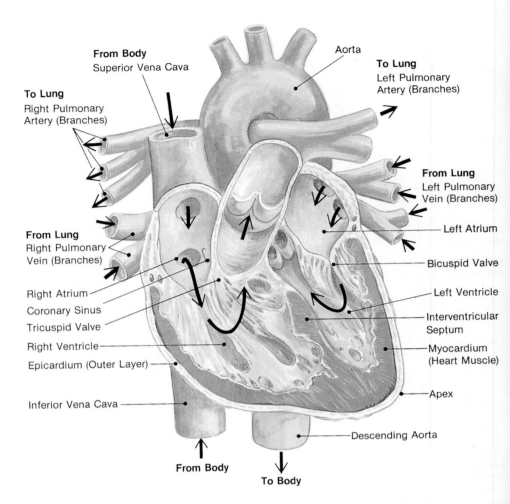

From Body
Superior Vena Cava

Aorta

To Lung
Left Pulmonary
Artery (Branches)

To Lung
Right Pulmonary
Artery (Branches)

From Lung
Left Pulmonary
Vein (Branches)

Left Atrium

Bicuspid Valve

From Lung
Right Pulmonary
Vein (Branches)

Right Atrium

Coronary Sinus

Tricuspid Valve

Right Ventricle

Epicardium (Outer Layer)

Inferior Vena Cava

Left Ventricle

Interventricular Septum

Myocardium
(Heart Muscle)

Apex

Descending Aorta

From Body

To Body

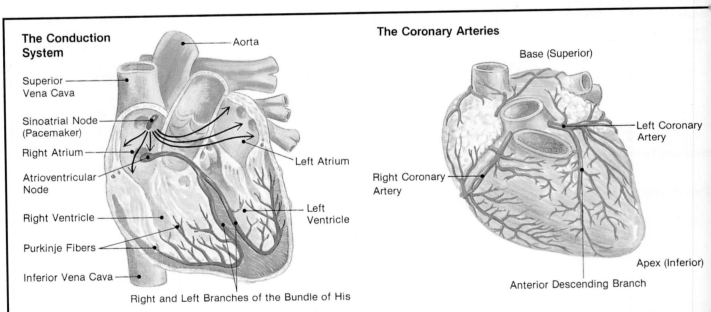

The Conduction System

Aorta

Superior Vena Cava

Sinoatrial Node
(Pacemaker)

Right Atrium

Atrioventricular Node

Right Ventricle

Purkinje Fibers

Inferior Vena Cava

Left Atrium

Left Ventricle

Right and Left Branches of the Bundle of His

The Coronary Arteries

Base (Superior)

Left Coronary Artery

Right Coronary Artery

Apex (Inferior)

Anterior Descending Branch

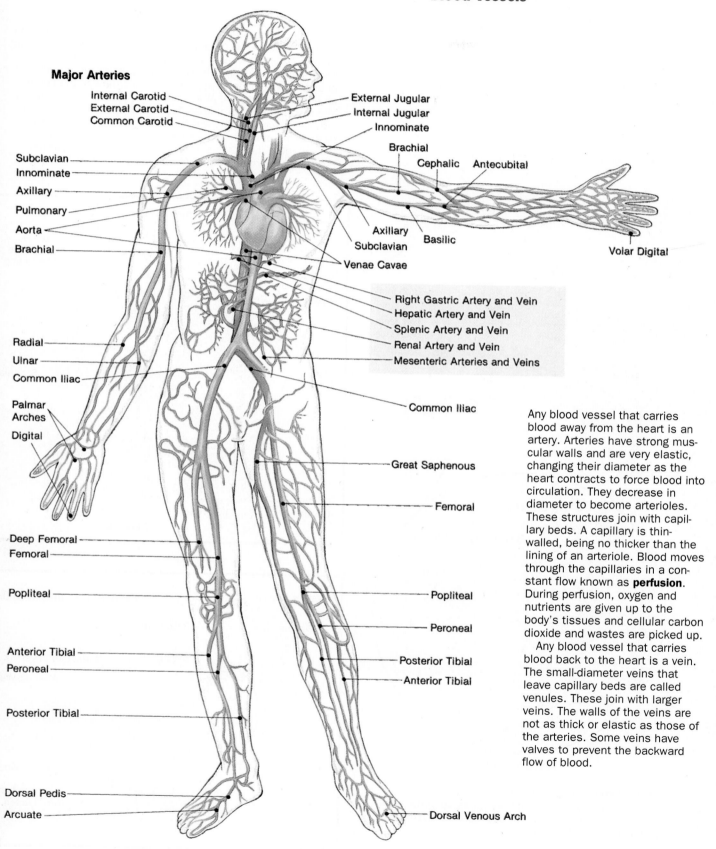

Major Arteries

Internal Carotid
External Carotid
Common Carotid

External Jugular
Internal Jugular
Innominate
Brachial
Cephalic   Antecubital

Subclavian
Innominate
Axillary
Pulmonary
Aorta
Brachial

Axillary
Subclavian
Basilic

Venae Cavae

Volar Digital

Right Gastric Artery and Vein
Hepatic Artery and Vein
Splenic Artery and Vein
Renal Artery and Vein
Mesenteric Arteries and Veins

Radial
Ulnar
Common Iliac

Palmar
Arches
Digital

Common Iliac

Great Saphenous

Femoral

Deep Femoral
Femoral

Popliteal

Popliteal

Peroneal

Anterior Tibial
Peroneal

Posterior Tibial
Anterior Tibial

Posterior Tibial

Dorsal Pedis
Arcuate

Dorsal Venous Arch

Any blood vessel that carries blood away from the heart is an artery. Arteries have strong muscular walls and are very elastic, changing their diameter as the heart contracts to force blood into circulation. They decrease in diameter to become arterioles. These structures join with capillary beds. A capillary is thin-walled, being no thicker than the lining of an arteriole. Blood moves through the capillaries in a constant flow known as **perfusion**. During perfusion, oxygen and nutrients are given up to the body's tissues and cellular carbon dioxide and wastes are picked up.

Any blood vessel that carries blood back to the heart is a vein. The small-diameter veins that leave capillary beds are called venules. These join with larger veins. The walls of the veins are not as thick or elastic as those of the arteries. Some veins have valves to prevent the backward flow of blood.

Respiratory System

The airway consists of structures involved with the conduction and exchange of air. Conduction is the movement of air to and from the exchange levels of the lungs. Air enters through the nose (primary) and mouth (secondary) and travels down the pharynx to enter the larynx. After passing through the larynx, air enters the trachea. At its distal end, the trachea branches into the left and right primary bronchi. These bronchi branch into secondary bronchi, which then branch into the bronchioles. Some of the bronchioles end as closed tubes. Air movement in them helps the lungs expand. The rest of the bronchioles carry the air to the exchange levels of the lungs.

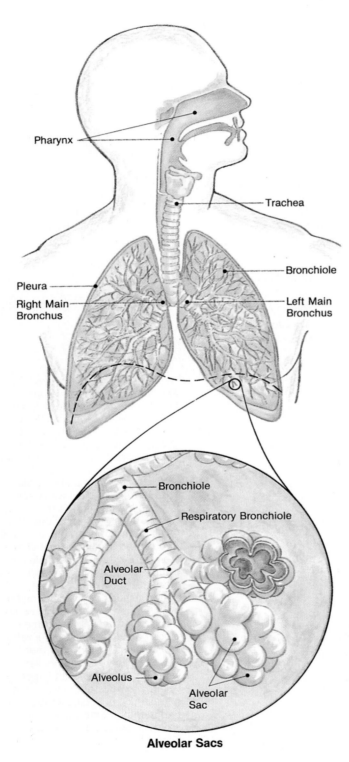

Pharynx
Trachea
Bronchiole
Pleura
Left Main Bronchus
Right Main Bronchus

Alveolar Sacs

Bronchiole
Respiratory Bronchiole
Alveolar Duct
Alveolus
Alveolar Sac

The respiratory bronchioles turn into alveolar ducts. These form alveolar sacs that are made up of the alveoli. Gas exchange takes place between the alveoli and the capillaries in the lungs.

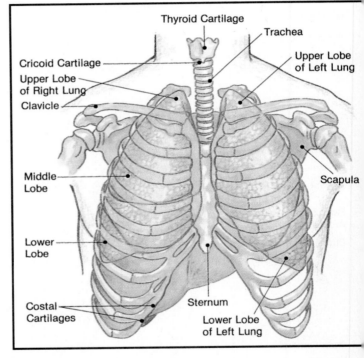

Thyroid Cartilage
Trachea
Cricoid Cartilage
Upper Lobe of Right Lung
Upper Lobe of Left Lung
Clavicle
Middle Lobe
Scapula
Lower Lobe
Costal Cartilages
Sternum
Lower Lobe of Left Lung

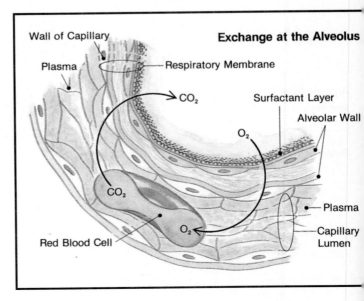

Exchange at the Alveolus

Wall of Capillary
Plasma
Respiratory Membrane
CO_2
Surfactant Layer
Alveolar Wall
O_2
CO_2
Plasma
O_2
Red Blood Cell
Capillary Lumen

The digestive system includes the digestive tract and various supportive structures and accessory glands. The tract begins at the oral cavity with the teeth and tongue. The salivary glands release saliva into the mouth to moisten food for swallowing. The tract continues down the throat to the esophagus, through the cardiac sphincter, and into the stomach. Acid and digestive enzymes are added to the food to produce chyme. The chyme passes through the pyloric sphincter to enter the small intestine. Digestive enzymes from the pancreas and bile from the liver are added to the chyme. The processes of digestion and absorption are completed in the small intestine. Wastes are carried through the ileoceccal valve into the large intestine. The wastes are moved to the rectum, from where they can be expelled through the anus.

Liver, Stomach, and Pancreas

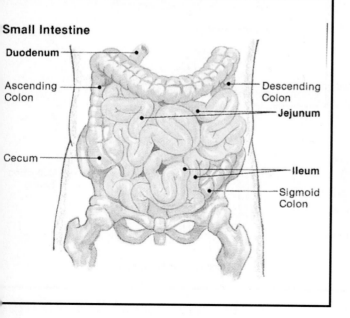

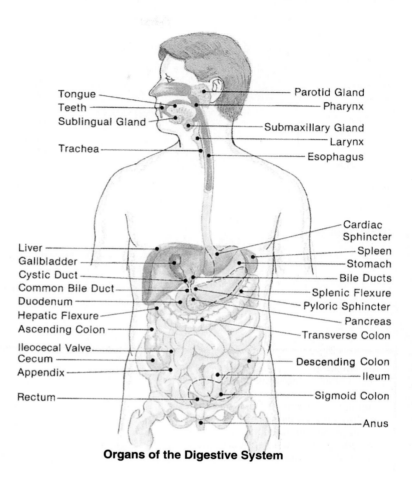

Organs of the Digestive System

Small Intestine

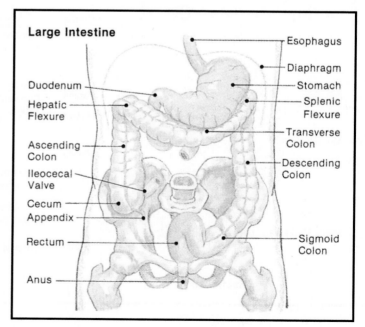

Large Intestine

Urinary System

Organs of the Urinary System

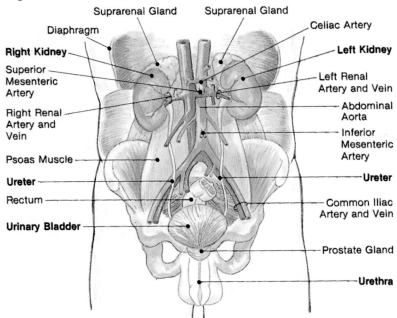

Suprarenal Gland
Suprarenal Gland
Diaphragm
Celiac Artery
Right Kidney
Left Kidney
Superior Mesenteric Artery
Left Renal Artery and Vein
Right Renal Artery and Vein
Abdominal Aorta
Inferior Mesenteric Artery
Psoas Muscle
Ureter
Ureter
Rectum
Common Iliac Artery and Vein
Urinary Bladder
Prostate Gland
Urethra

The urinary system is part of the body's excretory structures (urinary system, lungs, sweat glands, and intestine). The kidneys remove the wastes of chemical activities (metabolism) in the body. These wastes are removed from the blood to produce urine. At the same time, the kidneys remove certain excess compounds, regulate the blood pH (acid–base balance), and the concentration of sodium, potassium, chlorine, glucose, and other important chemicals.

The Nephron

Each kidney is made up of microscopic nephrons. Both wastes and needed chemicals are filtered from the blood. As these materials are passed through the nephron, the needed compounds (including water) are sent back into the blood. Wastes are collected as urine.

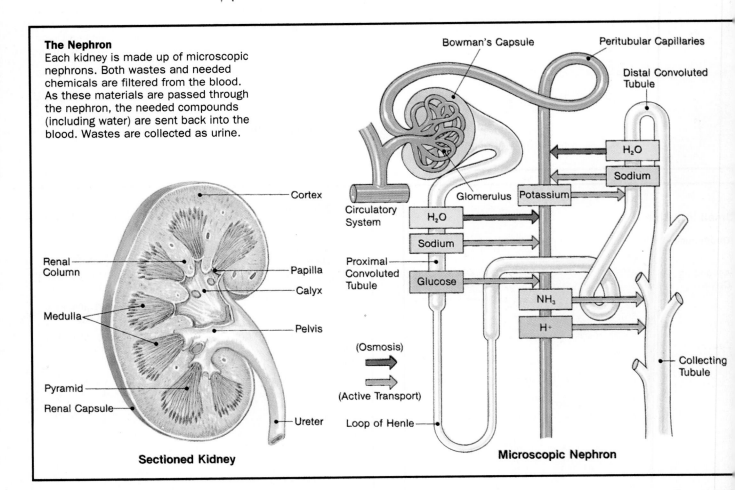

Bowman's Capsule
Peritubular Capillaries
Distal Convoluted Tubule
H_2O
Sodium
Potassium
Glomerulus
Circulatory System
H_2O
Sodium
Proximal Convoluted Tubule
Glucose
NH_3
H^+
Collecting Tubule
(Osmosis)
(Active Transport)
Loop of Henle

Microscopic Nephron

Cortex
Renal Column
Papilla
Calyx
Medulla
Pelvis
Pyramid
Renal Capsule
Ureter

Sectioned Kidney

The reproductive system consists of the organs, glands, and supportive structures that are involved with human sexuality and procreation. In the male, spermatozoa and the hormone testosterone are produced in the testes. The female produces ova (eggs) and the hormones estrogen and progesterone in her ovaries. The union of ovum and sperm produce a single cell called a zygote. Through growth, cell division, and cellular differentiation (the formulation of specialized cells) the new individual develops and matures.

Female

Fundus
Ovary
Uterus
Cervix
Vagina
Rectum
Fallopian (Uterine) Tube
Urinary Bladder
Symphysis Pubis
Urethra
Labium Minus
Clitoris
Labium Majus

Labium Minus (singular), Labia Minora (plural)
Labium Majus (singular), Labia Majora (plural)

Male

Symphysis Pubis
Prostate Gland
Urethra
Corpus Cavernosum
Corpus Spongiosum
Testis
Epididymis
Duct of Bulbourethral Gland
Ductus Deferens
Urinary Bladder
Seminal Vesicle
Rectum
Ejaculatory Duct
Bulb of Urethra

The Ovary

Suspensory Ligament of Ovary
End of Fallopian Tube
Released Ovum
Mature Follicle
Maturing Follicle
Primary Follicle (Ovum and Single Layer of Follicle Cells)
Ovarian Ligament
Ovum
Corpus Luteum (Produces Estrogen and Pregesterone)
Corpus Albicans
Egg Nest

The developing ovum and its supportive cells are called a follicle. Each month, follicle-stimulating hormone (FSH) from the pituitary gland starts the growth of several follicles. Usually, only one will mature and release an ovum (ovulation). During its growth, the follicle produces estrogen. After ovulation, the remaining cells of the follicle form a specialized structure that produces both estrogen and progesterone.

The Breast

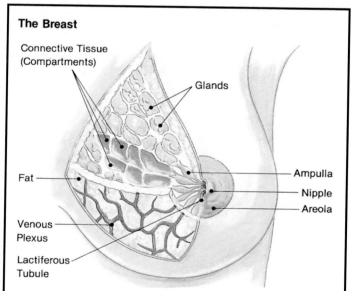

Connective Tissue (Compartments)
Glands
Fat
Venous Plexus
Lactiferous Tubule
Ampulla
Nipple
Areola

The breasts contain the mammary glands that produce milk (lactation). A mammary gland is a highly modified form of sweat gland. Estrogen stimulates the growth of the ducts, while progesterone stimulates the development of the secreting (milk-producing) cells. Lactic hormone from the pituitary stimulates milk production. Another pituitary hormone, oxytocin, stimulates the milk-producing cells to eject their milk into the ducts.

407

Integumentary System
Membranes

The Skin

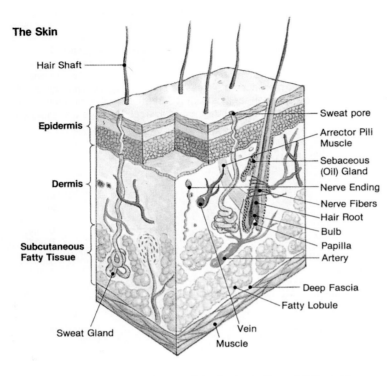

Epidermis

Dermis

Subcutaneous Fatty Tissue

Hair Shaft

Sweat pore

Arrector Pili Muscle

Sebaceous (Oil) Gland

Nerve Ending

Nerve Fibers

Hair Root

Bulb

Papilla

Artery

Deep Fascia

Fatty Lobule

Sweat Gland

Vein

Muscle

The skin is the largest organ of the body. In the adult the skin covers about 3000 square inches (1.75 square meters) and weighs about 6 pounds. It is involved with protection, insulation, thermal regulation, excretion, and the production of vitamin D.

Membranes

Membranes cover or line body structures to provide protection from injury and infection. There are four major classes of membranes. Mucous membranes line those structures that open to the outside world (for example, the mouth, the airway, digestive tract, urinary tract, and vagina). Serous membranes line the closed body cavities and cover the outsides of organs. The cutaneous membrane is the skin. Synovial membranes line joints to reduce friction during movement.

A serous membrane that covers an organ is called a visceral layer. The term parietal layer is used for the part of the serous membrane that lines a cavity. The serous membrane in the thoracic cavity is called pleura (for example, the parietal pleura lines the chest cavity). In the abdominal cavity, it is called peritoneum (for example, the parietal peritoneum). A double layer of peritoneum is called mesentery. The membrane that lines the sac surrounding the heart is pericardium.

Synovial Joint

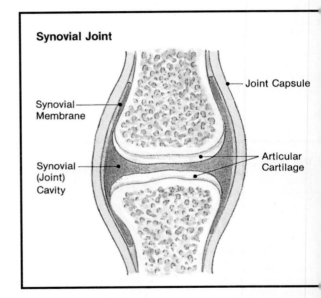

Synovial Membrane

Synovial (Joint) Cavity

Joint Capsule

Articular Cartilage

The Peritoneum

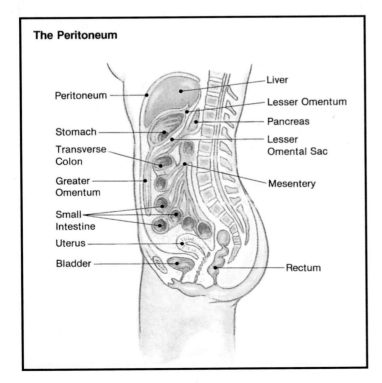

Peritoneum

Stomach

Transverse Colon

Greater Omentum

Small Intestine

Uterus

Bladder

Liver

Lesser Omentum

Pancreas

Lesser Omental Sac

Mesentery

Rectum

The Pleura

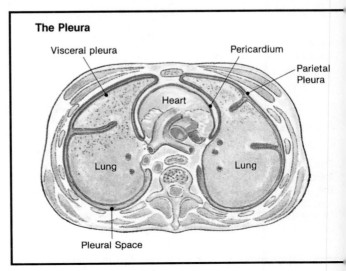

Visceral pleura

Pericardium

Parietal Pleura

Heart

Lung

Lung

Pleural Space

The Eye

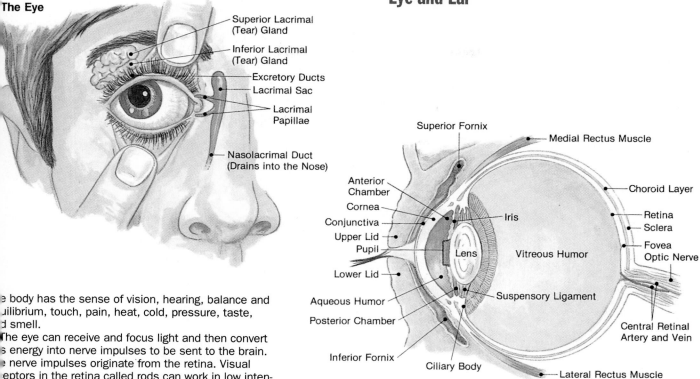

Superior Lacrimal (Tear) Gland

Inferior Lacrimal (Tear) Gland

Excretory Ducts

Lacrimal Sac

Lacrimal Papillae

Nasolacrimal Duct (Drains into the Nose)

Superior Fornix

Medial Rectus Muscle

Anterior Chamber

Cornea

Conjunctiva

Upper Lid

Pupil

Lower Lid

Aqueous Humor

Posterior Chamber

Inferior Fornix

Iris

Lens

Vitreous Humor

Suspensory Ligament

Ciliary Body

Choroid Layer

Retina

Sclera

Fovea

Optic Nerve

Central Retinal Artery and Vein

Lateral Rectus Muscle

[Th]e body has the sense of vision, hearing, balance and [eq]uilibrium, touch, pain, heat, cold, pressure, taste, [an]d smell.

[T]he eye can receive and focus light and then convert [thi]s energy into nerve impulses to be sent to the brain. [Th]e nerve impulses originate from the retina. Visual [rec]eptors in the retina called rods can work in low inten[sit]y light. They have no color function. The visual recep[tor]s called cones operate in high intensity light and do [perc]eive colors.

[T]he ear's functions include hearing, static equilibrium (balance while standing still), and dynamic [eq]uilibrium (balance when moving). The outer and middle ear are responsible for sound gathering [an]d its transmission. The inner ear has the nerve endings for hearing and equilibrium.

The Ear

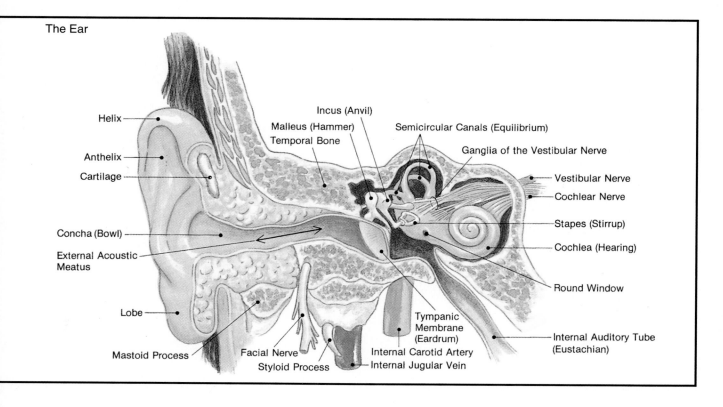

Helix

Anthelix

Cartilage

Concha (Bowl)

External Acoustic Meatus

Lobe

Mastoid Process

Incus (Anvil)

Malleus (Hammer)

Temporal Bone

Semicircular Canals (Equilibrium)

Ganglia of the Vestibular Nerve

Vestibular Nerve

Cochlear Nerve

Stapes (Stirrup)

Cochlea (Hearing)

Round Window

Internal Auditory Tube (Eustachian)

Facial Nerve

Styloid Process

Tympanic Membrane (Eardrum)

Internal Carotid Artery

Internal Jugular Vein

Glossary

Abbreviation: A shortened form of a word or phrase.

Abduction: Moving away from the midline of the body.

Abuse, Elderly: Mistreatment of older people.

Acceptance Stage: The last stage of grief, which is one of peace and acceptance.

Acetone: Ketones; the waste product produced by the breakdown of fat.

Acquired Immune Deficiency Syndrome (AIDS:) The last stage of HIV infection.

Activities of Daily Living (ADLs): The activities that a person does every day in order to live.

Acute Illness: An illness that begins suddenly and is not long lasting.

Adapt: To adjust or change in order to cope with a situation.

Adaptive Equipment: Equipment used to help adjust to a disability and to function as independently as possible.

Adduction: Moving toward the midline of the body.

ADLs: *See* Activities of Daily Living.

Administrator: The person who is responsible for the operation of the entire facility.

Adrenalin: Epinephrine; a hormone secreted by the adrenal glands that allows the body to produce great amounts of energy in an emergency.

Aggressive: Displaying forceful, attacking behavior.

AIDS: *See* Acquired Immune Deficiency Syndrome.

Airborne Transmission: The transmission of infection by inhaling pathogens that are floating in the air.

Alimentary Canal: The long continuous tube containing the primary organs of the digestive system.

Alveoli: Air sacs in the lungs where the exchange of oxygen and carbon dioxide takes place.

Alzheimer's Disease: A progressive nervous disorder that eventually destroys all mental function.

Ambulate: To walk.

Amnesia: A loss of memory.

Amputation: The removal of a body part, usually by surgery.

Anatomy: The study of body structure.

Anger Stage: Second stage of grief, which is nondirectional anger.

Angina: Chest pain caused by decreased blood flow to the heart muscle.

Antibody: A substance that is produced by the immune system of the body when a foreign body invades.

Anxiety: A state of being uneasy or worried.

Anus: The outer opening of the rectum.

Aphasia: The loss of ability to express oneself through the use of speech, writing, and/or gestures.

Apical Pulse: The heartbeat heard over the apex of the heart.

Apical-Radial Pulse: The pulse measurement that is taken simultaneously by two individuals, at the apex of the heart and at the wrist.

Appendage: An extension of a body part.

Appendicitis: Inflammation of the appendix.

Arteries: Blood vessels that carry blood away from the heart.

Arteriosclerosis: Narrowing of the arteries.

Arthritis: Chronic disease that causes inflammation of the joints.

Asepsis: Absence of pathogens.

Aseptic Practices: All the practices used to prevent the spread of infection.

Aspirate: To choke on food or fluid.

Aspiration: Choking or inhalation of food or fluid.

Aspiration Pneumonia: Pneumonia that results from food or fluid entering the airway.

Assault: A threat to do bodily harm.

Assertiveness: The ability to stand up for one's beliefs.

Assess: Check or evaluate.

Assistant Director of Nurses (A.D.O.N.): The person who helps the director of nurses.

Atherosclerosis: Clogging of the arteries by the buildup of substances and fat.

Atrium: One of the upper chambers of the heart.

Atrophy: Wasting or a decrease in size.

Auditory Canal: The tube that carries sound waves to the eardrum.

Auditory Nerve: The nerve that carries sound messages to the brain.

Auricle: The outer part of the ear that surrounds the opening to the auditory canal.

Axilla/Axillae: Underarm/underarms.

Bargaining Stage: The third stage of grief; an attempt to gain more time by promising something in return.

Battery: Touching another person's body without permission.

Bedpan: A pan that the resident uses for elimination.

Bed Scale: A scale to weigh a person who cannot get out of bed.

Bedside Commode: A portable chair with a toilet seat that fits over a pan or regular toilet.

Benign Tumor: A tumor that does not spread.

Biohazardous Waste: Waste matter that has been contaminated with blood or body fluids and may cause infection.

Bladder: A muscular sac that stores urine.

Blood/Body Fluids Isolation: Isolation to prevent the spread of pathogens by contact with blood or body fluids.

Blood Pressure (BP): The force of blood against the artery walls as it is circulated by the heart.

Body Alignment: Maintaining a normal or correct anatomical position.

Body Language: Body movements and posture that communicate a message.

Body Mechanics: The use of the body to produce motion.

Body Structure: Refers to how the body parts are arranged.

Body Temperature: The amount of heat in the body.

Bony Prominences: Places where bones are near the surface of the skin.

BP: *See* blood pressure.

Brachial Pulse: The pulse located in the bend of the elbow, which is used for taking the blood pressure.

Bruise: An injury that discolors the skin.

Bursa: Small sacs of fluid that lubricate and prevent friction in the joints.

C.A.D.: *See* Coronary artery disease.

Call Signal: A device that allows a resident to call for help from the patient unit.

Calorie: The amount of energy produced as the body burns food.

Cancer (CA): A disease in which body cells improperly grow and reproduce.

Capillaries: Small blood vessels that connect arteries to veins.

Carbohydrates: Nutrients that are primarily starch and sugar and are used for energy.

Carbon Dioxide: A gas that is a waste product of the body.

Carcinogens: Substances known or suspected of causing cancer.

Cardiac: A term that refers to the heart.

Cardiac Arrest: An absence of heartbeats.

Cardiopulmonary Resuscitation (CPR): Emergency care to restore heart and lung function.

Care Plan: The plan of care for the resident.

Carotid Pulse: The pulse felt on the carotid artery in the front of the neck.

Carrier: A person who has a pathogen in his or her body but no signs or symptoms of infection.

Cartilage: Fibrous connective tissue that provides padding between bones.

Cataract: A clouding of the lens of the eye.

CDC: *See* Centers for Disease Control.

Cell: The smallest unit of the body.

Centers for Disease Control (CDC): The federal agency that tracks infectious diseases.

Central Nervous System (CNS): The brain and spinal cord.

Cerebrovascular Accident (CVA): A stroke.

Certified Nursing Assistant (C.N.A.): A person who assists the nurses in providing care for the residents.

Chain of Command: The order of authority and problem solving within a facility.

Charge Nurse: The nurse who is responsible for one team or nursing station.

Charting: Recording information into the resident's medical record.

Chemotherapy: Treatment with medication; often refers to treatment of cancer.

Chest Compressions: A step that replaces the heart function in the procedure for CPR.

Cheyne-Stokes Respirations: An irregular breathing pattern that occurs shortly before death.

CHF: *See* Congestive Heart Failure.

Chronic Illness: An illness that begins slowly and lasts for a long time.

Chronic Obstructive Pulmonary Disease (COPD): A chronic disease that obstructs the airway and interferes with respiration.

Clean-Catch (Midstream) Urine Specimen: A urine specimen collected during the middle of the urinary stream.

Closed Bed: A bed that is fully made up with a blanket and bedspread.

Closed Fracture: A broken bone that is enclosed within the skin.

C.N.A.: *See* Certified Nursing Assistant.

Coccyx: A bone at the base of the spine.

Colon: The large intestine.

Colostomy: A surgical opening into the colon.

Comatose: Unconscious or unable to respond.

Combative: Ready to fight or struggle.

Communicable Disease: A disease or infection that spreads easily from one person to another.

Communication: The sharing of information.

Communication Barriers: Problems that interfere with communication.

Communication Impairment: Difficulty in communicating because of one or more disabilities.

Competency: The ability to perform a skill.

Complication: A problem that can result from a disease or other condition.

Confidentiality: Maintaining the privacy of resident information.

Congested: Filled with fluid.

Congestive Heart Failure (CHF): Pooling of blood and other fluids due to failure of the heart to pump efficiently.

Conjunctiva: Mucous membrane that protects the eyeball.

Constipation: The passage of hard, dry stool.

Contact Isolation: Isolation that is designed to prevent the spread of pathogens by direct or indirect contact.

Contagious: Easily spread from one person to another.

Contaminate: To dirty or expose to microorganisms.

Contracture: Permanent shortening of a muscle due to lack of use or lack of exercise.

Convulsion: *See* seizure.

COPD: *See* Chronic Obstructive Pulmonary Disease.

Cornea: Part of the eye that helps to focus light rays.

Coronary Artery Disease: Heart disease caused by narrowing of the coronary arteries.

CPR: *See* Cardiopulmonary resuscitation.

Cubic Centimeter (cc): A metric unit of fluid measurement.

CVA: *See* Cerebrovascular accident.

Cyanosis: A blue color of the lips, nails, and skin, caused by lack of oxygen.

Dangling: Sitting on the side of the bed.

Decubitus Ulcer (Pressure Sore; Bedsore): A breakdown of tissue that occurs when blood flow is interrupted.

Defecation: The elimination of solid wastes from the body.

Dehydration: The condition of having less than the normal amount of fluid in the body.

Dementia: An impairment of mental function.

Denial Stage: The first stage of grief in which the person refuses to believe what is happening.

Dentures: False teeth.

Depression: Feelings of sadness or hopelessness.

Depression Stage: The fourth stage of grief; sadness and quietness.

Dermis: The inner layer of the skin that contains blood vessels and nerve endings.

Developmentally Disabled: A person who has not developed normally due to a birth defect, an injury, or an illness.

Diabetes Mellitus: A chronic disease in which the body is unable to use insulin to break down sugar for energy.

Diaphragm: A muscle between the chest cavity and the abdominal cavity that assists in respiration.

Diarrhea: Loose, watery stool.

Diastole: The stage of the cardiac cycle when the heart is resting and filling with blood.

Diastolic Pressure: The pressure of blood flowing during the heart's relaxation (diastole).

Digestion: The process of preparing food for the body's use.

Direct Contact: Transmission of infection by touching an infected person.

Director of Nurses (D.O.N.): The person who is responsible for the nursing department.

Disability: A decrease in the ability to carry out daily activities.

Discharge Planning: The plans and arrangements for care of the resident after discharge.

Disinfection: The use of chemicals to destroy pathogens.

Disoriented: Confused as to person, place, or time.

Disorientation: Confusion about person, place, or time.

Disruptive Behavior: Behavior that interferes with normal routine.

Distended: Swollen; inflated.

D.O.N.: *See* Director of Nursing.

Double Bagging: An isolation procedure for disposing of contaminated items, in which two bags are used to prevent the spread of infection.

Douche (Vaginal Irrigation): A procedure in which fluid is allowed to flow into and out of the vagina.

Drainage/Secretion Precautions: Measures used to prevent the spread of infection by contact with a wound or drainage.

Droplet Transmission: The transmission of infection by breathing in fine drops of moisture exhaled by an infected person.

Draw Sheet: A small sheet that is placed across the middle of the bottom sheet (pull sheet, turning sheet).

Dyspnea: Difficult breathing.

Edema: Swelling of a body part with fluid.

Elimination: The process by which the body rids itself of waste.

Emergency Medical Services (EMS): A public service system that responds to emergencies.

Emesis: Vomitus.

Emesis Basin: Small kidney-shaped basin into which the resident spits or vomits.

Empathy: The ability to realize how you would feel if you were in the other person's place.

Emphysema: A chronic respiratory disease in which the lung tissue loses its elasticity.

Employability Skills: Skills that are necessary to get a job and to keep a job.

EMS: *See* Emergency Medical Services.

Enema: The introduction of fluid into the rectum and colon.

Enteric Isolation: Isolation designed to prevent the spread of pathogens by contact with feces.

Environment: All the conditions and influences around us.

Epidermis: The outer layer of the skin.

Epiglottis: Cartilage that covers the trachea to prevent food from entering the airway.

Epinephrine: Adrenalin; a hormone secreted by the adrenal glands that allows the body to quickly produce great amounts of energy in an emergency.

Esophagus: A tube that leads from the throat to the stomach for the passage of food and fluids.

Estrogen: Female hormone.

Ethics: Guidelines that are concerned with right or wrong behavior.

Ethnic: Refers to the cultural group to which an individual belongs.

Exocrine Glands: Glands that secrete substances into organs or outside the body.

Expectorate: To spit.

Extension: Straightening and extending.

External Catheter (Texas Catheter): A soft rubber sheath placed over the penis to collect urine.

Extremities: The arms and legs.

Fallopian Tubes: Tubes that carry the ovum from the ovary to the uterus.

False Imprisonment: The act of restraining or restricting a person's movements when the person is not in danger of harming himself or herself.

Fat: A nutrient used for energy.

Fecal Impaction: A large amount of hard, dry stool.

Feces: Solid wastes from the digestive system; stool; bowel movement; BM.

Fetus: The child in utero from three months to birth.

First Aid: Immediate care for injuries or sudden illness that is given to prevent further injury and save lives.

Flatus: Gas or air expelled from the digestive system.

Flex: To bend.

Flexion: A bending motion.

Flow Sheet: A chart form that is commonly used in

long-term care to record resident information.

Foley Catheter: A tube inserted and left in the bladder to drain urine; a retention catheter.

Foot Drop: A contracture of the foot caused by shortening of the muscles in the calf of the leg.

Fowler's Position: A sitting or semisitting position.

Fracture: A broken bone.

Fracture Pan: A bedpan with a flat end that goes under the resident.

Fresh-Fractional (Double-Voided) Urine Specimen: A small amount of urine that is collected within a few minutes of emptying the bladder.

Function: A purpose or action.

Gait: Manner of walking.

Gait/Transfer Belt: A piece of equipment used to assist unsteady residents to transfer or walk.

Gangrene: A serious infection that causes tissue death.

Gastrointestinal (GI) System: The digestive system.

Gastrostomy Tube: A tube that is placed directly into the stomach for feeding.

Gatch Handle: A crank that is used to change the position of the bed.

Geriatric Resident: An elderly person who lives in a long-term care facility.

Geriatrics: The branch of medicine that is concerned with the problems and diseases of the elderly.

Geri-chair (Geriatric Chair): A reclining chair on wheels; a type of wheelchair.

GI: *See* Gastrointestinal System.

Glaucoma: A disease in which pressure in the eye gradually destroys the optic nerve.

Glossary: A section of a book that contains definitions of many words that are found in the book.

Graduate: A container, marked with measurements, that is used to measure fluids.

Hands-On Care: Activities in which a person's hands touch a resident's body.

HBV (Hepatitis B Virus): The virus that causes Hepatitis B.

Health: A state of complete physical, mental, and social well-being, not merely absence of disease or infirmity.

Health Care Team: All the people who provide care and services for the residents.

Heart: A muscular pump that circulates blood throughout the body.

Heimlich Maneuver: Immediate first aid for a complete airway obstruction.

Hemiplegia: Paralysis of one side of the body.

Hemorrhage: Severe bleeding.

Hepatitis: A disease that affects the liver.

Heredity: The transmission of characteristics from parents or other ancestors.

HIV: *See* Human Immunodeficiency Virus.

HIV Infection (AIDS): A disease that destroys the immune system and leaves the body unable to fight infection.

Hormone: A chemical substance produced by the endocrine glands.

Hospice: A program that provides care for the terminally ill and their families.

Human Immunodeficiency Virus: The microorganism that causes HIV infection.

Hydration: Adequate supply of fluids.

Hyperglycemia: High blood sugar.

Hypertension: High or above-normal blood pressure.

Hypoglycemia: Low blood sugar.

Hypostatic Pneumonia: Pneumonia that results from fluid collecting in the lung.

Hypotension: Low or below-normal blood pressure.

Immobilize: To prevent movement.

Immunity: The body's resistance to injury and disease.

Impairment: A limitation caused by disease, injury, or a birth defect.

Incident Report: Written documentation of an incident.

Incision: A clean, smooth cut.

Incontinence: The inability to control urine or feces.

Incus: The middle of the three ossicles of the ear.

Inservice: Educational program for employees.

Independence: The ability to care for oneself and control one's life.

Indirect Contact: Transmission of infection by touching an object.

Infection: A disease condition that occurs when germs enter the body and cause damage.

Inflammation: Tissue reaction with redness, swelling, heat, and pain.

Intake and Output (I&O): All fluids taken into the body and all fluids that are eliminated.

Integument: Skin.

Integumentary System: The skin and its appendages.

Interdependent: Depending on one another.

Intravenous (IV): A needle into the vein for receiving fluids.

Invasion of Privacy: An occurrence when either the privacy of the resident's body or the privacy of personal information is not protected.

Iris: The colored part of the eye.

Islets of Langerhans: Cluster of cells in the pancreas that produce insulin and glucagon.

Isolation: Separating a person, using barriers to prevent the spread of pathogens.

Job Description: A list of the tasks and responsibilities of a nursing assistant.

Joint: A connection of two or more bones.

Kardex: A card file that summarizes the plan of care for a resident.

Ketones: Acetone; the waste product produced by the breakdown of fat as it is used for energy.

Kidney: The organ of the urinary system that filters and removes waste products from the blood.

Laceration: A rough skin tear.

Larynx: A structure in the respiratory system that contains the vocal cords.

Lateral Position: Lying on the side.

Lens: The part of the eye that focuses light images onto the retina.

Licensed Practical Nurse (L.P.N.)/Licensed Vocational Nurse (L.V.N.): A person who is educated and licensed to assist the registered nurse in planning, providing, and evaluating nursing care.

Ligament: Fibrous tissue that connects bone to bone.

Listening: Giving your attention to what you are hearing, while thinking about its meaning.

Long-Term Care Facility (LTCF): A facility that provides heath care to people who are not able to care for themselves at home but are not sick enough to be in a hospital.

Lungs: The major organ of respiration.

Malignant Tumor: A tumor that grows rapidly and spreads.

Malleus: The outer most and largest of the three ossicles.

Malnutrition: A condition of poor nutrition.

Meatus: Outside opening of the urethra.

Mechanical Diet: A diet in which the texture of the food is changed.

Menstruation: The discharge of the lining of the uterus which occurs at regular intervals.

Mental Retardation: Developmental disability characterized by low intellect and learning difficulties.

Metabolism: The combination of all body processes.

Metastasize: To spread to other parts of the body.

Methicillin-Resistant Staphylococcus Aureus (MRSA): An infectious disease caused by a pathogen that is resistant to many antibiotics.

MI: *See* Myocardial Infarction.

Microorganisms: Small living things that cannot be seen without the aid of a microscope.

Milliliter: A metric unit for measuring fluid.

Mitered Corner: A squared corner used in bedmaking to anchor the linen.

Mobility: The ability to move.

Motivation: An inner feeling that causes a person to take action.

MRSA: *See* Methicillin-resistant Staphylococcus Aureus.

MS: *See* Multiple Sclerosis.

Mucous Membranes: Thin sheets of tissue that line certain parts of the body.

Mucus: Fluid secreted by mucous membranes and glands.

Multiple Sclerosis (MS): A progressive disease that interferes with the transmission of nerve impulses.

Myocardial Infarction (MI): A major heart attack that causes the death of heart muscle tissue.

Nasogastric (NG) Tube: A tube that is inserted through the nose into the stomach.

Negligence: Failure to give proper care, which results in physical or emotional harm to the resident.

Nephron: The basic filtering unit of the kidney.

Neuron: A nerve cell.

NG Tube: *See* Nasogastric Tube.

Nocturia: The need to urinate frequently during the night.

Nonpathogens: Microorganisms that do not cause infection.

Nonverbal Communication: Sharing information without the use of words.

Normal Flora: Microorganisms that are necessary for health, and are usually found in specific locations.

NPO: The abbreviation for "nothing by mouth."

Nutrients: Food elements that are necessary for metabolism.

Nutrition: The intake and use of food by the body.

Obese: Very fat.

Objective Reporting: Reporting specific, factual information.

OBRA: *See* Omnibus Budget Reconciliation Act.

Observation: Using the senses of sight, smell, hearing, and touch to gather information.

Occupational Safety and Health Administration (OSHA): A governmental agency that is concerned with the health and safety of workers.

Occupational Therapy: A restorative program that supports residents' indepen-dence in performing activities of daily living.

Occupied Bed: A bed that is made while the resident is in it.

Olfactory Nerve: Carries impulses for smell to the brain.

Ombudsmen Committee: A committee that investigates complaints of resident abuse in health care facilities.

Omnibus Budget Reconciliation Act (OBRA): A law that focused on the care of the elderly in long-term care facilities.

Open Bed: A bed that is made with the linen turned down.

Open Fracture: A broken bone with an open skin injury.

Opportunistic Disease: A disease that develops in a person who has a weakened immune system.

Optic Nerve: The nerve that carries sight messages to the brain.

Oral: Pertaining to the mouth.

Oral Hygiene: Mouth care.

Orderly: A male nursing assistant.

Organ: A group of tissues that work together to perform a certain function.

Orthopneic Position: An upright sitting position in which the resident is leaning forward with the arms supported in front, at chest level.

OSHA: *See* Occupational Safety and Health Administration.

Ossicles: The three bones of the ear.

Osteoarthritis: Inflammation of the bones and joints.

Ostomy: A surgical opening into the body.

Ovaries: Female reproductive organs that produce hormones and ova.

Oxygen: A gas required for respiration.

Pancreas: The gland that produces hormones necessary for the metabolism of sugar.

Paralysis: The inability to move a body part.

Paraplegia: Paralysis of the lower limbs of the body.

Parenteral: Not in or through the digestive system.

Parkinson's Disease: A chronic disease that causes loss of control of motor function.

Pathogens: Microorganisms that are harmful and cause infection.

Penis: A male reproductive organ through which urine is passed.

Perineal Care (Peri-care): Cleansing of the genital and anal areas of the body.

Peripheral Nervous System (PNS): All the nerves that are outside of the brain and spinal cord.

Peristalsis: The muscular contractions that move food through the digestive system.

Personal Hygiene: Cleanliness and care of health.

Petechiae: Patches of surface bleeding due to fragile blood vessels.

Pharynx: The throat; a passageway for food and air.

Physical Needs: Needs of the body.

Physical Therapy: A restorative program that helps residents strengthen muscles and regain physical independence.

Physiology: The study of body function.

Pneumonia: Acute infection of the lungs.

PO: The abbreviation for "by mouth."

Pollution: Contamination of the environment.

Postmortem Care: Care of the body after death.

Prefix: A word element that is placed at the beginning of a word.

Pressure Sore (Decubitus Ulcer; bedsore): A breakdown of tissue that occurs when blood flow is interrupted.

Priority: The process of rating each task in its order of importance.

Procedure: Steps to be taken in performing a task.

Procedure Book: Contains the steps required for all procedures that are performed within the facility.

Pronation: A turning down motion.

Prone Position: Lying on the abdomen.

Prostrate: A gland that surrounds the urethra in the male.

Prosthesis: An artificial body part.

Prosthetic Device: Replaces or assists a body part to perform its function.

Protein: A nutrient used to build and repair body tissue.

Protective (Reverse) Isolation: Isolation in which the isolated person is protected from pathogens that are present in the normal environment.

Psychosocial Needs: Emotional, social, and spiritual needs.

Pulmonary: Refers to the lungs.

Pulse: Heartbeat.

Pupil: A round, dark opening in the iris that changes size to control the amount of light that can enter the eye.

Quadriplegia: Paralysis of both arms and legs.

Radial Pulse: The pulse located on the inner aspect of the wrist, at the base of the thumb.

Range-of-Motion Exercises: Exercises that are performed to put each joint through its normal area of movement.

Rapport: A mutually trusting relationship.

Reality Orientation: A technique that helps to maintain awareness of person, place, and time.

Receptors: Nerve endings that receive and transmit messages to the brain.

Recording: Writing information about the resident.

Reflex: An automatic response to a stimuli.

Registered Nurse (R.N.): A person who is educated and licensed to plan, provide, and evaluate nursing care.

Regular Diet: A diet in which there are no restrictions.

Rehabilitation: A method that is used to bring the resident back to as nearly normal function as possible.

Rehabilitation Nursing Assistant (R.N.A.): *See* Restorative Nursing Assistant.

Report: The communication of resident assignments and information to those who are coming on duty.

Reproductive System: The system through which humans reproduce themselves.

Rescue Breathing: The procedure of ventilating a person who is not breathing.

Resident: A person who lives in a long-term care facility.

Residents' Bill of Rights: A list of the rights and freedoms of the residents.

Respirations: Breathing.

Respiratory Arrest: Breathing stops.

Respiratory Isolation: Isolation to prevent the spread of airborne pathogens.

Responsibility: A duty or obligation to do something.

Restorative Attitude: An attitude that includes positive feelings and beliefs that a restorative measure will help the resident.

Restorative Care: The nursing care that is given to help the resident attain and maintain the highest level of function and independence.

Restorative Environment: An environment that promotes independence.

Restorative Nursing Assistant (R.N.A.): A certified nursing assistant who has completed additional training in rehabilitation.

Restraint/Safety Device: A device that is used to restrict a person's freedom of movement.

Retina: The inner layer of the eyeball that contains sight receptors.

Reverse (Protective) Isolation: Isolation in which the isolated person is protected from pathogens that are present in the normal environment.

Rheumatoid Arthritis: A form of arthritis that often causes crippling.

R.N.A.: *See* Restorative Nursing Assistant.

Rods and Cones: Sight receptors in the eye.

Root: The foundation of a word; it contains the basic meaning.

S&A Test: The urine test for sugar and acetone.

Sacrum: Bone above the coccyx at the base of the spine.

Safety Device/Restraint: A device that is used to restrict freedom of movement.

Sclera: The white part of the eye.

Scrotum: A double sac that holds the testes.

Seizure: A convulsion; a sudden spasm of muscles caused by abnormal brain activity.

Self-actualization: The need to prove oneself by accepting challenges and meeting goals.

Self-esteem: The opinion one has of ones self.

Self-worth: The value a person puts on himself or herself.

Semicircular Canals: Part of the inner ear.

Semen: The fluid that contains sperm and is released from the penis during sexual intercourse.

Shearing: A force upon the skin that stretches it between the bone inside and a surface outside the body.

Shower Chair: A wheeled chair used for showering weak residents.

Shroud: A cover for wrapping a dead body.

Sim's Position: A lateral position in which the lower arm is behind the resident and the upper leg is bent or flexed in a knee-chest position.

Slander: A false statement that damages another person's reputation.

Specimen: A sample of material from a person's body.

Sperm: A male reproductive cell.

Sphygmomanometer: The blood pressure cuff; an instrument for measuring blood pressure.

Sputum: Mucus from the lungs or deep in the respiratory system.

Stapes: The inner most of the three ossicles.

Sterile: Free of all microorganisms.

Sternum: Breastbone.

Stethoscope: An instrument used for listening to body sounds.

Stimuli: Factors that cause a reaction.

Stoma: Mouth of a surgical opening.

Stool: Feces, bowel movement, or BM; solid waste material from the digestive system.

Stress: Mental and physical tension or strain.

Subcutaneous Fat: The inner layer of the skin that provides a shock absorbing cushion for insulation and protection.

Suffix: A word element that is placed at the end of a word.

Suffocation: Interruption of respiration, preventing the intake of oxygen.

Sundowner's Syndrome: An increase in behavior problems, confusion and agitation as evening occurs.

Supination: A turning up motion.

Supine Position: Lying on the back.

Susceptibility: A condition of being likely to catch a disease if exposed.

Symptom: Evidence of disease that cannot be observed.

System: A group of organs that work together to perform a function.

Systole: The stage of the cardiac cycle when the heart is contracting and pumping blood.

Systolic Pressure: The pressure of blood flowing during the heart's contraction (systole).

Tactile: Refers to the sense of touch.

Team Leader: The nurse responsible for one area of a nursing unit.

Tendon: Fibrous tissue that connects muscle to bone.

Terminal Illness: An illness that is expected to end in death.

Testes: The male reproductive organs that produce sperm and testosterone.

Testosterone: A male hormone.

Texas Catheter (External Catheter): A soft rubber sheath placed over the penis to collect urine.

Therapeutic Diet: Any of the special diets used to treat disease.

Tissue: A group of cells that work together to perform a certain function.

Toothettes: Small sponges on sticks, to be used for oral care.

Toxic: Poisonous.

Transfer/Gait Belt: Equipment used to assist unsteady residents to transfer or walk.

Trauma: Physical or emotional injury or upset.

Tremors: Shaking or trembling.

Tumor: A mass of tissue that grows in the body and performs no useful function.

Twenty-four (24)-Hour Urine Specimen: Collecting all the urine that is voided during a 24-hour period.

Universal Precautions: A method of infection control based on the belief that any contact with certain body fluids will cause infection.

Ureter: A tube that leads from the kidney to the bladder.

Urethra: The tube that leads from the bladder to the outside of the body.

Urinal: A container that the male resident uses when urinating.

Urinary Frequency: The need to urinate often.

Urinary Meatus: The outer opening of the urethra.

Urinary Urgency: A sudden strong urge to urinate.

Urinate: Void; micturate; expel urine from the body.

Uterus: The female reproductive organ that protects and nourishes the developing baby during pregnancy.

Vagina: The female reproductive organ and birth canal.

Vaginal Irrigation (Douche): A procedure in which fluid is allowed to flow into and out of the vagina.

Validation Therapy: A technique that creates a climate of acceptance by encouraging the confused resident to explore thoughts.

Vehicle Transmission: The transmission of infection by food, water, blood, or medication that contains pathogens.

Veins: Blood vessels that carry blood back to the heart.

Ventilate: To blow breaths into the airway of a person who is not breathing.

Ventricle: One of the lower chambers of the heart.

Verbal Communication: The use of words to share information.

Villi: Hairlike projections in the small intestine that absorb food and fluids and release them into the bloodstream.

Virus: The smallest known microorganism.

Vital Signs: Measurement of heart function, breathing, and temperature regulation.

Void: To urinate; to eliminate liquid body wastes.

Wellness: The ability to adapt or change in order to live life to the fullest.

Whole-Person Approach: An approach that assists the resident to meet physical, emotional, social, sexual, and spiritual needs.

Will: A written document that states how a person wants his property divided when he dies.

Index